Organ-specific Parasites in Cattle

Edited by

Tanmoy Rana
Department of Veterinary Clinical Complex
West Bengal University of Animal & Fishery Sciences
Kolkata, India

Organ-specific Parasites in Cattle

Editor: Tanmoy Rana

ISBN (Online): 978-981-5322-10-1

ISBN (Print): 978-981-5322-11-8

ISBN (Paperback): 978-981-5322-12-5

First published in 2025.

need for a court order if at any point you breach any terms of this License Agreement. In no event will any delay or failure by Bentham Science Publishers in enforcing your compliance with this License Agreement constitute a waiver of any of its rights.

3. You acknowledge that you have read this License Agreement, and agree to be bound by its terms and conditions. To the extent that any other terms and conditions presented on any website of Bentham Science Publishers conflict with, or are inconsistent with, the terms and conditions set out in this License Agreement, you acknowledge that the terms and conditions set out in this License Agreement shall prevail.

Bentham Science Publishers Pte. Ltd.
80 Robinson Road #02-00
Singapore 068898
Singapore
Email: subscriptions@benthamscience.net

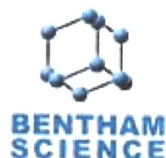

BENTHAM SCIENCE

CONTENTS

FOREWORD i

PREFACE ii

LIST OF CONTRIBUTORS iii

CHAPTER 1 INTRODUCTION 1
Sirigireddy Sivajothi, Bhavanam Sudhakara Reddy, Syed Afreen and *Tanmoy Rana*
   INTRODUCTION 1
      Nematodes 4
         Life Cycle of the Nematode 5
      Lungworms 6
      Trematodes 7
         Fasciolosis 7
      Cestodes 7
         Taeniasis 7
   PROTOZOAN INFECTIONS 8
      Coccidiosis 8
      Cryptosporidiosis 8
      Giardiasis 9
      Neosporosis 9
      Echinococcosis (Hydatidosis) 10
      Haemoprotozoan Parasites 10
      Babesiosis 11
      Oriental Theileriosis 11
      Anaplasmosis 12
   EXTERNAL PARASITES 12
      Some Examples of External Parasites Include 13
         Blood-Sucking Flies 13
         Non-Blood Sucking Flies 16
         Infestations of Fly Maggots (Myiasis) 17
      Seasonal Parasite Pressure 20
      Diagnosis 20
   PREVENTION AND CONTROL 22
      Colostrum Importance in Calves 23
      Anti-Parasitic Medications 23
      Pasture Management 24
      General Considerations for Parasite Control Include 25
      Important Factors to Consider for Preventing Both Internal and External Parasite Infections Include 25
         Source Negative Cattle 25
         Minimize Dose or Eliminate Exposure Completely 25
         Monitoring Program to Ensure Early Identification 25
         Therapeutic Prevention Programs 25
      Environmental Management 25
   CONCLUSION 26
   REFERENCES 26

CHAPTER 2 PARASITES OF THE GASTROINTESTINAL TRACT INFECTION 29
K.P. Shyma, Ajit Kumar, Jay Prakash Gupta and *Gyan Dev Singh*
   INTRODUCTION 29

COMMON GI PARASITES OF CATTLE 30
    Ostertagia ostertagi 30
    Trichostrongylus spp. 30
    Cooperia sp. 30
    Haemonchus spp. 30
    Paramphistomum spp. 31
    Strongyloides papillosus 31
    Bunostomum phlebotomum 31
    Toxocara vitulorum 32
    Moniezia spp. 32
    Oesophagostomum spp. 33
    Schistosoma spp. 33
    Trichuris spp. 34
ECONOMIC IMPACT DUE TO GASTROINTESTINAL PARASITISM 34
    Reduced Growth Rates 34
    Decreased Milk Production 34
    Morbidity and Mortality 34
    Treatment Costs 35
    Labor Costs 35
    Reduced Fertility 35
    Increased Feed Costs 35
    Trade Restrictions 35
MANAGEMENT OF GI PARASITISM 35
    Pasture Management 35
    Strategic Deworming 36
    Fecal Egg Count Monitoring 36
    Nutrition and Herd Health 36
    Quarantine and New Animal Introduction 36
    Genetic Selection 36
    Manure Management 36
    Minimize Stress 36
    Environmental Modifications 37
    Consultation with Veterinarian 37
    CONCLUSION 37
    REFERENCES 37

CHAPTER 3 PARASITES IN THE UROGENITAL TRACT INFECTION 39
Farhat Bano, Muhammad Tahir Aleem, Muhammad Mohsin, Muhammad Asmat
Ullah Saleem and *Furqan Munir*
    INTRODUCTION 39
        Trichomonas Foetus 42
        Stephanurus Dentatus 45
        Neospora Caninum 46
        Trypanosoma Brucei Brucei 48
        Dioctophyma Renale 50
    FUTURE PERSPECTIVES 52
    CONCLUSION 53
    REFERENCES 53

CHAPTER 4 PARASITES IN THE CIRCULATORY SYSTEM 57
Pallabi Pathak and *Joken Bam*
    INTRODUCTION 57

Schistosoma 57
Onchocerca 60
Theileria 60
Babesia 62
Anaplasma 64
Trypanosoma 65
CONCLUSION 67
REFERENCES 67

CHAPTER 5 PARASITES IN THE INTEGUMENTARY SYSTEM 68
Bhupamani Das, Niral Patel, Dhyanjyoti Sarma and *R. M. Patel*
INTRODUCTION 68
EFFECT OF PARASITIC DISEASE ON INTEGUMENTARY SYSTEM 68
Helminth Parasite Affecting Integumentary System 69
Ectoparasites Affecting Integumentary System 73
FLIES 74
Effect of fly larvae on skin: Myiasis 81
TICK 82
LICE 83
MITE 85
FLEA 87
LEACH 88
Miscellaneous 88
Protozoa Affecting Integumentary System 89
CONCLUSION 90
REFERENCES 91

CHAPTER 6 PARASITES IN THE NERVOUS SYSTEM 94
Muhammad Mohsin, Muhammad Tahir Aleem, Muhammad Zahid Farooq,
Muhammad Asmat Ullah Saleem and *Furqan Munir*
INTRODUCTION 94
Taenia Multiceps 97
Thelazia rhodesi 100
Thelazia gulosa 102
Thelazia skrjabini 104
Hypoderma bovis 106
Trypanosoma brucei brucei 108
FUTURE PERSPECTIVE 110
CONCLUSION 110
REFERENCES 110

CHAPTER 7 PARASITES IN THE EYE AND EAR 115
Muhammad Mohsin, Muhammad Tahir Aleem, Muhammad Zahid Farooq,
Muhammad Asmat Ullah Saleem and *Furqan Munir*
INTRODUCTION 115
Raillietia auris 117
Rhabditis species 120
Thelazia rhodesii 120
Thelazia gulosa 122
Thelazia skrjabini 123
Otobius megnini 124
Significance of Parasites of Eye and Ear on Cattle 125

    FUTURE PERSPECTIVES 126
    CONCLUSION 127
    REFERENCES 127

CHAPTER 8 PARASITES OF THE RESPIRATORY SYSTEM 132
    Fathy Ahmad Osman
    INTRODUCTION 132
        Primary Parasite of the Respiratory System 134
            Husk Disease 134
            Anthelmintic Prophylaxis 139
        Nasal Schistosomiasis in Cattle 139
            Snoring disease 139
        Mammomonogamiasis 142
            Syngamoniasis 142
        Parasites of another Organ System that Produces Respiratory Symptoms Toxocariasis 145
            Neoascaris vitulorum 145
            Strongyloidiasis 146
            Bunostomosis 149
        Parasite affecting the respiratory system through larvae migration and/or proliferation 151
            Hydatid disease (Echinococcosis) Definition 151
            Sarcocystosis 153
    CONCLUSION 157
    REFERENCES 157

CHAPTER 9 PARASITES OF LIVER AND PANCREAS 160
    Bhupamani Das, Ayushi Nair, Mayank Prajapati and *Pallabi Pathak*
    INTRODUCTION 160
        Parasites that Directly Affect the Liver and Pancreas 161
            Fasciola gigantica 161
            Fasciola hepatica 164
            Fascioloides magna 165
            Dicrocoelium dentriticum 167
            Eurytrema pancreaticum 169
        Parasites that Indirectly affect the Liver and Pancreas 170
            Schistosoma spindale 170
            Gigantocotyle explanatum 172
            Paramphistomum spp. 173
            Echinococcus granulosus 174
            Toxocara vitulorum 176
            Toxoplasma gondii 177
            Babesia bigemina 178
            Theileria annulata 180
            Anaplasma marginale 181
    CONCLUSION 183
    REFERENCES 183

CHAPTER 10 PARASITES OF THE MUSCULOSKELETAL SYSTEM 192
    Bhupamani Das and *Ayushi Nair*
    INTRODUCTION 192
        Transmission of Parasites through Musculoskeletal System 193
            Horizontal Transmission 193
            Vertical Transmission 194

Impact on the Musculoskeletal System 194
Parasitic Diseases that Directly Affect the Musculoskeletal System 194
    Taenia Saginata 194
    Sarcocystis Species 196
    Toxoplasma Gondii 198
    Ecchninococcus Granulosus 200
    Besnoitia Species 201
    Neospora Caninum 203
    Hypoderma Species 206
Parasitic Diseases that Indirectly Affect the Musculoskeletal System 208
    Toxocara Vitulorum 208
    Bunostomum Radiatum 210
    Ascaris Suum 210
CONCLUSION 211
REFERENCES 211

CHAPTER 11 FAECAL EXAMINATION FOR DIAGNOSIS OF PARASITIC DISEASES 218
Joken Bam, Pallabi Pathak, Nitika Sharma and *Doni Jini*
INTRODUCTION 218
FAECAL SAMPLING, PRESERVATION AND TRANSPORTATION TO LABORATORY 219
METHODS OF FAECAL EXAMINATION 220
Qualitative Method 223
    Direct Method 223
Concentration Method 223
Floatation Method 223
Sedimentation Method 224
Quantitative Method 225
    Modified McMaster Test 225
    Modified Stoll Test 226
    Cornell-Wisconsin Egg-counting Test 226
    Formol-Ether technique 226
FAECAL CULTURE TECHNIQUES 227
Baermann Test 228
FAECAL STAINING METHOD FOR DIAGNOSIS OF CRYPTOSPORIDIUM 229
CONCLUSION 229
REFERENCES 229

CHAPTER 12 HISTOPATHOLOGICAL DIAGNOSIS OF PARASITIC DISEASES 230
Paras Saini, Sushma Kajal, Surbhi Gupta and *Snehil Gupta*
INTRODUCTION 230
Trematodes 233
    Fasciola hepatica and F. gigantica 233
    Schistosomiasis 234
    Amphistomiasis 234
Cestodes 234
Nematodes 236
    Toxocara vitulorum Identification 238
    Strongyle Worm Identification 239
    Nodular Worm Identification 239
    Lungworm Identification 240
    Hookworm Identification 240
    Gongylonema Identification 240

     Onchocerca Identification 241

     Parafilaria bovicola Identification 241

     Trichuris Identification 242

   Specific Histopathological Diagnostic Features of Commonly Found Cattle Arthropods 242

   Specific Histopathological Diagnostic Features of Commonly found Pentastomids Parasites in Cattle 243

   Specific Histopathological Diagnostic Features of Commonly Found Protozoan Parasites in Cattle 243

   Histopathological Techniques for Parasitic Diagnosis 244

  CONCLUSION 247

  REFERENCES 248

CHAPTER 13 ANTI-PARASITIC DRUGS 249

Muhammad Asmat Ullah Saleem, Muhammad Asif Wisal, Muhammad Waqas, Muhammad Mohsin and *Muhammad Tahir Aleem*

  INTRODUCTION 249

  ANTI-PROTOZOAL DRUGS 253

   Non-sulfonamides 253

     Amprolium 253

     Decoquinate 254

     Diclazuril 255

     Imidocarb 255

     Lasalocid 255

     Metronidazole 255

   Sulfonamides 256

     Sulfadimethoxine 256

     Sulfamethazine 257

     Sulfaquinoxaline 257

  ANTHELMINTICS 257

   Ivermectin 257

   Albendazole 258

   Fenbendazole 259

   Levamisole 259

  ECTOPARASITIC DRUGS 260

   Pyrethrins 260

   Carbamates and Organophosphates 261

   Foramidines 262

  RESISTANCE TO ANTIPARASITIC DRUGS 263

  CONCLUSION 264

  REFERENCES 265

CHAPTER 14 HOST RESISTANCE TO PARASITIC DISEASES 270

Farhat Bano, Muhammad Ahsan, Muhammad Asmat Ullah Saleem, Muhammad Mohsin and *Muhammad Tahir Aleem*

  INTRODUCTION 271

   Evolution of Resistance 272

   Host-parasite Relationship 273

   Role of Innate and Acquired Immunity 276

   Resistance against Ecto and Endoparasites 278

   Cellular Response to Parasitic Attack 279

   The Sources of Variation in Resistance to Parasitic Diseases 281

   The Process of Parasite Rejection 282

How Parasites Escape Host Immune System 284
Parasitic Infections in the Compromised Host 286
FUTURE PERSPECTIVES 288
CONCLUSION 289
REFERENCES 289

CHAPTER 15 ANTIPARASITIC VACCINES 298
P. Ramadevi, J. Jayalakshmi1 and Snehil Gupta
INTRODUCTION 298
Development of Parasitic Vaccines and Challenges 300
   Helminth Vaccines 300
   Echinococcus Granulosus 303
   Oesophagostomum 304
   Ostertagia Ostertagi and Cooperia Oncophora 304
   Haemonchus Placei and H. Similis 304
   Dictyocaulus Viviparus 305
   Protozoal Vaccines 307
   Neospora Caninum 307
   Tritrichomonas Foetus 308
   Theileria 308
   Babesia 310
   Eimeria 311
   Cryptosporidium 311
   Anaplasma Marginale 312
   Arthropod Vaccines 313
CONCLUSION 317
REFERENCES 317

CHAPTER 16 PREVENTIVE MEASURES AND CONTROL OF PARASITES 325
Muhammad Tahir Aleem, Fakiha Kalim, Azka Kalim, Furqan Munir and Jazib Hussain
INTRODUCTION 326
COMPREHENDING CATTLE PARASITES 328
PASTURE MANAGEMENT APPROACH FOR EFFECTIVE PARASITIC CONTROL ... 331
Pasture Rotation 331
Pasture Resting Period 332
Waste Management and Removal 333
Fecal Examination and Deworming Practices 334
GRAZING MANAGEMENT STRATEGIES 338
Grazing Intensity or Stocking Rate 338
Age Group Distribution for Grazing 338
Multi-species Grazing 338
Zero Grazing 339
MANAGEMENT OF DWELLING PLACES OR SHEDS 339
MANAGEMENT OF NUTRITION AND DEVELOPING IMMUNITY 339
Intake of Vitamin Supplements 340
Consumption of Mineral Supplements 341
Immunization 341
BIOLOGICAL CONTROL 341
CONCLUSION 343
REFERENCES 344

SUBJECT INDEX 357

FOREWORD

The well-being and health of livestock constitute crucial pillars for implementing sustainable agricultural practices within the intricate domain of animal husbandry and agriculture. Cattle, recognized as key components of global agriculture, play an essential role in supplying meat, milk, and other indispensable by-products. Despite their significance, various challenges often undermine the optimal productivity of cattle, and among these concerns, parasitic infections emerge as a noteworthy issue.

The book titled "Organ-specific Parasites of Cattle" delves into the intricate realm of parasitism, centering its attention on those elusive organisms that target specific organs within the host bovine. This thorough inquiry, undertaken by a team of experts in parasitology, veterinary medicine, and animal health, seeks to elucidate the intricacies of the biology, impacts, and control measures associated with these organ-specific parasites.

This groundbreaking publication provides valuable perspectives for cattle farmers contending with the persistent challenge of parasite-related diseases, while also serving as a repository of information for veterinary professionals, researchers, and students. The book's concentration on organ-specific parasites contributes to a deeper understanding of the intricate dynamics between hosts and parasites, enriching our comprehension of these complex interactions.

The pages that follow are evidence of the contributors' unwavering commitment as they have painstakingly collected and synthesized the most recent findings from research and field observations and practical experiences. We sincerely hope that this compilation will prove to be a useful tool, promoting a more thorough understanding of the intricacies related to organ-specific parasites and, in the process, aiding in the creation of more robust and long-lasting control methods.

"Organ-specific Parasites of Cattle" serves as a beacon in the constantly changing field of agriculture and animal health, pointing the way toward a more sophisticated and all-encompassing strategy for reducing the negative effects of these parasitism on the well-being and output of the bovine species. In the continuous search for the welfare of cattle and the resilience of our agricultural systems, may this work serve as an inspiration for more research, creativity, and cooperation.

Samuel Uchenna Felix
National Animal Production Research Institute/Ahmadu
Bello University Nigeria/Department of Food and Animal Science
Alabama A&M University, USA

PREFACE

Parasitic infections, a major global concern, adversely affect cattle health as well as production by losing the economic status of the farmers significantly in terms of declined milk production, inferior meat quality, depreciation of hide, loss of manure production, and draught power. A significant pinpoint evaluation of diseases as well as confirmatory diagnosis is required for specific treatment of both ecto- and endo-parasites. In addition, morphological identification of parasites is a basic important tool for the standard methods for diagnosis. Histopathological analysis of parasitic diseases may play an important role in the diagnosis as well as in providing knowledge of the severity of complications of parasitic diseases. It also provides insights into the interactions between parasites and animal hosts and their impact on infected animals. Interestingly, parasites in cattle can cause delayed growth rates, poor physical development and fertility, serious health-related issues, and death in infected cattle. Besides, several parasites may infect both animals and humans, causing public health concerns. The pathological changes are also observed through toxic, subtractive, inflammatory, allergic, obstructive, traumatic, necrotic, and immunosuppressive pathogenic mechanisms caused by parasites in cattle in a wide diverse host/parasite relationships. Parasites may also have the ability to cause tumors or tumor-like lesions in infected cattle.

The present book is organized with the aim to provide a comprehensive approach used in the identification of various images of parasites, the diagnosis of parasites, and prevention and control strategies to counteract parasitic diseases of cattle. It also provides knowledge of its distribution, epidemiology, lifecycle, morphology, clinical manifestations, diagnosis, prophylaxis, and therapeutic measures of parasitic diseases of cattle. The book also covers numerous informative tables and color images for the easy identification of parasites, their induced diseases, and updated information on suitable prevention and control measures. The book is well acceptable as both a textbook and a reference guide for students, academicians, researchers, field veterinarians, veterinarian nurses, laboratory staff, farm managers and also livestock owners. The book is systematically arranged and provides high-quality literature of international standards on organ-specific parasites and parasitic diseases in cattle and their diagnosis and therapeutic management. The book serves as a useful basic resource for all researchers, academics, and postgraduates wishing to gather knowledge on parasitic diseases, diagnosis, treatment, and prevention of cattle parasites and parasitic diseases with an aim to develop new antiparasitic drugs.

Tanmoy Rana
Department of Veterinary Clinical Complex
West Bengal University of Animal & Fishery Sciences
Kolkata, India

List of Contributors

Azka Kalim	Faculty of Medical Sciences, Government College University, Faisalabad-38000, Pakistan
Ajit Kumar	Bihar Veterinary College, Bihar Animal Sciences University, Patna, India
Ayushi Nair	Department of Medicine, College of Veterinary Science & A.H., Kamdhenu University, Sardarkrushinagar, Gujarat, India-385506
Bhavanam Sudhakara Reddy	College of Veterinary Science - Proddatur, Sri Venkateswara Veterinary University, Andhra Pradesh, India
Bhupamani Das	Department of Clinics (Veterinary Parasitology), College of Veterinary Science & Animal Husbandry, Kamdhenu University, Sardarkrushinagar, Gujarat, India
Dhyanjyoti Sarma	Department of Clinics (Veterinary Parasitology), College of Veterinary Science & Animal Husbandry, Kamdhenu University, Sardarkrushinagar, Gujarat, India
Doni Jini	ICAR-Research Complex for North-eastern Hill Region Arunachal Pradesh Centre, Basar, India
Farhat Bano	College of Veterinary Medicine, Northeast Agricultural University, Harbin, 150030, P.R. , China
Furqan Munir	Department of Parasitology, Faculty of Veterinary Science, University of Agriculture, Faisalabad 38040, Pakistan
Fathy Ahmad Osman	Animal Health Research Institute, Department of Parasitology, Agricultural Research Center, Egypt
Fakiha Kalim	Department of Parasitology, Faculty of Veterinary Science, University of Agriculture, Faisalabad 38040, Pakistan
Gyan Dev Singh	Bihar Veterinary College, Bihar Animal Sciences University, Patna, India
Jay Prakash Gupta	Bihar Veterinary College, Bihar Animal Sciences University, Patna, India
Joken Bam	ICAR-Research Complex for the Northeastern Hill Region, Arunachal Pradesh Centre, Basar, India
J. Jayalakshmi	Department of Veterinary Parasitology, Sri Venkateswara Veterinary University, Tirupati-517101, India
Jazib Hussain	DNRF Center for Chromosome Stability, Department of Cellular and Molecular Medicine, Faculty of Health and Medical Sciences, University of Copenhagen, Denmark
K.P. Shyma	Bihar Veterinary College, Bihar Animal Sciences University, Patna, India
Muhammad Tahir Aleem	MOE Joint International Research Laboratory of Animal Health and Food Safety, College of Veterinary Medicine, Nanjing Agricultural University, Nanjing 210095, China Center for Gene Regulation in Health and Disease, Department of Biological, Geological, and Environmental Sciences, College of Sciences and Health Professions, Cleveland State University, Cleveland, OH 44115, USA
Muhammad Mohsin	Shantou University Medical College, Shantou, Gunagdong, 515045, China
Muhammad Asmat Ullah Saleem	College of Veterinary Medicine, Northeast Agricultural University, Harbin, 150030, P.R. , China

Muhammad Zahid Farooq Department of Animal Science, University of Veterinary and Animal Sciences (Jhang Campus), Lahore 54000, Pakistan

Mayank Prajapati College of Veterinary Science & Animal Husbandry, Kamdhenu University, Sardarkrushinagar, Gujarat, India

Muhammad Asif Wisal College of Animal Sciences and Technology, Jilin Agricultural University, Changchun, China

Muhammad Ahsan Faculty of Veterinary Sciences, University of Agriculture, Faisalabad, Pakistan

Muhammad Waqas Ondokuz Mayıs University, Samsun, Turkey

Niral Patel Department of Clinics (Veterinary Parasitology), College of Veterinary Science & Animal Husbandry, Kamdhenu University, Sardarkrushinagar, Gujarat, India

Nitika Sharma ICAR-Centre Institute for Research on Goat, Makhdoom, Mathura, Uttar Pradesh, India

Pallabi Pathak Lakhimpur College of Veterinary Science, Assam Agricultural University, Joyhing, Lakhimpur, Assam, India

Paras Saini Department of Veterinary Pathology, Lala Lajpat Rai University of Veterinary and Animal Sciences, Hisar, India

P. Ramadevi Department of Veterinary Parasitology, Sri Venkateswara Veterinary University, Tirupati-517101, India

R. M. Patel Department of Clinics (Veterinary Parasitology), College of Veterinary Science & Animal Husbandry, Kamdhenu University, Sardarkrushinagar, Gujarat, India Department of Veterinary Medicine, College of Veterinary Science & Animal Husbandry, Kamdhenu University, Sardarkrushinagar, Gujarat, India

Sirigireddy Sivajothi College of Veterinary Science - Proddatur, Sri Venkateswara Veterinary University, Andhra Pradesh, India

Syed Afreen College of Veterinary Science - Proddatur, Sri Venkateswara Veterinary University, Andhra Pradesh, India

Sushma Kajal Department of Veterinary Pathology, Lala Lajpat Rai University of Veterinary and Animal Sciences, Hisar, India

Surbhi Gupta Department of Veterinary Physiology and Biochemistry, Lala Lajpat Rai University of Veterinary and Animal Sciences, Hisar, India

Snehil Gupta Department of Veterinary Parasitology, Lala Lajpat Rai University of Veterinary and Animal Sciences, Hisar, India

Tanmoy Rana Department of Veterinary Clinical Complex, West Bengal University of Animal & Fishery Sciences, Kolkata, India

CHAPTER 1

Introduction

Sirigireddy Sivajothi[1,*], **Bhavanam Sudhakara Reddy**[1], **Syed Afreen**[1] and **Tanmoy Rana**[2]

[1] *College of Veterinary Science - Proddatur, Sri Venkateswara Veterinary University, Andhra Pradesh, India*

[2] *Department of Veterinary Clinical Complex, West Bengal University of Animal & Fishery Sciences, Kolkata, India*

Abstract: Bovine parasitism presents a complex and variable disease condition affecting grazing cattle, encompassing both internal and external parasites. Internal parasites reside within the animal, while external parasites inhabit the animal's exterior. Both types can significantly impact cattle health. Understanding internal parasites and their control in natural field conditions necessitates awareness of external parasites and their role in cattle production cycles. The economic significance of different parasitic worms in cattle hinges on factors such as parasite species, the damage they cause, and parasite numbers within the animals at any given time.

Keywords: Cattle, Control, Diagnosis, External parasites, Internal parasites.

INTRODUCTION

Livestock is a crucial part of the agricultural sector, significantly contributing to the rural economy, especially for small and marginal farmers. Parasites are organisms that inhabit or feed on another species, known as the host, for sustenance. Typically, helminths and protozoa are endoparasites, residing within the host's body, while ectoparasites present over the host's external surface (Fig. 1) [1, 2]. Haemoparasites, on the other hand, inhabit the host's bloodstream, often causing clinical or subclinical parasitic infection.

The impact of internal parasites (Table **1**) on cattle is influenced by factors such as the severity of infection, the age of the animal, and its stress levels. Typically, younger animals and those experiencing stress are more prone to displaying signs of parasitic infection. Mature cows tend to develop a degree of immunity against parasites residing in the lower gastrointestinal tract. However, parasite burdens

[*] **Corresponding author Sirigireddy Sivajothi:** College of Veterinary Science - Proddatur, Sri Venkateswara Veterinary University, Andhra Pradesh, India; E-mail: sivajothi579@gmail.com

can be particularly detrimental to mature cows nearing parturition due to suppressed immunity during this critical period [3, 4]. Parasitism's effects can be categorized into two types: subclinical and clinical. Subclinical effects encompass losses in animal productivity such as reduced milk production, weight gain, altered carcass composition, and conception rates. On the other hand, clinical effects manifest as visible disease-like symptoms including roughness of coat, anemia, edema, and diarrhea. The subclinical effects hold significant economic importance for producers. In dairy animals, subclinical gastrointestinal parasitic infections represent the primary health challenges limiting productivity [5, 6]. and is considered one of the major challenges in the development of dairy cattle globally [7, 8]. Subclinical infections result in illness and death among young animals, along with significant production losses in adults. While parasitic infections may not always manifest as apparent diseases, they lead to decreased production, including stunted growth, decreased appetite, and poor feed efficiency. The severity of the disease depends on factors such as the type of parasite or the number of parasites present [9, 10]. It is undeniable that, whether mild or severe, the disease causes infected animals to experience slower growth rates, preventing them from reaching their full growth potential. This inevitably results in economic losses for producers [11, 12]. Calf diarrhea stands out as a prevalent animal health issue among dairy farmers, with high mortality rates observed within the first year of life. In numerous cases, gastrointestinal parasite infections are a leading cause of this mortality. The economic impact of calf diarrhea can reach up to a 20% loss, significantly reducing dairy net profits by 38% [13, 14]. The repercussions extend to the loss of future breeding stock and dairy cows, ultimately affecting milk production. It is estimated that the cattle industry invests approximately USD 2.5 billion in pharmaceutical products for parasite control [15, 16].

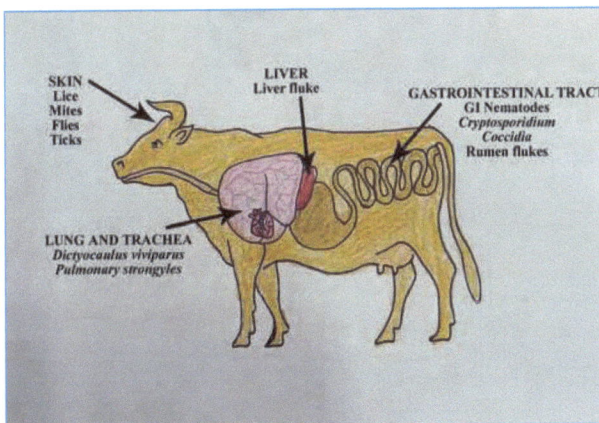

Fig. (1). Types of parasites and location.

Table 1. Major classes of internal parasites.

Roundworms or Nemathelminthes
Strongyles.
Gastrointestinal worms
Abomasum worms: *Haemonchus, Trichostrongylus, Ostertagia.*
Duodenum worms: *Trichostrongylus, Nematodirus, Cooperia, Strongyloides.*
Large intestine worms: *Oesophagostomum, Trichuris.*
Small intestine worms or Ancylostomatidae (hookworm): *Ancylostoma, Necator, Bunostomum.*
Lungworm or metastrongyles: *Dictyocaulus, Metastrongylus, Protostrongylus.*
Flatworms or platyhelminthes
Cestodes (tapeworm): *Moniezia, Stilesia, Avitellina.*
Trematodes (Flukes): *Fasciola, Dicrocoelium* (liver), *Paramphistomum, Schistosoma nasale.*

More than 2000 years ago, Hippocrates proposed that "all disease begins in the gut." While modern science has revealed this statement to be not entirely accurate, substantial evidence supports the significant association between many diseases and the intestine. Cattle can contract infections from various internal parasites, including roundworms (nematodes), tapeworms (cestodes), and flukes (trematodes) (Fig. **2**). Protozoans, such as coccidia, represent another category of internal parasites [17, 18].

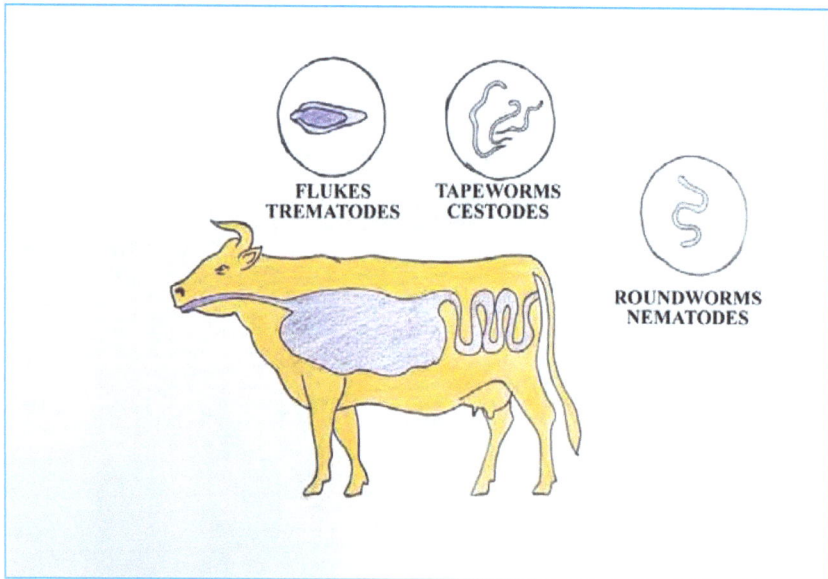

Fig. (2). Types of internal parasites.

Roundworms are widely recognized as the most economically impactful internal parasites affecting livestock. While cattle may also suffer from tapeworm infections, their impact on animal performance is relatively minor compared to roundworms. Challenges with flukes typically arise in environments conducive to snail populations, such as poorly drained pastures and stagnant water bodies like ponds or ditches within pasture areas. Snails play a crucial role in the life cycle of flukes [19, 20].

Nematodes

Nematodes (Table 2) are cylindrical worms with bilateral symmetry and tapered ends. They have an outer cuticle layer, lack circular muscles, and contain a pseudo coelom that houses all major systems, including the digestive, excretory, nervous, and reproductive systems. In cattle, trichostrongyles are the most common nematodes, comprising several genera that inhabit the abomasum, small intestine, and large intestine [21, 22]. The genera that produce the trichostrongyle type of eggs are *Bunostomum, Chabertia, Cooperia, Haemonchus, Oesophagostomum, Ostertagia* and *Trichostrongylus* sp. They have similar life cycle and produce oval, thin-shelled eggs.

Table 2. Characteristics of main Nematodes in cattle.

Parasite	Description	Infected Organ	Life Cycle	Symptoms
Haemonchus spp.	M: 10-20 mm red F: 18-30 mm red and white	Abomasum	IS: 4-6 days PP: 3 weeks	Anemia, soft swelling under jaw and abdomen, weakness, no weight gain.
Ostertagia spp.	M: 6-9 mm, brown F: 8-12 mm	Abomasum	IS: 4-6 days PP: 3 weeks	Same as *Haemonchus* and also lack of appetite, diarrhea.
Trichostrongylus spp.	M: 4-5.5 mm F: 5-7 mm light brown	Abomasum, duodenum	IS: 3-4 days PP: 2-3 weeks	Same as *Haemonchus* and also diarrhea and weight loss.
Cooperia spp.	red M: 5-7 mm F: 6-9 mm	Duodenum	IS: 5-6 days PP: 15-20 days	Same as *Haemonchus*.
Bunostomum spp.	10-30 mm	Duodenum	IS: ? PP: 30-56 days	Edema, anemia, weight loss, diarrhea.
Chabertia spp	M: 13-14 mm F: 17-20 mm	Large intestine	IS: 5-6 days PP: 42 days	Anemia, diarrhea with blood.
Oesophagostomum spp.	M: 12-17 mm F: 15-22 mm	Large intestine	IS: 6-7 days PP: 41-45 days	Dark green diarrhea edema.
Protostrongylus spp.	M: 16-28 mm F: 25-35 mm	Lungs	IS: 12-14 days PP: 30-37 days	Pneumonia.

Parasite	Description	Infected Organ	Life Cycle	Symptoms
Dictyocaulus spp.	M: 30-80 mm F: 50-100 mm	Lungs	IS: 6-7 days PP: 3-4 weeks	Sticky nasal discharge, difficulty breathing, cough.

Life Cycle of the Nematode

Fig. (**3**) illustrates the life cycle of the nematode. Within the host animal, adult nematodes lay eggs, which are then excreted from the host *via* feces, subsequently contaminating the pasture. From the egg, a first-stage larva emerges, which undergoes two molts before developing into a third-stage larva. At this stage, the larva gains the ability to migrate from dung pats and soil onto moist grass. Larvae can persist on pasture for up to a year [23, 24]. Infection occurs when the third-stage larvae are ingested with the grass. Inside the host's gastrointestinal tract, the larvae complete their life cycle. Once they reach adulthood, reproduction takes place, beginning the cycle again [25, 26]. In contrast to other nematodes, the medium stomach worm has the ability to enter a state of hypobiosis, akin to hibernation, during part of its parasitic life cycle. This phase typically commences in the spring, with the "hibernating" larvae remaining dormant until summer before emerging.

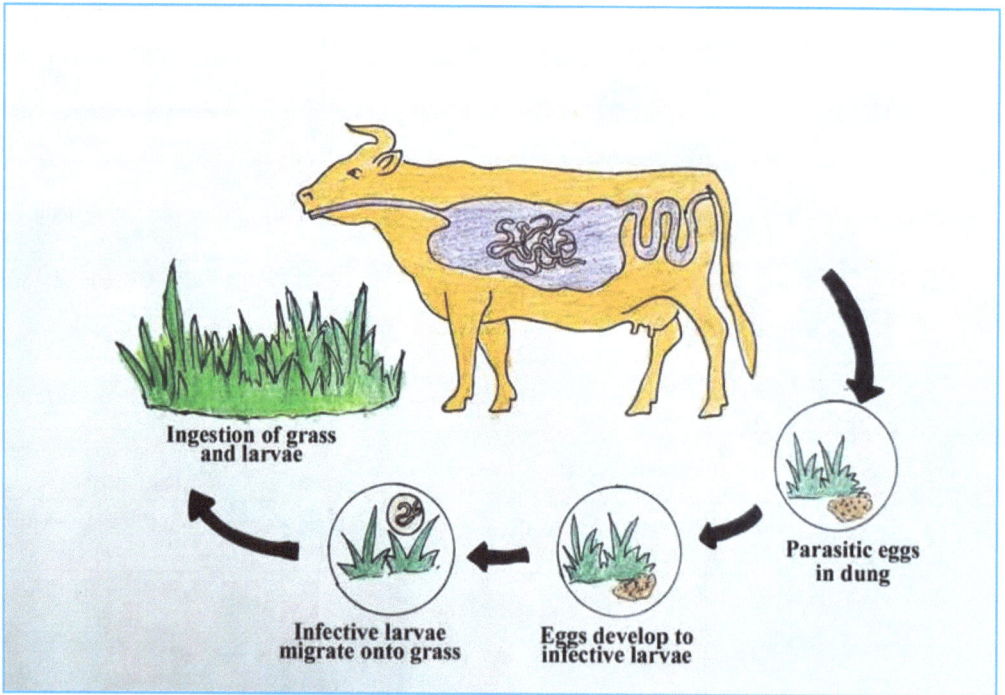

Fig. (3). Life cycle of nematodes.

Lungworms

Parasitic bronchitis, commonly known as husk, stands as a significant parasite infection affecting the bovine respiratory tract, caused by the nematode *Dictyocaulus viviparus* (Fig. **4**). While primarily impacting cattle, this species has also been documented in other ruminants, such as deer. The parasite is widespread, with higher infection rates observed in wetter regions, particularly in the western areas of the British Isles. Severe lungworm outbreaks in growing cattle can result in average losses ranging from £50 to £100 per head, while lost milk production in adults may reach up to £3 per cow per day [27, 28]. Similar to numerous other parasitic nematodes, infection with lungworms is acquired through the ingestion of infective larvae from contaminated pasture. The epidemiology of this infection is intricate, with outbreaks frequently proving unpredictable. Symptoms typically manifest in first-year grazing cattle during late summer and autumn, although they can also occur earlier in the year and affect older animals. The hallmark clinical sign of lungworm infection is widespread coughing within a herd, and mortality may occur in cases of heavy infections [29].

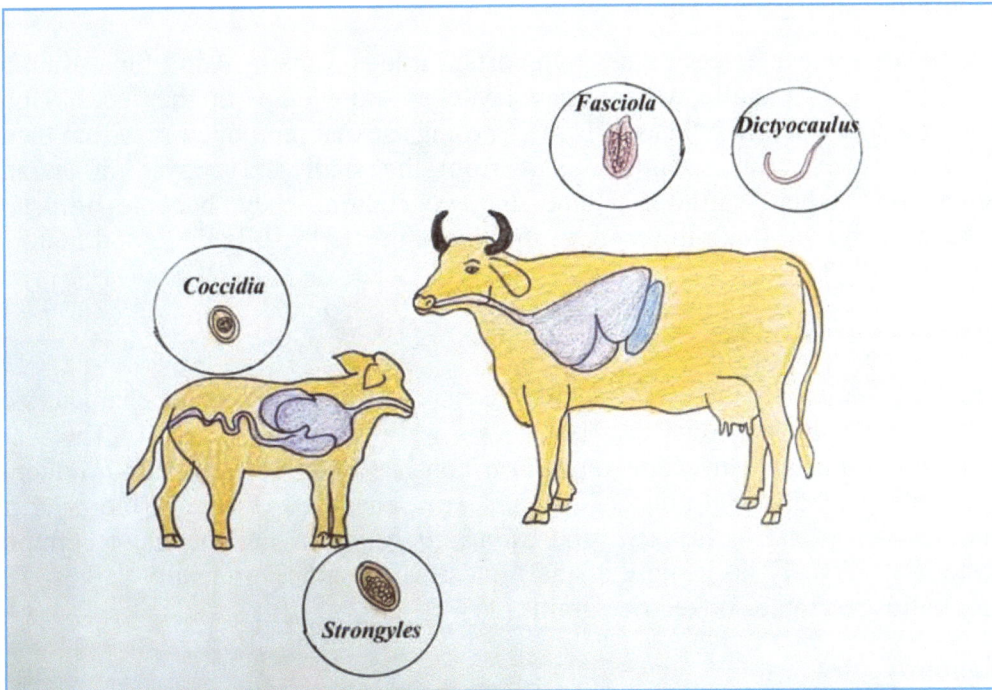

Fig. (4). Endoparasites.

Trematodes

Trematodes, also known as flukes, possess a dorsoventrally flattened, unsegmented, leaf-like body structure. They are equipped with suckers, hooks, or clamps to attach to the host. With the exception of *Schistosoma*, trematodes are hermaphrodites. Among the common trematodes affecting cattle are *Paramphistomes*, colloquially referred to as 'rumen flukes'. These flukes have an oral sucker at the front and a large ventral sucker at the rear. While adult flukes are generally non-pathogenic, their pathogenicity stems from the migration of their juvenile forms within the small intestine [30].

Fasciolosis

The condition is caused by the flukes *Fasciola hepatica* and *Fasciola gigantica*, which affect various mammalian hosts, including families such as Bovidae, Cervidae, Capridae, Equidae, and others. These flukes can also infect humans. *F. hepatica* is common in temperate regions worldwide, while *Fasciola gigantica* is primarily found in tropical and subtropical areas. In India, *Fasciola gigantica* is mainly prevalent in cattle [31].

The fluke's life cycle necessitates two hosts: cattle and snails. Adult flukes inhabit the bile ducts of cattle, where they lay eggs expelled with the feces. Upon hatching, larval stages infect snails, undergoing asexual reproduction within them. Certain juvenile fluke stages depart from the snail and encyst on aquatic vegetation. When cattle consume the vegetation, they become infected. Subsequently, the fluke migrates to the liver, infects the bile duct, and matures into an adult [32].

Cestodes

Cestodes, commonly known as tapeworms, have a ribbon-like shape characterized by a flat body that lacks a body cavity or alimentary canal. They are hermaphroditic, and the adult tapeworm consists of a series of egg-producing segments called proglottids. Nutrients are absorbed through the worm's integument. *Moniezia expansa* and *Moniezia benedeni* are the most common cestodes, primarily infesting the small intestine of cattle, especially calves. The proglottids resemble cooked rice grains [33].

Taeniasis

Taeniasis is a true zoonosis in which humans act as the definitive hosts and spread the infection, while cattle serve as intermediate hosts. The adult tapeworm *Taenia saginata* resides in the small intestine of humans, measuring approximately 5 to

12 meters in length. Eggs or gravid segments are excreted with feces onto the ground. Cattle become infected by ingesting these eggs while grazing, leading to the development of the larval stage *Cysticercus bovis* in their skeletal and cardiac muscles. Transmission from humans to animals can occur either directly or indirectly, although direct transmission is rare [34]. Transmission can also occur when hands contaminated with *Taenia* eggs are used to feed or handle calves. However, the most common mode of transmission is indirect, involving the contamination of food, soil, and sewage, as well as transmission by birds or flies. Sewage plays a significant role in spreading *Taenia* infections between humans and animals. Additionally, human habits, behaviors, religious practices, and beliefs influence dietary choices and cooking methods, affecting the transmission dynamics between animals and humans. Taeniasis is more prevalent in areas where people consume inadequately cooked or smoked meat or where open defecation is practiced [35].

PROTOZOAN INFECTIONS

Coccidiosis

Coccidiosis is one of the most pathogenic intestinal diseases, caused by various species of *Eimeria* within the phylum Apicomplexa [36]. The disease primarily affects confined animals raised under intensive husbandry practices and is more common in housed animals than in those on pasture. When combined with other enteropathogens, coccidia has been recognized as a major contributor to diarrhea in calves (Fig. **4**) [12].

Cryptosporidiosis

Cryptosporidium is a widely distributed intracellular apicomplexan protozoan parasite that can infect a variety of hosts, including humans, domestic animals, wild animals, birds, rodents, and reptiles. In cattle, the earliest reported cases of *Cryptosporidium* infection date back to the early 1970s [15]. However, because of its association with other viral or bacterial enteropathogens, the status of *Cryptosporidium* species as primary enteropathogens remained uncertain until 1980, when Tzipori *et al.* reported an outbreak of neonatal diarrhea attributed solely to *Cryptosporidium* infection. Bovine cryptosporidiosis is common among newborn calves and is characterized by acute gastrointestinal disturbances, including mucoid or hemorrhagic watery diarrhea, along with symptoms such as fever, lethargy, anorexia, and weight loss. These symptoms result in significant economic losses in farm animals and increased neonatal morbidity in cattle. Shedding intensity is notably higher in calves with diarrhea. Furthermore, *Cryptosporidium parvum*, an emerging zoonotic protozoan parasite affecting calves, is associated with diarrhea in children (Muraleedharan 2009).

Cryptosporidium infection rates have been observed to be notably elevated in urban slum areas [1, 32] and in patients with diarrhea [3]. *Cryptosporidium parvum* has been documented as the predominant parasite found in individuals who test positive for human immunodeficiency virus (HIV) [8]. In Sheather's sucrose flotation method, the oocysts appear as round or oval-shaped, refractile bodies with a thin cytoplasmic membrane. In contrast, when using modified Ziehl-Neelsen staining, the oocysts exhibit a spherical to ellipsoidal shape and are stained pink to red, containing four sporozoites against a pale green background.

Giardiasis

Giardiasis in dairy cattle stems from the flagellate protozoa *Giardia duodenalis* (also known as *G. lamblia* or *G. intestinalis*), belonging to the Class Mastigophora and Family Hexamitidae. It ranks among the most prevalent enteroparasites globally and has been recognized under the WHO's neglected disease initiative [10]. The disease is most commonly found in developing countries and areas with poor sanitation and hygiene practices. The parasite has two distinct morphological forms: the vegetative trophozoite and the thin-walled cyst. The cyst, which is the infective stage, encysts immediately upon being released into feces. *Giardia* cysts can spread directly between hosts or through various fomites, including contaminated water and food. Trophozoites are released from ingested cysts in the small intestine, where they multiply. In cattle, *Giardia* infection often presents as subclinical or asymptomatic; however, symptoms such as anorexia, watery and foul-smelling diarrhea, reduced weight gain, and poor health may occasionally occur in young calves. Infections are associated with a reduced microvillus surface area, decreased intestinal enzyme activity, and increased intestinal transit, ultimately resulting in malabsorptive diarrhea [23].

Neosporosis

Neospora caninum, a protozoan parasite, is emerging as a significant infectious agent causing weak calves and abortion in cattle. Reported infections span most parts of the world, with estimates indicating that 12-45% of aborted fetuses from dairy cattle are infected with the organism. A distinctive characteristic of the disease is abortion occurring at 4-6 months of gestation, a timeframe unique among infectious causes of bovine abortion. *N. caninum* demonstrates highly efficient transmission rates, with infection rates reaching up to 90% within certain herds. Cows acquire this parasite through two primary routes: 1) "Horizontal" transmission, by consuming feed or water contaminated with eggs (oocysts) from infected dogs and other canids, or 2) "Vertical" transmission, from cow to fetus during pregnancy. Once infected, *N. caninum* establishes a lifelong infection in adult cows, bulls, calves, or fetuses. Infected cows can transmit the organism to their calves through the placenta in every pregnancy, with the vast majority of congenitally infected calves (95%) appearing normal but remaining infected for life. Heifer calves born with the infection can pass it on to the next generation when they become pregnant, thus perpetuating the infection within the herd. While vertical transmission is the primary mode of transmission in cattle, both horizontal and vertical transmission are crucial for parasite survival [21, 27].

Echinococcosis (Hydatidosis)

Echinococcosis/hydatidosis is acknowledged as the foremost helminth zoonosis, bearing profound economic and public health implications, especially in developing countries [8, 11]. Echinococcosis is caused by a small taeniid tapeworm from the genus *Echinococcus*. This genus includes four recognized species: *E. granulosus, E. multilocularis, E. oligarthrus,* and *E. vogeli.* Their infective larval stages, known as metacestodes, form large cysts - either hydatid or alveolar cysts - in various mammalian hosts, including humans. The eggs of these tapeworms are usually found on the surface of dog feces and can accumulate in the perianal region of dogs. Dogs may carry these eggs on their tongues and snouts to various parts of their bodies. Direct contact with infected dogs is a significant mode of transmission to humans; however, consuming vegetables and water contaminated with infected dog feces can also lead to infection. It is important to note that humans serve as accidental intermediate hosts and are not capable of transmitting the disease.

Haemoprotozoan Parasites

Haemoprotozoan parasites present significant challenges to improving livestock production. The primary haemoprotozoan diseases affecting livestock in our country are trypanosomiasis, theileriosis, babesiosis, and anaplasmosis, all of which lead to substantial economic losses for livestock owners. Among these, babesiosis, theileriosis, and anaplasmosis are transmitted through ticks and are commonly referred to as tick-borne diseases (TBD). These diseases have been prevalent in our country for a considerable period. However, with the introduction of exotic breeds of cattle to enhance the productivity of indigenous stock and improve milk yield, the significance of these diseases has increased. Losses attributed to haemoprotozoan diseases include mortality, reduced milk yield, weight loss, abortion, infertility, diminished draft power, and the cost of treating affected animals [25]. The estimated annual loss due to tick-borne diseases (TBD) reaches 364 million USD, impacting approximately 1.3 million cattle through mortality. Theileriosis is responsible for 68% of these losses. Mortality-related costs comprise 49% of the overall losses, while chemotherapy expenses account for 21%, and the use of acaricides contributes 14% to the estimated annual losses from TBD. Additionally, infection and treatment methods account for 1% of the total losses, with reduced milk production and weight loss contributing 6% and 9%, respectively [31]. It is important to highlight those asymptomatic infections constituted a substantial portion (50.8%) of these costs. Among subclinical infections, those linked to anemia caused the highest losses in live weight. Disease cases contributed to 23.64% of the losses, with mortality being the most significant factor [29].

Babesiosis

In cattle, it is caused by two species affecting cattle: *Babesia bovis* and *Babesia bigemina*, which have a wide distribution and are particularly significant in Africa, Asia, Australia, and Central and South America. Vectors for *Babesia* transmission, with *Boophilus microplus* being the principal vector for *B. bigemina* and *B. bovis*, prevalent in tropical and subtropical regions. *B. bovis* generally exhibits greater pathogenicity compared to *B. bigemina* or *B. divergens*. Infections typically manifest with elevated rectal temperature, absence of feed intake, neurological signs and circulatory shock, occasionally accompanied by nervous signs due to the sequestration of infected erythrocytes in cerebral capillaries. In acute cases, the maximum parasitemia (percentage of infected erythrocytes) in circulating blood is usually less than 1% for *B. bovis* infections. In contrast, *B. bigemina* infections often exhibit parasitemia exceeding 10%, sometimes reaching as high as 30%, with major signs including fever, haemoglobinuria, and anaemia. Unlike *B. bovis*, intravascular sequestration of infected erythrocytes does not occur with *B. bigemina* infections. The parasitemia and clinical presentation of *B. divergens* infections resemble those of *B. bigemina* infections to some extent [27].

Oriental Theileriosis

Theileria are obligate intracellular protozoan parasites that infect both wild and domestic Bovidae worldwide, with some species also affecting small ruminants. They are transmitted by ixodidae ticks and have complex life cycles involving both vertebrate and invertebrate hosts. In India, bovine tropical theileriosis is primarily caused by *Theileria annulata*, which is also prevalent in large parts of the Mediterranean coast of North Africa, extending to northern Sudan, southern Europe, southeastern Europe, the Near and Middle East, China, and Central Asia. The parasite group referred to as the *T. sergenti/ T. buffeli/ T. orientalis* complex is now recognized to consist of two species: *T. sergenti*, found in the Far East, and *T. buffeli / T. orientalis* (commonly referred to as *T. buffeli*) with a global distribution. The infective stage of *T. annulata* is the sporozoite stage, which is transmitted by various species of *Hyalomma* ticks while feeding on bovine hosts. Several species of *Hyalomma*, including *H. anatolicum anatolicum* (found in

Eurasian countries including India and African countries), *H. dromedarii* (found in Central Asia), *H. marginatum* (found in India and the Middle East), and *H. detritum* (found in North Africa and Russian countries), are responsible for the transmission of *T. annulata* [22].

Anaplasmosis

Anaplasmosis, also known as gall sickness, yellow bag, or yellow fever, is an infectious parasitic disease that affects cattle, caused by the microorganism *Anaplasma marginale*. This obligate intraerythrocytic parasite belongs to the order Rickettsiales, family Anaplasmataceae, and genus *Anaplasma*. It primarily targets red blood cells, resulting in severe anemia, weakness, fever, loss of appetite, depression, constipation, decreased milk production, jaundice, abortion, and, in severe cases, death. The incubation period for the disease varies from 2 weeks to over 3 months, with an average duration of 3 to 4 weeks [27]. Adult cattle are more susceptible to infection than calves. The disease generally presents as mild in calves under one year of age, is rarely fatal in cattle up to two years old, can be fatal in animals up to three years old, and is often fatal in older cattle. After recovering from the infection, whether naturally or through standard treatment, animals typically become lifelong carriers of the disease. While carriers may not exhibit symptoms, they can transmit the infection to other susceptible cattle. Occasionally, some animals may spontaneously clear the infection completely and regain susceptibility to the disease. Anaplasmosis is prevalent in tropical and subtropical regions worldwide [21].

EXTERNAL PARASITES

External parasites (Fig. **5**) are parasites that live on the outside of an animal's body. They can attach to the skin of the animal and feed on its blood. External parasites can be very irritating and can cause serious skin problems or disease.

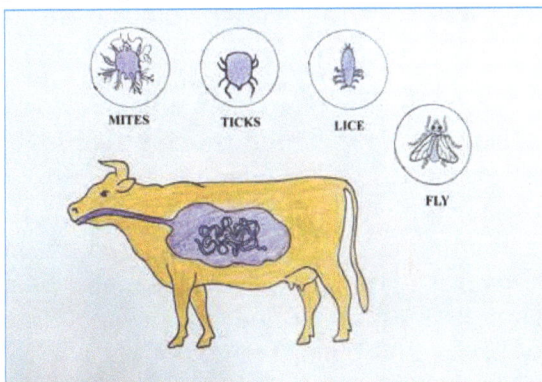

Fig. (5). Types of external parasites.

Some Examples of External Parasites Include

Fleas, Ticks, Mites, Lice, Stable flies, House flies, Horn flies, Face flies, Mosquitoes.

Blood-Sucking Flies

Black Flies

Black flies are small, dark, stout-bodied insects with a distinctive humpbacked appearance. Adult females primarily feed on blood during daylight hours and are not particular about their hosts. They often hover around the eyes, ears, and nostrils of animals, landing to inflict irritating bites by puncturing the skin. When bitten in large numbers, animals may experience weakness due to blood loss, anaphylactic shock, or even death. The life cycle of black flies begins with the deposition of eggs on logs, rocks, or other solid surfaces in the eddies of flowing streams. Larvae attach themselves to rocks or vegetation using a posterior sucker or threads. The duration of the larval stage varies significantly depending on the species and environmental conditions. Once pupation is complete, adults emerge and display strong flying abilities, capable of traveling distances of 7 to 10 miles from their breeding sites.

Horn Flies

The horn fly stands out as one of the most significant pests affecting cattle, inflicting pain, irritation, and disruption to their normal activities. This persistent biter pierces the skin to feed on blood, causing discomfort to the host. During periods of high summertime populations, horn flies contribute to weight loss and reduced milk production in cattle. Additionally, their presence may lead to the formation of open sores on the head and underline, increasing the risk of secondary infections. These flies tend to congregate at specific sites on the host, particularly the withers and back [20].

Horn fly populations reaching 50 or more per animal are considered economically significant, although there have been reports of counts as high as 10,000 to 20,000 per animal. In such extreme cases, considerable blood loss can occur. Eggs are laid exclusively in fresh cattle manure, typically within 10 minutes of deposition. Larvae hatch within approximately 18 hours and feed on the dung, progressing through three stages over 3 to 5 days. The pupal stage lasts 3 to 5 days before adults emerge, with a preoviposition period of 3 days. Mating occurs on the host, and females can lay about 200 eggs throughout their lifetime. The entire life cycle, from egg to adult, typically spans 10 to 14 days [28].

Adult horn flies feed intermittently, typically around 20 times a day, and remain on the host continuously throughout both day and night, except during oviposition. This behavior makes them susceptible to chemical control methods. When used consistently, dust bags provide optimal control of horn flies, although sprays, ear tags, and dips can also be effective. While back rubbers and pour-on treatments may offer some control, they are generally less effective. Larval control can be achieved with feed additives; however, adult populations may not see a significant decrease in fly migration and continue to sustain high infestation levels [30].

Horse and Deer Flies

Horse flies and deer flies, also known as Tabanids, are robust insects known for their strong flying abilities. Similar to mosquitoes, only female flies bite. They are typically active during the daytime and are known for their aggressive biting behavior. Their attacks can lead to reduced weight gain and decreased milk production in affected animals. Due to the painful nature of their bites and the frequency of their attacks, horseflies often induce frenzied behavior in their hosts, sometimes prompting them to run long distances in an attempt to evade the flies [6].

Tabanids inject an anticoagulant into the wound when they bite, causing blood to ooze. These wounds create favorable conditions for secondary invasion by other insects and diseases, potentially leading to further blood loss. Due to their intermittent feeding pattern, tabanids can act as significant mechanical vectors for diseases such as anthrax, tularemia, and anaplasmosis. Most tabanid species are aquatic or semi-aquatic during their immature stages, while some develop in moist soil, leaf mold, or decaying logs. Typically, eggs are laid in layers on vegetation, objects above water, or in moist areas that promote larval growth. Eggs hatch within 5 to 7 days, after which the larvae descend to the water's surface or moist areas to begin feeding on organic matter [2].

Many species of horse and deer flies feed on insect larvae, crustaceans, snails, and earthworms. Once the larvae reach the pupal stage, they migrate to drier soil, usually one to two inches below the surface. The pupal stage typically lasts 2 to 3 weeks before the adults emerge. The duration of the life cycle varies significantly among species, ranging from 70 days to 2 years.

In Florida alone, there are over 122 species of horse and deer flies, with some present throughout most of the year. These flies present significant challenges for pest control. While daily mist applications can provide protection for animals, they are often impractical for most cattle farmers to implement [8].

Sand Flies and Biting Midges

Sand flies, also referred to as punkies, no-see-ums, or biting midges, are small biting flies. They breed in wet or aquatic habitats, making them difficult, if not impossible, to control. These flies are primarily a nuisance and can cause significant irritation. In large numbers, they may even lead to suffocation. One species of sand fly is recognized as a vector for the bluetongue virus in cattle, while some species act as intermediate hosts for helminths. However, there is limited knowledge regarding the life cycle of sand flies that affect livestock [11].

Stable Flies

The stable fly, also known as the dog fly, shares similarities with the house fly in size and color, but it can be distinguished by its bayonet-like mouthparts. Unlike other discussed flies, both male and female stable flies are aggressive biters. They are capable of flying long distances from their breeding sites.

Stable flies cause irritation and weakness in animals, leading to significant blood loss in severe cases. Bite wounds can also become sites for secondary infections. These flies are easily disturbed while feeding and can mechanically transmit diseases such as anthrax and anaplasmosis. In 2012, their economic impact on the US cattle industry was estimated to exceed $2.2 billion annually.

Stable flies breed in areas with soggy hay, grain, or feed, fermenting weed or grass cuttings, spilled green chop, peanut litter, seaweed deposits along beaches, and manure mixed with hay. When depositing eggs, females often crawl into loose materials to lay eggs in small pockets. A single female may lay up to 500 to 600 eggs in four separate batches. Eggs hatch within 2 to 5 days, and the newly emerged larvae bury themselves, feed, and mature within 14 to 26 days. While the average life cycle is around 28 days, this duration can vary from 22 to 58 days depending on weather conditions [25].

Adult stable flies can remarkably fly up to 80 miles from their breeding sites. When there are more than 10 flies per animal, it is considered economically detrimental, indicating significant fly breeding in the area. Effective control of stable flies primarily depends on cultural control measures. Since the larvae thrive in moist breeding environments, it is essential to identify and eliminate these breeding sources to promote drying. Animal treatments are limited to insecticide applications through fogging or misting to reduce fly populations [4].

Non-Blood Sucking Flies

Cattle Grubs

The common cattle grub typically lays its eggs on the hair of cattle, attaching clusters of 5 to 15 eggs to a single hair. The process of oviposition does not inflict pain on the host animal. In the spring months (February, March, April, May), cattle may exhibit frenzied behavior, running for water or shade to escape the northern cattle grub, often known as "gadding." This behavior seems to be triggered by the bee-like sound produced by the fly in flight.

Eggs hatch within about 4 days, and the newly hatched maggots burrow into the skin. The first-stage larvae of the common cattle grub migrate through connective tissue, aided by enzyme secretion, and usually settle in the mucous membrane of the gullet. In contrast, the larvae of the northern cattle grub are typically located in the spinal cord. During the early fall months in Florida (October to November), the migrating first-stage larvae begin to reach the backs of cattle. At this point, they create a breathing hole by cutting or digesting through the skin, resulting in a distinctive warble [7].

After molting in the warble formed on the host's back, the first-stage larvae transition to the second stage within 3 to 4 days. The second-stage larva then undergoes another molt to become the third stage, during which it experiences rapid growth. The larva feeds on pus, necrotic cells, and secretions from the wall of the warble or cyst, spending approximately one to two months inside the warble to reach full development. Once fully grown, the grub exits through the breathing hole in the skin and falls to the ground to pupate. Pupation occurs within 2 to 3 days, and the pupal stage lasts between 20 to 60 days, depending on ambient temperature. The entire life cycle takes about one year. The larvae cause two types of injury to the host. First, there is irritation from the larval migrations within the host's body, followed by irritation when the larva emerges from beneath the skin. Second, the larva's exit from the warble leaves an open, oozing wound that is persistent and susceptible to secondary infection [9].

However, the economic losses are considerably greater. Milk production can drop by 10 to 20 percent, and the animals' frantic attempts to escape from the flies can lead to significant weight loss. Furthermore, the carcass value diminishes substantially, as the flesh takes on a greenish-yellow, jelly-like appearance at the sites where the grubs are located, making it unfit for consumption. Additionally, the value of the hide decreases due to the holes created in the skin [30].

During the treatment period, which begins after the egg hatch has ceased and continues until the larvae have moved up to, but not into, the back or gullet region, various methods can be employed for cattle grub control. These methods include sprays, dips, feed additives, and pour-on, with pour-on generally yielding the most effective results.

Infestations of Fly Maggots (Myiasis)

Myiasis refers to the infestation of living tissue by fly larvae in a host. While several types of maggots can invade the wounds of warm-blooded animals, the primary screwworm is the only species that exclusively feeds on live flesh. Efforts to eradicate the primary screwworm from the Southeast, such as releasing sterile male flies, have been successful; however, the risk of reinfestation persists [2].

Other species, such as the secondary screw-worm and certain blowflies, can also infest wounds. These species typically lay their eggs on the carcasses of deceased animals and occasionally on dead tissue within open wounds. While they primarily feed on dead flesh and wound secretions, their presence can result in additional tissue damage, leading to further necrosis, which they subsequently feed upon [7].

Differentiating between primary screwworms and other fly larvae is not straightforward. Samples of eggs and maggots should be preserved in a container filled with 70% alcohol. Wounds should be treated with insecticidal ointments, sprays, or dusts to prevent and manage infestations.

<u>Lice</u>

Lice are generally permanent ectoparasites, meaning they spend their entire life cycle on the host animal. Both immature and adult lice stages are parasitic, requiring them to remain on their host to survive. Each species of louse typically prefers a specific host, although some may infest multiple breeds of cattle. However, lice species that affect cattle are usually not found on other animals, such as swine or horses. Additionally, most sucking lice are specific to certain areas on the host's body [11].

In Florida, cattle are vulnerable to five types of sucking lice and one type of biting louse. The sucking lice, which feed on blood, include the long-nosed cattle louse and the short-nosed cattle louse, both found on the head, neck, and brisket during winter to early spring. The cattle tail louse is primarily found in the tail brush as adults, while immatures can be located on various body parts during the summer to late fall, and sometimes year-round. The biting louse, known as the cattle biting louse, feeds on skin and hair, causing itching, irritation, and hair loss. This louse can become a significant problem during the fall, winter, or spring.

Lice populations experience seasonal fluctuations largely influenced by the condition of the host animal. The biting louse and most sucking lice typically start to proliferate in the fall, reaching their peak populations in late winter or early spring. During the summer, louse populations are usually minimal, often resulting in no noticeable symptoms. Several factors related to the host's environment - such as skin temperature, moisture levels, hair thickness, oil content on the skin, and grooming habits - can significantly affect the size of the louse population. Additionally, animals under stress are generally more susceptible to harboring larger louse populations compared to those in normal conditions [12].

Lice are typically transmitted between animals through direct contact. Transmission from one herd to another usually occurs when carrier animals are introduced, although some lice may hitch a ride on flies (phoresy) and move from place to place.

Feeding lice irritate host animals, and infestations can be detected through changes in behavior. Sucking lice pierce the skin to draw blood, while biting lice use their chewing mouthparts to feed on hair particles, scabs, and skin secretions. This feeding irritation causes animals to rub and scratch, resulting in raw areas on the skin and hair loss. Nervousness and inadequate nutrition may lead to weight loss, and affected animals may appear listless. In severe cases, blood loss from sucking lice can result in anemia and even abortion [15].

Female lice attach their eggs to the hair of the host, near the skin surface. These eggs hatch within 8 to 12 days, depending on the species and environmental temperature. The nymphs undergo three stages of development and reach maturity in approximately three weeks. The typical duration from egg to adult capable of laying eggs is about 25 to 28 days.

Controlling louse infestations is essential whenever animals excessively scratch and rub. However, louse control is challenging because most pesticides do not effectively kill louse eggs. Since eggs usually hatch 8 to 12 days after pesticide application, retreatment is necessary approximately two weeks after the initial treatment. To prevent new louse infestations, it is crucial to treat any new animals introduced into the herd [17].

Cattle tail lice present a distinct challenge, as their eggs can remain viable and hatch up to 40 days after being laid. To effectively manage this issue, it is advisable to wait three weeks between treatments to ensure that most eggs have hatched by the time the second application is given. Cattle tail lice are particularly problematic during the summer and fall seasons. The most effective method for controlling lice is the use of forced dust bags. Additionally, residual sprays, dips, and pour-on treatments can also provide satisfactory control.

Follicular mites, on the other hand, are microscopic, cigar-shaped organisms that live within the skin, specifically in the hair follicles. All life stages of these mites occur within the follicles, leading to the formation of nodular lesions on the skin. These lesions can sometimes rupture, resulting in holes in the hide and making the skin susceptible to secondary infections. Controlling follicular mites is challenging due to their deep penetration into the skin [19].

Mosquitoes

Mosquitoes are tiny insects equipped with piercing-sucking mouthparts and characteristic scales on their wings. Although female mosquitoes are known for feeding on blood, they do not always need it for the initial egg-laying process. Many mosquito species target livestock, causing painful bites that result in discomfort, reduced vitality, and, in severe cases, potential suffocation or significant blood loss. Furthermore, their relentless attacks can lead to weight loss and decreased milk production in affected animals.

The mosquito life cycle consists of four distinct stages. Eggs are typically laid directly on the water's surface or on moist soil and container sides that are likely to be flooded soon. Common breeding sites include drainage ditches, ponds, discarded cans, old tires, and tree holes. Most mosquito species' eggs hatch within 2 to 3 days, resulting in larvae, commonly known as "wigglers," which feed on organic matter in the water. These larvae go through four developmental stages over approximately 7 to 10 days. Following this, they enter the pupal stage, lasting 2 to 3 days, before the adult mosquito emerges from the pupal skin at the water's surface.

In regions where mosquitoes present a significant threat to livestock, implementing control measures is crucial. The most effective strategy is source reduction, which involves eliminating or draining mosquito breeding sites. Additionally, daily fogging or aerosol treatments targeting adult mosquitoes can provide temporary relief, though their long-term effectiveness is limited [8].

Ticks

Ticks are readily discernible from insects due to their undivided body structure, which creates a sac-like, leathery appearance resulting from the firm fusion of the thorax and abdomen. While ticks lack a distinct head, they possess a head-like structure equipped with recurved teeth that enable them to firmly attach to their host. Female ticks can significantly swell in size, assuming a bean-like form when fully engorged. The developmental cycle of ticks comprises four stages: egg, 6-legged seed or larval stage, 8-legged nymphal stage, and 8-legged adult [11].

A fully engorged female tick can lay between 100 and 18,000 eggs on the ground. The larval or seed ticks that hatch from these eggs typically climb onto grasses or other low vegetation to wait for passing animals. These larvae then molt into nymphs and progress through three to five nymphal stages (specific to soft ticks). Ticks retain their eight-legged structure throughout both the nymphal and adult stages. After feeding, most ticks drop off the host to molt. All life stages - males, females, and immature ticks - feed on blood and lymph. The effects of ticks on the host include inflammation, itching, and swelling at the bite site, blood loss, wounds that may become infected, obstruction of body openings, and paralysis due to the injection of toxic fluids. Moreover, ticks transmit numerous diseases, including anaplasmosis, bovine piroplasmosis, and tularemia. Some ticks have the capability to transmit diseases to their offspring without feeding on an infected animal. Tick-borne diseases contribute to economic losses in terms of livestock mortality and morbidity worldwide. Tick control efforts may include premise control using insecticides, which target engorged ticks or those on foliage awaiting a host. On animals, tick control is best achieved with insecticide sprays or dips.

Parasitism presents a major challenge to production, significantly hindering animal productivity and growth, with important zoonotic implications. Although parasitic diseases are rarely fatal, the long-term debilitating effects of subclinical parasitism are crucial in terms of production losses for affected animals. Various epidemiological factors contribute to parasitic infections in cattle in this region. Therefore, there is an urgent need for proper monitoring of parasitic infections in local cattle using modern techniques to ensure accurate diagnosis, treatment, and control of these infections [12, 15].

Seasonal Parasite Pressure

Parasite pressure in pastures fluctuates according to season and management practices. The burden of parasites typically reaches its peak during the spring and diminishes during the hot, dry summer months. Conversely, cattle in drylot systems generally experience fewer worms and exhibit less seasonal variation in parasite load. Effective herd management, including robust nutrition and health programs, contributes to reduced parasite pressure under favorable conditions.

Diagnosis

Diagnostic tests for parasites in livestock play a crucial role in management practices and assessing both individual and herd health. Among these tests, fecal examination stands out as the primary method for detecting parasites residing in the gastrointestinal tract, which comprise the majority of economically and clinically significant parasites in livestock. Fecal parasitology tests are broadly categorized as qualitative or quantitative. Qualitative tests identify specific parasite taxa based on the distinctive morphology of their diagnostic stages, such as eggs, oocysts, cysts, or larvae. On the other hand, quantitative tests aim to measure the occurrence of targeted parasite taxa by enumerating their diagnostic stages. Faecal samples are typically analyzed for helminthic eggs, worms, and coccidial oocysts using techniques like the modified McMaster method. Identification of characteristic helminthic eggs from *Trichuris* and *Moniezia* species, nematode larvae, and coccidial oocysts was performed at the genus level only, relying on morphological features for classification [4]. Tapeworm segments were identified during the collection of fecal samples by observing the appearance of segments in the feces. For Moniezia species eggs, tapeworm segments were ground in a small amount of water, and the material was examined to identify the eggs. The quantification of eggs per gram of feces (epg) was performed exclusively for gastrointestinal nematodes using the modified McMaster technique [34]. Animals with over 500 eggs per gram (epg) of gastrointestinal nematodes (GIN) were categorized as having a high intensity of infection, while those with less than 500 epg were classified as having a low intensity of GIN infections [32].

Recent research has concentrated on developing and validating innovative molecular techniques to identify gastrointestinal nematodes (GIN) at the species level using eggs or larvae obtained from coproculture. This approach holds promise as a potential tool for routine GIN diagnostics in livestock. In the future, it may become the preferred option over coproculture and microscopic identification [37].

Regular utilization of parasite diagnostics is crucial for implementing efficient parasite control programs and for assessing the effectiveness of these programs [36].

Various epidemiological, clinical, immunodiagnostic, and molecular techniques are employed for diagnosing haemoprotozoan diseases. While laboratory diagnosis predominantly relies on morphological identification of the causative agent for most diseases, other advanced methods are also utilized. Films derived from capillary or venous blood play a pivotal role in diagnosing theileriosis, babesiosis, acute stages of trypanosomiasis, and microfilariasis. Although blood smear analysis is a common method for evaluating hematologic conditions, its use in diagnosing infectious diseases is limited due to the rarity of diseases requiring this approach. Nevertheless, blood smear examination provides valuable insights, often offering more information than other hematologic procedures. In veterinary emergency practice, interpreting blood smears is frequently employed for swiftly assessing animals in need of laboratory evaluation [22]. Microscopic examination of blood smears is regarded as a crucial method for diagnosing blood parasites in cattle. At times, it serves as the primary step for definitively identifying infectious agents such as blood protozoa, rickettsia, trypanosomes, and microfilariae. Morphological alterations in erythrocytes, leukocytes, and platelets are often associated with infections caused by these blood parasites. These changes can be either specific or nonspecific to the disease. Nonspecific alterations may encompass morphological changes in leukocytes and erythrocytes (*e.g.*, toxic granulations, macrocytosis), or the detection of certain pathogens (such as blood parasites) in a peripheral blood smear facilitates rapid diagnosis. Among the most significant blood parasites affecting cattle are *Theileria, Babesia*, and *Anaplasma* [2, 4].

PREVENTION AND CONTROL

Parasites can exert significant detrimental effects, especially on calves, ranging from subclinical immune suppression and appetite reduction to decreased production and even severe clinical illness leading to death. Managing parasites is a crucial component of a comprehensive preventive health program. This program should also include immunity management through vaccinations, effective management practices, proper handling techniques, and nutritional strategies tailored to meet the specific challenges and goals of the farm [25]. Temperature and rainfall are the primary climatic elements that affect the prevalence of internal parasites, and they can serve as indicators for predicting outbreaks of endoparasitic infections. Control strategies should take into account factors such as the age and class of cattle, their nutritional status, stress levels, seasonal variations, and the probability of environmental contamination by parasites. Implementing pasture management techniques along with the administration of anthelmintic (dewormer) products for treatment are essential components of effective parasite control practices [10, 21].

The main goal of a prevention strategy for parasitic infections is to reduce animals' exposure to parasites and their infectious stages. Since multiple animals are usually at risk, preventive measures are aimed at entire groups rather than individual animals. This strategy is similar to those used for preventing other infectious diseases on the farm. However, when addressing parasite infection prevention, veterinarians must be aware of the specific infectious forms of the parasite (such as eggs or larvae) and consider whether other hosts are involved in the parasite's life cycle [25]. Next, the most effective parasiticidal treatment is selected, and management protocols, such as grazing rotations, are meticulously planned to reduce exposure to infectious parasite stages in the environment. Essentially, prevention strategies focus on maintaining good on-farm hygiene practices and using timely, appropriate deworming agents alongside pasture management techniques, as recommended for beef cattle. Additionally, various formulations of deworming medications are available for dairy cattle [22].

Colostrum Importance in Calves

Passive immunity is crucial for young calves, primarily acquired from their mothers, comprising mainly of antibodies. This immunity is transferred across the placenta during gestation and through colostrum, the first milk produced after birth. Colostrum is rich in antibodies, vital for bolstering the immunity of young animals, shielding them from diseases, and aiding in combating infections. Beyond antibody transfer, colostrum intake initiates anabolic processes in various tissues, fostering postnatal growth and organ development. Given that newborn calves possess limited antibodies and an immature immune system incapable of antibody production for several weeks, colostrum plays a pivotal role in providing protection during this critical phase of immune system development. Hence, effective colostrum management emerges as a paramount factor influencing calf health and survival [11].

The significance of colostrum in facilitating passive immunity and safeguarding offspring is widely acknowledged, given that antibodies are unable to traverse the cow's placenta to reach the fetus. Colostrum is enriched with high levels of nutrients, hormones, cytokines, antibodies, and various maternal leukocytes. Neonatal calves possess remarkable capability in absorbing immunoglobulins and growth factors from the gastrointestinal tract, including IgA, IgM, IgG, IGF-1, lactoferrin, and lysozyme. Hence, the quality of colostrum is paramount, ensuring an adequate supply of antibodies for absorption by the calves [22].

Anti-Parasitic Medications

Anthelmintics utilized for controlling intestinal parasites in calves are available in various formulations, including oral preparations, injections, syrups, external applications, and as feed mixing components. These products belong to two main classes: benzimidazoles and macrocyclic lactones.

Benzimidazoles, often referred to as white dewormers, contain active ingredients such as albendazole, fenbendazole, or oxfendazole. They are effective against most major adult gastrointestinal parasites and numerous larval stages. However, they typically have a short duration of efficacy and come in various oral formulations.

Macrocyclic lactones, including avermectins and milbemycins, are commonly used in commercial products such as ivermectin, doramectin, eprinomectin, and moxidectin. These compounds offer a broad antiparasitic spectrum at low doses, targeting multiple larval stages, including hypobiotic larvae, as well as various external parasites. Available in oral, subcutaneous, and pour-on formulations for calves, their efficacy can last up to 35 days, depending on the specific product [25].

Strategic deworming in calves involves timing treatments to benefit both the animal and the herd while minimizing environmental contamination for a period matching the parasites' life cycle. The key is to treat calves before they begin shedding eggs and to move them to parasite-free pastures. Deworming typically starts at 10-14 days of age and continues monthly until the calves reach six months old. These deworming treatments can be coordinated with other management tasks, such as summer vaccinations for calves and fall processing of both calves and cows. Treatment schedules may vary based on geographic factors, such as moisture levels in regions like the southern areas [23].

Calves and stockers should be incorporated into a strategic deworming program while on pasture. Key treatment periods include pre-weaning during nursing and intensive grazing as stockers. Deworming should not coincide with weaning, as treating calves before separation helps reduce stress-related impacts on immune function and improves overall performance.

Some parasites may survive even the most effective drug treatments due to genetic selection for resistant worms in treated populations. Although modern dewormers are broad-spectrum, safe, effective, and affordable, over-reliance on them, rather than emphasizing proper husbandry practices, has contributed to rising parasite resistance. To prevent this, deworming treatments should be applied selectively and strategically.

Similar concepts apply to the control of other types of internal parasites such as tapeworms (cestodes), flukes (trematodes), and protozoans (such as coccidia). It is crucial to comprehend the distinct life cycles of these various types of parasites, as well as the efficacy of products used to treat them.

Pasture Management

Effective pasture management is key to controlling parasites. To break the parasite life cycle, remove calves from pastures for 3-6 months, allowing worm larvae to die off. Practice pasture rotation or co-grazing with horses or adult cattle to further reduce parasite presence. Maintaining proper stocking rates is also essential for promoting pasture health and minimizing the risk of parasite transmission [21].

General Considerations for Parasite Control Include

- Avoid overgrazing pastures; most infective nematode larvae reside in the top 2 inches of vegetation.
- Spread manure during hot, dry conditions to eliminate worm eggs and larvae present in the feces.
- Implement crop and livestock rotation practices.
- Maintain a high level of nutrition for the animals.
- Monitor flock health using body condition scores and other clinical indicators [21, 22].

Important Factors to Consider for Preventing Both Internal and External Parasite Infections Include

Source Negative Cattle

Ensure replacement breeding stock tests negative for parasites before purchase, and avoid introducing infected animals into parasite-free herds.

Minimize Dose or Eliminate Exposure Completely

Adopt indoor production methods to limit access to common infection sources. Implement an all-in-all-out system, ensuring facilities are fully emptied between production groups. Maintain cleanliness by regularly cleaning facilities with appropriate detergents and disinfectants between groups. Eliminate environments that support external parasite breeding, such as removing standing water to reduce mosquito populations.

Monitoring Program to Ensure Early Identification

Establishing a comprehensive monitoring program allows for early detection of parasite issues and prompt intervention. This can include regular fecal sampling, monitoring for clinical symptoms, and identifying visible signs of infection during routine post-mortems or slaughter inspections.

Therapeutic Prevention Programs

Strategic preventive therapy programs are frequently employed to treat parasite infections, aiming to minimize both the parasite burden on individual animals and the risk of transmission to herd mates through shedding.

Environmental Management

In cattle, as with other livestock species, administering anti-parasitic drugs is periodically considered as one aspect of parasite elimination methods. Cattle premises regularly sanitized with suitable sanitizers play crucial roles. Another efficient method involves removing manure from paddocks and pastures, with a recommended frequency of twice a week. Using dragging or harrowing to break up manure pats is less effective and should only be done in areas where the manure dries quickly. Composting manure and soiled bedding, on the other hand, generates enough heat to kill parasite larvae and eggs. It is crucial to avoid spreading non-composted manure on pastures, as this can increase parasite contamination. To minimize parasite exposure, reducing animal numbers, lowering stocking density, and preventing overgrazing are essential. Rotating pastures and grazing with different livestock on rested pastures also help reduce risks. New animals should be tested for fecal egg counts (FEC) upon arrival and dewormed, if necessary before being introduced to the herd [27].

CONCLUSION

Parasites remain a persistent concern in both conventional and organic farming systems. Understanding parasitic diseases is fundamental for implementing effective control strategies and enhancing farm profitability. The epidemiological landscape of parasites has been dynamic, influenced by various factors of human and environmental origin. Advancements in diagnostic methods have facilitated the identification of parasite strains, aiding in disease etiology determination. Additionally, the zoonotic risk associated with consuming cattle meat underscores the importance of accurate diagnosis and robust control measures. Therefore, prevention and control efforts must be carefully evaluated to mitigate parasitic infections by minimizing or preventing animals' exposure to parasites and their infectious forms.

REFERENCES

[1]   Allison RW, Meinkoth JH. Anemia caused by Rickettsia, Mycoplasma, and protozoa ch.31. in Weiss, D.G and Ward, K.J. Schalm's of Veterinary Hematology 6th (ed.). WILEY-BLACKWELL, A john Wiley & Sons, Ltd, Puplication. 2010; pp. 199-200.

[2]   Almeida VA, Magalhães VCS, Muniz Neta ES, Munhoz AD. Frequency of species of the Genus Eimeria in naturally infected cattle in Southern Bahia, Northeast Brazil. Rev Bras Parasitol Vet 2011; 20(1): 78-81.
        [http://dx.doi.org/10.1590/S1984-29612011000100017] [PMID: 21439239]

[3]   Alsaad KM. Clinical, hematological and biochemical study of Anaplasmosis in local cattle Master thesis, College of Veterinary Medicine, University of Mosul, Iraq 1990.

[4]   Awash HD, Abera C, Gemechu MY, Tolasa T. Gastrointestinal helminth infections in small-scale dairy cattle farms of Jimma town, Ethiopia. Ethiopian J ApplSci Tech 2011; 2: 31-7.

[5]   Blevins SM, Greenfield RA, Bronze MS. Blood smear analysis in babesiosis, ehrlichiosis, relapsing fever, malaria, and Chagas disease. Cleve Clin J Med 2008; 75(7): 521-30.
        [http://dx.doi.org/10.3949/ccjm.75.7.521] [PMID: 18646588]

[6] Buret A, denHollander N, Wallis PM, Befus D, Olson ME. Zoonotic potential of giardiasis in domestic ruminants. J Infect Dis 1990; 162(1): 231-7.
[http://dx.doi.org/10.1093/infdis/162.1.231] [PMID: 2355197]

[7] Census Office of the Registrar General and Census Commissioner, India. Ministry of Home Affairs, Government of India. 2011.

[8] Charlier J, Höglund J, von Samson-Himmelstjerna G, Dorny P, Vercruysse J. Gastrointestinal nematode infections in adult dairy cattle: Impact on production, diagnosis and control. Vet Parasitol 2009; 164(1): 70-9.
[http://dx.doi.org/10.1016/j.vetpar.2009.04.012] [PMID: 19414223]

[9] Chowdhury N, Tada I. Helminths of domesticated animals in Indian subcontinent. Helminthology. Springer-Verlag, Narosa Publishing House 1994; pp. 73-120.
[http://dx.doi.org/10.1007/978-3-642-78838-3_3]

[10] Das M, Deka DK, Sarmah PC. Cryptosporidium infection in cattle of sub-tropical region of Assam, India. Int J Sci Res 2015; 4: 10-2.

[11] Das P, Roy SS, MitraDhar K, *et al.* Molecular characterization of Cryptosporidium spp. from children in Kolkata, India. J Clin Microbiol 2006; 44(11): 4246-9.
[http://dx.doi.org/10.1128/JCM.00091-06] [PMID: 16971647]

[12] Eckert J, Gemmell MA, Soulsby EJ. Surveys on prevalence and geographic Distribution of echinococcosis. In: Eckert J, Gemmell MA, Soulsby EJ (Edn), Echinococcosis/hydatidosis Surveillance, Prevention and Control: FAO/UNEP/WHO Guidelines. 1982; pp. 36-45.

[13] Ezatpour B, Hasanvand A, Azami M, Mahmoudvand H, Anbari K. A slaughterhouse study on prevalence of some helminths of cattle in Lorestan provience, west Iran. Asian Pac J Trop Dis 2014; 4(5): 416-20.
[http://dx.doi.org/10.1016/S2222-1808(14)60599-5]

[14] Georgie atton. Calf Diseases: The Importance of Colostrum., Ridgeway science. 2020.

[15] Gharbi M, Sassi L, Dorchies P, Darghouth MA. Infection of calves with Theileria annulata in Tunisia: Economic analysis and evaluation of the potential benefit of vaccination. Vet Parasitol 2006; 137(3-4): 231-41.
[http://dx.doi.org/10.1016/j.vetpar.2006.01.015] [PMID: 16481113]

[16] Gibbs HC. Mechanisms of survival of nematode parasites with emphasis on hypobiosis. Vet Parasitol 1982; 11(1): 25-48.
[http://dx.doi.org/10.1016/0304-4017(82)90119-4] [PMID: 6891524]

[17] Goory AA. Experimental study of *Theileria annulata* in calves by *Hyalomma anatolicum.* Master thesis, College of Veterinary Medicine, University of Mosul, Iraq 1981.

[18] Grace D, Himstedt H, Sidibe I, Randolph T, Clausen PH. Comparing FAMACHA© eye color chart and Hemoglobin Color Scale tests for detecting anemia and improving treatment of bovine trypanosomosis in West Africa. Vet Parasitol 2007; 147(1-2): 26-39.
[http://dx.doi.org/10.1016/j.vetpar.2007.03.022] [PMID: 17498880]

[19] Hasson RH. Study of hematological changes in experimentally infected cattle by Babesia Master thesis, College of Veterinary Medicine, University of Mosul, Iraq 1980.

[20] Keyyu JD, Kassuku AA, Msalilwa LP, Monrad J, Kyvsgaard NC. Cross-sectional prevalence of helminth infections in cattle on traditional, small-scale and large-scale dairy farms in Iringa district, Tanzania. Vet Res Commun 2006; 30(1): 45-55.
[http://dx.doi.org/10.1007/s11259-005-3176-1] [PMID: 16362610]

[21] Keyyu JD, Kyvsgaard NC, Monrad J, Kassuku AA. Epidemiology of gastrointestinal nematodes in cattle on traditional, small-scale dairy and large-scale dairy farms in Iringa district, Tanzania. Vet Parasitol 2005; 127(3-4): 285-94.

[http://dx.doi.org/10.1016/j.vetpar.2004.10.014] [PMID: 15710529]

[22] Kroft SH. Infectious diseases manifested in the peripheral blood. Clin Lab Med 2002; 22(1): 253-77.
[http://dx.doi.org/10.1016/S0272-2712(03)00074-X] [PMID: 11933578]

[23] Lefkaditis M, Mpairamoglou R, Sossidou A, Spanoudis K, Tsakiroglou M, Györke A. Importance of colostrum IgG antibodies level for prevention of infection with *Cryptosporidium parvum* in neonatal dairy calves. Prev Vet Med 2020; 176: 104904.
[http://dx.doi.org/10.1016/j.prevetmed.2020.104904] [PMID: 32066023]

[24] Manual of Veterinary Parasitological Laboratory Techniques, Ministry of Agriculture, Fisheries and Food (MAFF). London: Her Majesty's Stationary Office 1986; pp. 1-67.

[25] Kustritz MR. Parasite Control., Veterinary Preventive Medicine. Vet Med 2022.

[26] Martin SW, Wiggins AD. A model of the economic costs of dairy calf mortality. Am J Vet Res 1973; 34(8): 1027-31.
[PMID: 4755771]

[27] Arnold M. Neospora caninum abortion in cattle. Lexington (KY): Department of Animal & Food Sciences, Cooperative Extension Service; 2012.

[28] Mohandass K, Sehgal R, Sud A, Malla N. Prevalence of intestinal parasitic pathogens in HIV seropositive individuals in Northern India. Japan. J Infect Dis 2002; 55: 83-4.

[29] Muraleedharan K. *Cryptosporidium parvum*: an emerging protozoan parasite of calves in India associated with diarrhea among children. Curr Sci 2009; 96: 1562.

[30] Nath G, Singh TB, Singh SP. Prevalence of *Cryptosporidium* associated diarrhea in a community. Indian Pediatr 1999; 36(2): 180-3.
[PMID: 10713814]

[31] Radostits OM, Blood DC, Gay CC. Veterinary medicine: a textbook of the diseases of cattle, sheep, pigs, goats, and horses. 8th ed. Philadelphia: Bailliere Tindall 1994. p. 1181-99.

[32] Savioli L, Smith H, Thompson A. Giardia and *Cryptosporidium* join the Neglected Diseases Initiative. Trends Parasitol 2006; 22(5): 203-8.
[http://dx.doi.org/10.1016/j.pt.2006.02.015] [PMID: 16545611]

[33] Sloss M, Kemp R, Zajac AM. Veterinary Clinical Parasitology. Ames, Iowa, United States: Iowa State University Press 1995.

[34] Soulsby EJL. Helminths, arthropods and protozoa of domesticated animals. 7th ed., London: ELBS and Bailliere Tindall 1982.

[35] Urquhart GM, Armour J, Duncan JL, Dunn AM, Jennings FW. Veterinary Parasitology. 2nd ed., Blackwell Science Ltd. 1996.

[36] Williams JC, Loyacano AF. Internal parsites of cattle in Louisiana and other southern states. Louisiana State Universit. Agcenter Res Info Sheet 2001; 104: 1-19.

[36] Tiele D, Sebro E, H/Meskel D, Mathewos M. Epidemiology of Gastrointestinal Parasites of Cattle in and Around Hosanna Town, Southern Ethiopia. Vet Med (Auckl). 2023 Jan 17;14:1-9

CHAPTER 2

Parasites of the Gastrointestinal Tract Infection

K.P. Shyma[1,*], Ajit Kumar[1], Jay Prakash Gupta[1] and **Gyan Dev Singh[1]**

[1] *Bihar Veterinary College, Bihar Animal Sciences University, Patna, India*

Abstract: Gastrointestinal parasites pose a significant threat to cattle health, welfare, and productivity worldwide. This chapter describes the major gastrointestinal parasites affecting cattle, their impact on the industry, current management strategies, and potential future directions for effective control. The economic implications of parasite infections in cattle production systems are explored, highlighting the need for integrated approaches to combat these parasites. Key aspects, such as grazing management, anthelmintic treatment, genetic selection, and emerging research, are discussed in the context of sustainable parasite control. The chapter underscores the importance of continued research and collaboration to mitigate the impact of gastrointestinal parasites on cattle populations.

Keywords: Aanthelmintics, Cattle, Control, Economic impact, Gastrointestinal parasites, Management.

INTRODUCTION

Cattle play a crucial role in the global food supply, providing meat and dairy products for human consumption. However, their productivity is threatened by a diverse range of gastrointestinal parasites. These parasites, including *Ostertagia spp., Cooperia spp., Haemonchus contortus, Trichostrongylus spp., Oesophagostomum spp., Bunostomum spp., Strongyloides spp.* Infections with these parasites are the major cause of monetary loss on farms globally. The losses are mainly caused by clinical disease or reduced growth rates in young animals and milk yield losses in adult cattle [1, 2]. The adverse effects of Gastrointestinal (GI) parasitism on production are attributed to a reduction in feed intake and the energy requirements of the immune response raised against these infections [3]. Understanding the impact of these parasites and implementing effective management strategies is imperative for sustaining cattle production systems.

---

* **Corresponding author Shyma K.P:** Department of Veterinary Parasitology, Bihar Veterinary College, Patna, India; E-mail: dr.shymakpvet@gmail.com

Tanmoy Rana (Ed.)

COMMON GI PARASITES OF CATTLE

Ostertagia ostertagi

This is one of the most economically important gastrointestinal nematodes affecting cattle. It resides in the abomasum and can lead to weight loss, decreased feed intake, and even death in severe cases. This disease is most common in late summer and autumn and often causes profuse watery diarrhea in calves in grass. The infective L3 are ingested and they migrate to the abomasum, where they borrow into the gastric glands where they moult to L4 and L5 and erupt out of the gland as an adult [4].

Trichostrongylus **spp.**

These nematodes can be found in the abomasum and small intestine of cattle. They can lead to reduced growth rates and overall poor health. *Trichostrongylus* infection can include weight loss, poor growth, reduced feed efficiency, anemia, diarrhea, and overall poor condition. Severe infections can lead to significant economic losses in terms of decreased milk production and meat quality [5].

Cooperia **sp.**

These nematodes also inhabit the gastrointestinal tract, specifically the small intestine. They can cause diarrhea, weight loss, and reduced feed efficiency. *Cooperia* parasites have a direct lifecycle. Ingested L3 exsheath, migrate into the intestinal crypts for two moults, and then the adults develop on the surface of the intestinal mucosa. The prepatent period is around 3 weeks [6].

Haemonchus **spp.**

While more commonly associated with sheep and goats, this blood-sucking nematode can also affect cattle. It causes anemia, and weakness, and can be fatal in heavy infections. *Haemonchus contortus* is a blood-sucking gastrointestinal parasite that resides in the abomasum of cattle and other ruminants. It feeds on blood, causing anemia, weakness, and potentially death in severe cases. Cattle become infected by ingesting the infective larvae of *Haemonchus contortus*, which are present in contaminated pastures. These larvae can survive for weeks to months in the environment under suitable conditions. Common clinical signs include anemia, weakness, decreased appetite, weight loss, bottle jaw, diarrhea, lethargy, and in severe cases, death. Various dewormers are effective against *Haemonchus contortus*, however, resistance to these drugs has been reported in some regions, so proper drug rotation and use are crucial [7].

Paramphistomum spp.

Paramphistomosis, caused by various species of the genus *Paramphistomum*, affects cattle and other ruminants. *Paramphistomum spp.* are flatworms known as rumen flukes or amphistomes. These parasites primarily inhabit the rumen and reticulum of the host's stomach and can cause significant health issues if left unchecked. Cattle become infected when they ingest aquatic plants contaminated with the infective cercariae released by infected snails. The clinical signs of *Paramphistomum spp.* infection in cattle can vary in severity. Common symptoms include reduced appetite, weight loss, decreased milk production, diarrhea, abdominal discomfort, anemia, in severe cases, dehydration and death [8].

Strongyloides papillosus

Strongyloides papillosus is a parasitic nematode that can infect cattle. This nematode primarily affects the small intestine of cattle and can cause a condition known as strongyloidosis. The life cycle of *Strongyloides papillosus* involves both direct and indirect transmission. The parasitic females release larvae in the host's faeces, and these larvae can develop into either free-living male or female adults or infective larvae, depending on environmental conditions. The infective larvae can directly penetrate the skin of the host or be ingested by the host. If ingested, the larvae migrate to the small intestine, where they develop into adults, lay eggs, and continue the cycle. Clinical signs of *Strongyloides papillosus* infection in cattle can vary and may include diarrhea, weight loss, reduced growth rate, decreased appetite, rough hair coat, lethargy, and suboptimal milk production. Diagnosing *Strongyloides papillosus* infections can be challenging due to the intermittent shedding of larvae and the variable clinical signs. Fecal examination to detect larvae or eggs may help confirm the presence of the parasite [9, 10].

Bunostomum phlebotomum

Bunostomum phlebotomum, commonly known as the hookworm, is a parasitic nematode that can affect cattle and other ruminant animals. This parasite primarily inhabits the small intestine of its host and can cause significant health issues, including anemia and decreased growth rates. The life cycle of *Bunostomum phlebotomum* involves several stages. Adult worms live in the small intestine of cattle, where they attach to the intestinal wall and feed on blood. Female worms lay eggs that are passed out in the host's feces. Under suitable environmental conditions, the eggs hatch, and the resulting larvae develop into the infective stage. Cattle become infected by ingesting these infective larvae while grazing. The clinical signs of *Bunostomum phlebotomum* infection in cattle include anemia, decreased appetite, weight loss, rough hair coat, diarrhea, and decreased growth rates especially in young animals. Diagnosis is often based on clinical signs, history of exposure to contaminated pastures, and detection of parasite eggs in fecal samples using a fecal flotation or sedimentation technique. Treatment of *Bunostomum phlebotomum* infections involves the use of anthelmintic drugs like benzimidazole compounds [11 - 14].

Toxocara vitulorum

Toxocara vitulorum, also known as the "large roundworm of cattle," is a parasitic nematode that primarily affects young calves. This roundworm is a significant concern in some regions and can cause health problems in cattle herds. Adult worms reside in the small intestine of cattle, where they lay eggs. These eggs are passed out in the host's feces. After shedding into the environment, the eggs embryonate and become infective. Cattle become infected by ingesting the infective eggs, which hatch into larvae in the intestines and then migrate through various tissues, causing damage. Pregnant cows can also transmit larvae to their calves through the placenta or milk. *Toxocara vitulorum* infections are most commonly seen in calves less than six months of age. Clinical signs include pot-bellied appearance, poor growth, diarrhea, rough hair coat, dehydration, weakness, coughing, and anemia. Diagnosing *Toxocara vitulorum* infections involves clinical signs, history of exposure, and detection of parasite eggs in fecal samples using a fecal flotation or sedimentation technique. Larvae might also be detected in various tissues during post-mortem examinations [15, 16].

Moniezia spp.

Moniezia spp., commonly known as tapeworms, are a group of parasitic flatworms that can infect cattle and other ruminant animals. These tapeworms primarily reside in the small intestine of their hosts and can cause various health issues if left untreated. There are several species within the *Moniezia* genus, and they share similar life cycles and characteristics. The life cycle of *Moniezia spp.* tapeworms involves several stages. Adult tapeworms attach to the intestinal wall of cattle, where they produce egg-filled segments called proglottids. These proglottids are shed in the host's faeces and can be seen in the manure. Once in the environment, the proglottids release eggs. These eggs are ingested by oribatid mites, which act as intermediate hosts. Cattle become infected by ingesting oribatid mites containing tapeworm cysticercoids. Once inside the host's intestine, the cysticercoids develop into adult tapeworms. *Moniezia spp.* infections in cattle are often considered to be less pathogenic compared to other gastrointestinal parasites. Clinical signs include weight loss, decreased appetite, reduced feed efficiency, and potentially, mild diarrhea. Praziquantel and albendazole are common drugs used to target these parasites [17, 18].

Oesophagostomum spp.

Oesophagostomum venulosum and *Oesophagostomum radiatum* mainly infect the large intestine and occasionally the distal small intestine, causing nodule worm disease, or simply gut in cattle. These nematodes may affect cattle from 3 months to 2 years of age, and the prepatent period is about 6 weeks. The life cycle of *O. radiatum* involves eggs being passed into the faeces of infected cattle. These eggs develop into larvae within the faeces and then hatch. The infective larvae are consumed by cattle as they graze on contaminated pastures. Larvae infiltrate the large intestinal mucosa but seldom move into the deeper areas of the intestinal wall near the serosa. The subsequent inflammatory reaction may lead to the formation of a caseous nodule that may mineralize over time. Clinical signs include weakness, unthriftiness, alternating episodes of diarrhea and constipation, and severe weight loss. Nodular lesions are typical at necropsy [19].

Schistosoma spp.

Schistosoma spp. are a group of parasitic trematode worms that cause the disease schistosomiasis, also known as bilharzia or snail fever, in several animal species. The disease is prevalent in areas with freshwater bodies where specific snail species act as intermediate hosts for the parasite. In cattle, *Schistosoma bovis, S. spindale, S. nasale, S. indicum* are the primary species of concern. Cattle can become infected by coming into contact with water sources that contain cercariae released by infected snails. The life cycle of *Schistosoma* involves several stages. Adult worms reside in the blood vessels around the intestines and reproductive organs of the host. They release eggs that pass through the host's intestines and are excreted in the feces. The eggs then immediately hatch in freshwater, releasing miracidia, which infect specific freshwater snails. Inside the snail, the parasites multiply and develop into cercariae, which are then released into the water. Cattle become infected when they come into contact with water containing these cercariae. *Schistosoma* infections in cattle can lead to various clinical signs depending on the severity of the infection. Common signs include weight loss, reduced appetite, decreased milk production, lethargy, anemia, and potentially even death in severe cases. The parasites can cause damage to blood vessels and liver tissue. Diagnosis of *Schistosoma* infections in cattle involves detecting eggs in fecal samples through fecal egg counts or microscopic examination. Blood tests can also indicate the presence of antibodies against the parasites. Anthelmintic treatment can be used to control *Schistosoma* infections in cattle. However, treatment may need to be repeated periodically due to the potential for reinfection from water sources [20, 21]

Trichuris spp.

Trichuris spp. commonly known as whipworms, are parasitic nematode worms that can infect various mammals, including cattle. Whipworm infections in cattle are caused by species such as *Trichuris ovis* and *Trichuris discolor*. These worms primarily inhabit the large intestine and cecum of their hosts and can lead to health issues if present in large numbers. The life cycle of Trichuris involves the adult worms residing in the large intestine of the host, where they attach to the intestinal wall and lay eggs. The eggs are passed in the feces and, after being deposited on pasture or bedding, embryonate and become infective. Cattle ingest these infective eggs while grazing or consuming contaminated feed or water. Once ingested, the eggs hatch in the small intestine, and the larvae migrate to the large intestine, where they mature into adult worms and continue the cycle. Clinical signs include weight loss, reduced appetite, and diarrhea. However, the symptoms are often less severe compared to other more pathogenic parasites. Diagnosis of Trichuris infections in cattle involves fecal egg counts to detect the presence of eggs in the faeces [18, 22].

ECONOMIC IMPACT DUE TO GASTROINTESTINAL PARASITISM

Gastrointestinal parasites, such as nematodes, cestodes, and trematodes, can have significant economic impacts on livestock industries worldwide. The economic burden of gastrointestinal parasites on cattle production cannot be understated. Reduced feed efficiency, anemia, and production losses result in substantial financial losses for cattle producers. These parasites affect animal health and productivity, leading to various losses including:

Reduced Growth Rates

Infected animals often have reduced feed efficiency and growth rates. Gastrointestinal parasites can cause damage to the intestinal lining, leading to malabsorption of nutrients and subsequent poor weight gain [23].

Decreased Milk Production

In dairy cattle, gastrointestinal parasite infections can result in decreased milk production due to compromised nutrient absorption and overall health.

Morbidity and Mortality

Severe parasite infections can lead to illness and even death, especially in young or immunocompromised animals. This increases veterinary costs and reduces the number of productive animals.

Treatment Costs

Treating parasitic infections requires medication and veterinary intervention, incurring costs for farmers. Frequent deworming can also lead to the development of drug-resistant parasites, further complicating control measures.

Labor Costs

Managing parasite infections may require additional labor for monitoring, treatment administration, and general animal care.

Reduced Fertility

Parasite infections can affect reproductive performance, leading to reduced fertility rates, longer calving intervals, and economic losses due to delayed or decreased reproduction.

Increased Feed Costs

Infected animals often require more feed to maintain their body condition, which increases feed expenses for farmers.

Trade Restrictions

Some parasitic infections can lead to trade restrictions, impacting international livestock trade and the economic opportunities for affected regions.

MANAGEMENT OF GI PARASITISM

Managing gastrointestinal parasites in cattle involves a combination of strategic practices aimed at preventing parasitic infestations, reducing their impact, and promoting overall herd health [24]. Effective parasite management requires a multifaceted approach and ongoing monitoring to adapt to changing conditions and challenges [25]. Here are some key management strategies:

Pasture Management

Rotational Grazing: Regularly moving cattle to fresh pastures helps break the parasite lifecycle by minimizing exposure to infective larvae in contaminated areas.

Rest Periods: Allowing pastures to rest after grazing can help reduce parasite burdens as larvae on the pasture become less infective over time.

Strategic Deworming

Targeted Treatment: Use fecal egg counts to determine the level of parasite burden in individual animals. Treat only those with significant egg counts to prevent overuse of anthelmintic drugs.

Rotate Anthelmintics: Regularly rotate between different classes of dewormers to reduce the risk of developing drug-resistant parasites.

Fecal Egg Count Monitoring

Regularly collect and analyze fecal samples from animals to monitor parasite burdens and adjust deworming strategies accordingly.

Nutrition and Herd Health

Proper Nutrition: Maintain cattle in good body condition to help them resist the negative effects of parasitic infections.

Adequate Water Supply: Ensure access to clean water, as dehydration can worsen the impact of parasites.

Quarantine and New Animal Introduction

Quarantine Period: Isolate new animals before introducing them to the herd to prevent introducing new parasite species or resistant strains.

Parasite Testing: Perform fecal exams on new animals to assess their parasite status before introducing them to the herd.

Genetic Selection

Select for Resistance: Some cattle breeds show natural resistance to certain parasites. Consider incorporating resistant genetics into the herd through breeding.

Manure Management

Composting: Properly composting manure can help reduce the viability of parasite eggs and larvae.

Minimize Stress

Stress Reduction: Minimize stressors such as abrupt changes in diet, extreme weather conditions, and transportation, which can weaken the immune system and make cattle more susceptible to parasites.

Environmental Modifications

Drainage: Improve drainage in pastures to reduce the presence of standing water, which can create favorable conditions for parasite development.

Consultation with Veterinarian

Comprehensive parasite management should be developed with the help of veterinarians tailored to the specific needs of the herd.

CONCLUSION

Recent advancements in genomics and immunology have paved the way for innovative parasite control strategies. Integrated management approaches are very much essential. Additionally, a deeper understanding of host-parasite interactions and the development of diagnostic tools could enable more accurate and timely interventions. Collaborative efforts among researchers, veterinarians, and cattle producers are essential to translate scientific findings into practical solutions.

REFERENCES

[1]   Githiori JB, Höglund J, Waller PJ, Baker RL. Evaluation of anthelmintic properties of some plants used as livestock dewormers against *Haemonchus contortus* infections in sheep. Parasitology 2004; 129(2): 245-53.
[http://dx.doi.org/10.1017/S0031182004005566] [PMID: 15376783]

[2]   Khan T, Khan W, Iqbal R, Maqbool A, Fadladdin AJ, Sabtain T. Prevalence of gastrointestinal parasitic infection in cows and buffaloes in Lower Dir, Khyber Pakhtunkhwa, Pakistan. Braz J Biol 2023; 83: e242677.
[http://dx.doi.org/10.1590/1519-6984.242677] [PMID: 35137844]

[3]   Asif Raza M, Iqbal Z, Jabbar A, Yaseen M. Point prevalence of gastrointestinal helminthiasis in ruminants in southern Punjab, Pakistan. J Helminthol 2007; 81(3): 323-8.
[http://dx.doi.org/10.1017/S0022149X07818554] [PMID: 17711599]

[4]   Fox MT. Pathophysiology of infection with Ostertagiaostertagi in cattle. Veterinary Parasitology 1993; 46: 1-143-158.

[5]   O'Connor LJ, Walkden-Brown SW, Kahn LP. Ecology of the free-living stages of major trichostrongylid parasites of sheep. Vet Parasitol 2006; 142(1-2): 1-15.
[http://dx.doi.org/10.1016/j.vetpar.2006.08.035] [PMID: 17011129]

[6]   Taylor MA, Coop RL, Wall RL. Veterinary Parasitology. Wiley-Blackwell 2015.
[http://dx.doi.org/10.1002/9781119073680]

[7]   Sutherland I, Scott I. Gastrointestinal nematodes of sheep and cattle: biology and control. Wiley-Blackwell 2010; p. 242.

[8]   Rolfe P F, Boray J C, Nichols P, Collinsi G H. Epidemiology of paramphistomosis in cattle. International Journal for Parasitology 1991; 2 I(7): 813-9.
[http://dx.doi.org/10.1016/0020-7519(91)90150-6]

[9]   Thamsborg SM, Ketzis J, Horii Y, Matthews JB. *Strongyloides* spp. infections of veterinary importance. Parasitology 2017; 144(3): 274-84.
[http://dx.doi.org/10.1017/S0031182016001116] [PMID: 27374886]

[10]   Swarnakar G, Bhardawaj B, Sanger B, Roat K. Prevalence of gastrointestinal parasites in cow and buffalo of Udaipur district, India. Int J Curr Microbiol Appl Sci 2015; 4(6): 897-902.

[11]   Squire SA, Yang R, Robertson I, Ayi I, Squire DS, Ryan U. Gastrointestinal helminths in farmers and their ruminant livestock from the Coastal Savannah zone of Ghana. Parasitol Res 2018; 117(10): 3183-94.
[http://dx.doi.org/10.1007/s00436-018-6017-1] [PMID: 30030626]

[12]   Ola-Fadunsin SD, Ganiyu IA, Rabiu M, *et al.* Helminth infections of great concern among cattle in Nigeria: Insight to its prevalence, species diversity, patterns of infections and risk factors. Vet World 2020; 13(2): 338-44.
[http://dx.doi.org/10.14202/vetworld.2020.338-344] [PMID: 32255977]

[13]   Charlier J, Höglund J, Morgan ER, Geldhof P, Vercruysse J, Claerebout E. Biology and epidemiology of gastrointestinal nematodes in cattle. Vet Clin North Am Food Anim Pract 2020; 36(1): 1-15.
[http://dx.doi.org/10.1016/j.cvfa.2019.11.001] [PMID: 32029177]

[14]   Hildreth MB, McKenzie JB. Epidemiology and control of gastrointestinal nematodes of cattle in Northern climates. Vet Clin North Am Food Anim Pract 2020; 36(1): 59-71.
[http://dx.doi.org/10.1016/j.cvfa.2019.11.008] [PMID: 32029189]

[15]   Jones JR, Mitchell ESE, Redman E, Gilleard JS. *Toxocara vitulorum* infection in a cattle herd in the UK. Vet Rec 2009; 164(6): 171-2.
[http://dx.doi.org/10.1136/vr.164.6.171] [PMID: 19202170]

[16]   Roberts JA. The life cycle of *Toxocara vitulorum* in Asian buffalo (*Bubalus bubalis*). Int J Parasitol 1990; 20(7): 833-40.
[http://dx.doi.org/10.1016/0020-7519(90)90020-N] [PMID: 2276859]

[17]   Terfa W, Kumsa B, Ayana D, Maurizio A, Tessarin C, Cassini R. Epidemiology of Gastrointestinal Parasites of Cattle in Three Districts in Central Ethiopia. Animals (Basel) 2023; 13;13(2): 285.
[http://dx.doi.org/10.3390/ani13020285]

[18]   Soulsby EJL. Helminths, Arthropods, and Protozoa of Domesticated Animals. 7th ed. London, UK: Bailliere Tindall 1989; pp. 136-41.

[19]   Urquhart G, Armour J, Ducan J, Dunn A, Jennings F. Veterinary Parasitology. Oxford, UK: Blackwell Science 1996; p. 307.

[20]   Aula OP, McManus DP, Jones MK, Gordon CA. Schistosomiasis with a Focus on Africa. Trop Med Infect Dis 2021; 6(3): 109.
[http://dx.doi.org/10.3390/tropicalmed6030109] [PMID: 34206495]

[21]   Liang S, Ponpetch K, Zhou YB, *et al.* Diagnosis of *Schistosoma* infection in non-human animal hosts: A systematic review and meta-analysis. PLoS Negl Trop Dis 2022; 16(5): e0010389.
[http://dx.doi.org/10.1371/journal.pntd.0010389] [PMID: 35522699]

[22]   García-Sánchez AM, Rivero J, Callejón R, *et al.* Differentiation of *Trichuris* species using a morphometric approach. Int J Parasitol Parasites Wildl 2019; 9: 218-23.
[http://dx.doi.org/10.1016/j.ijppaw.2019.05.012] [PMID: 31194117]

[23]   Strydom T, Lavan RP, Torres S, Heaney K. The Economic Impact of Parasitism from Nematodes, Trematodes and Ticks on Beef Cattle Production. Animals (Basel) 2023; 13(10): 1599.
[http://dx.doi.org/10.3390/ani13101599] [PMID: 37238028]

[24]   Keyyu JD, Kyvsgaard NC, Monrad J, Kassuku AA. Effectiveness of strategic anthelmintic treatments in the control of gastrointestinal nematodes and Fasciola gigantica in cattle in Iringa region, Tanzania. Trop Anim Health Prod 2009; 41(1): 25-33.

[25]   van der Voort M, Van Meensel J, Lauwers L, *et al.* Economic modelling of grazing management against gastrointestinal nematodes in dairy cattle. Vet Parasitol 2017; 236(236): 68-75.
[http://dx.doi.org/10.1016/j.vetpar.2017.02.004] [PMID: 28288768]

CHAPTER 3

Parasites in the Urogenital Tract Infection

Farhat Bano[1], Muhammad Tahir Aleem[2,3,*], Muhammad Mohsin[4], Muhammad Asmat Ullah Saleem[1] and Furqan Munir[5]

[1] *College of Veterinary Medicine, Northeast Agricultural University, Harbin 150030, P.R. China*

[2] *MOE Joint International Research Laboratory of Animal Health and Food Safety, College of Veterinary Medicine, Nanjing Agricultural University, Nanjing 210095, China*

[3] *Center for Gene Regulation in Health and Disease, Department of Biological, Geological, and Environmental Sciences, College of Sciences and Health Professions, Cleveland State University, Cleveland, OH 44115, USA*

[4] *Shantou University Medical College, Shantou, Gunagdong 515045, China*

[5] *Department of Parasitology, Faculty of Veterinary Science, University of Agriculture, Faisalabad 38040, Pakistan*

Abstract: Gastrointestinal parasites pose a significant threat to cattle health, welfare, and productivity worldwide. This chapter describes the major urogenital parasites affecting cattle, their impact on the industry, current management strategies, and potential future directions for effective treatment and control measures. The economic implications of parasite infections in cattle production systems are also elaborately explored by highlighting the need for integrated approaches to combat parasitic diseases. Key aspects including proper grazing management, treatment of anthelmintic drugs, selection of genetic variables, and emerging research, are properly discussed in the chapter. The chapter also underscores the importance of continued updated research and collaboration to mitigate the impact of urogenital parasites on cattle populations.

Keywords: Anthelmintics, Cattle, Control, Economic impact, Management, Urogenital parasites.

INTRODUCTION

The term "parasite" refers to a creature that inhabits or lives on another organism and depends on it for sustenance and other benefits, frequently at the host's expense. There are many different kinds of parasites, including protozoa, helm-

---
* **Corresponding author Muhammad Tahir Aleem:** MOE Joint International Research Laboratory of Animal Health and Food Safety, College of Veterinary Medicine, Nanjing Agricultural University, Nanjing 210095, China Center for Gene Regulation in Health and Disease, Department of Biological, Geological, and Environmental Sciences, College of Sciences and Health Professions, Cleveland State University, Cleveland, OH 44115, USA;
E-mail: dr.tahir1990@gmail.com

inths (worms), insects, and even some plants. By spreading illnesses, impairing the host's immune system, and interfering with regular physiological processes, they may harm the host [1]. In a biological connection known as parasitism, one organism gains while the other suffers consequences. The host gives the parasite a home and access to nutrients, and the parasite in exchange may impede the host's well-being, development, or reproduction. In order to take advantage of their hosts, parasites have developed a variety of tactics, from subtle interactions to dangerous pathogenic effects [2].

Cattle urinary system parasites present serious problems for the livestock business. *Trichomonas foetus* (*T. foetus*), a protozoan that causes trichomoniasis, is one such parasite. It mostly affects the reproductive tract but has the potential to spread to the urinary system (Fig. **1**). This can cause infertility and miscarriages in cows, which has an effect on the productivity of the herd [3]. Strongyle nematodes, such as *Haemonchus placei* and *Oesophagostomum radiatum*, which are typically linked to digestive issues, can also infiltrate the ureters and bladder, resulting in irritation and potential obstructions [4]. Flukes, especially *Fasciola hepatica* and *Fasciola gigantica*, have the ability to spread from the liver to nearby organs, including the urinary tract, and can harm those tissues as they do so [5]. Another genus of protozoan parasites, *Sarcocystis* spp., can indirectly affect the urinary system by causing inflammation and subsequent problems in neighboring organs. Even though coccidian infections predominantly affect the intestinal tract, they can cause considerable stress, which has unintended effects on the urine system. Increased urination, painful urination, and blood in the urine are some of the signs of these infections, and severe instances can result in renal failure [6]. Strategies like biosecurity precautions, routine deworming, pasture management, and selective breeding are used to manage these parasites. Combining these methods helps keep the cow herds healthy and productive by preventing the entrance and spread of these parasites.

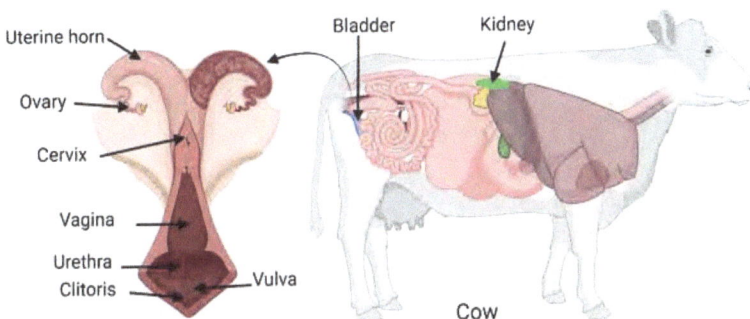

Fig. (1). Urogenital system of cattle.

Urinary parasites can have a significant negative influence on cattle farming, affecting the production, health, and overall economics of the farm. Despite not receiving as much attention as gastrointestinal parasites, urine parasites can nonetheless have serious repercussions (Table **1**). The effects of urinary parasites on cows include cattle can get urinary tract infections and other related health problems as a result of urinary parasites including *T. foetus* and certain nematodes [7]. These infections may cause discomfort, irritation, and inflammation in the urinary tract, which may have an impact on the animals' general health. *Trichomonas foetus* is one of the urinary tract parasites that specifically affect cattle reproduction. Trichomoniasis can impair a cow's ability to conceive and induce miscarriages, which can result in severe financial losses for breeding herds. Reduced reproductive success can impede the herd's growth and development [8]. Due to discomfort and the overall physiological stress brought on by the infection, cattle with urinary parasites may consume less feed, lose weight, and produce less milk. The farm's overall production and profitability suffer as a result. Increased veterinary expenses may result from the treatment and control of urinary parasite infections. The financial capacity of the livestock enterprise may be strained by diagnostic procedures, treatments, and probable problems resulting from these infections. Cattle with persistent urinary parasite infections might not be as healthy or productive, which would lower their market value [9]. When purchasing cattle from farms with a history of parasite problems, buyers are likely to be cautious. Urinary parasite control entails more work and management efforts. To reduce the risk of new infections, this entails locating affected animals, putting treatment plans into place, and modifying herd management procedures. Animals' overall welfare may be impacted by stress, which can also weaken their immune systems and increase their susceptibility to other illnesses. The normal dynamics of the herd can be changed by parasite infections. The requirement for treatment and quarantine procedures to prevent the spread of infections to other animals may make management challenges worse [10].

A proactive strategy for the prevention and management of urinary parasites is essential to reducing their negative effects on cow production. It can be useful to regularly check the herd for symptoms of urinary parasite infections, including changes in urination patterns and general health. The introduction of urinary parasites to the farm can be avoided by putting biosecurity procedures in place. If infections are found, it is crucial to collaborate with a veterinarian to create efficient treatment and control plans [11]. The danger of urinary parasite infections can be decreased by using proper herd management techniques, such as keeping clean and dry living conditions. Cattle farmers may protect the wellbeing, productivity, and financial success of their herds by being aware of the possible effects of urinary parasites and adopting proactive measures to avoid, identify, and treat these diseases [12].

Table 1. Parasites in the urogenital tract, site of predilection, symptoms, diagnosis, and treatment.

Parasite	Predilection Site	Symptoms	Diagnosis	Treatment	References
Trichomonas foetus	Prepuce, uterus	No clinical signs in the bull. Abortion, irregular oestrus cycle, and repeated service in cattle.	Clinical history, microscopic confirmation of parasite in placental fluids, uterine washings, vaginal mucus, pyometra discharge, and stomach content of aborted faetus. Alternatively laboratory tests for the presence of specific agglutinin.	Culling of bull, symptomatic treatment and sexual rest for 3 months in females. Dimetridazole intravenous or orally.	[13 - 16]
Stephanus dentatus	Kidney, perirenal fat	Kidney dysfunction, such as increased thirst, decreased hunger, weight loss, or aberrant posture.	Clinical signs and microscopy.	Anthelmintic drugs.	[22 - 26]
Neospora caninum	Blood	Abortion, exophthalmia, mummification, weak calves with ataxia.	Histological examinations, ELISA, PCR.	No effective treatment in cattle.	[27 - 33]
Trypanosoma brucei brucei	Blood, central nervous system, reproductive tract, or myocardium	Intermittent fever, anemia, abortion, edema, decreased fertility.	Clinical history, microscopy, ELISA, PCR.	Isometamidium and diminazene aceturate.	[36 - 40]
Dioctophyma renale	Kidney	Hematuria, nephritis, renal enlargement, loin pain.	Clinical signs, microscopy.	Anthelmintic drugs.	[42 - 45]

Trichomonas Foetus

Some parasites manage to establish themselves in the most unexpected areas within the complex web of livestock health issues, posing special difficulties for both farm management and animal health. It has been discovered that *T. foetus*, a microscopic protozoan has effects on cattle reproduction, and also has an impact on these animals' urinary systems. This is a flagellated protozoan that flourishes in the reproductive systems of these animals. It is mostly known for its harmful effects on cattle reproduction. Recently discovered cases of this parasite invading the urinary system and creating unanticipated health issues have been revealed [13] (Fig. **2**).

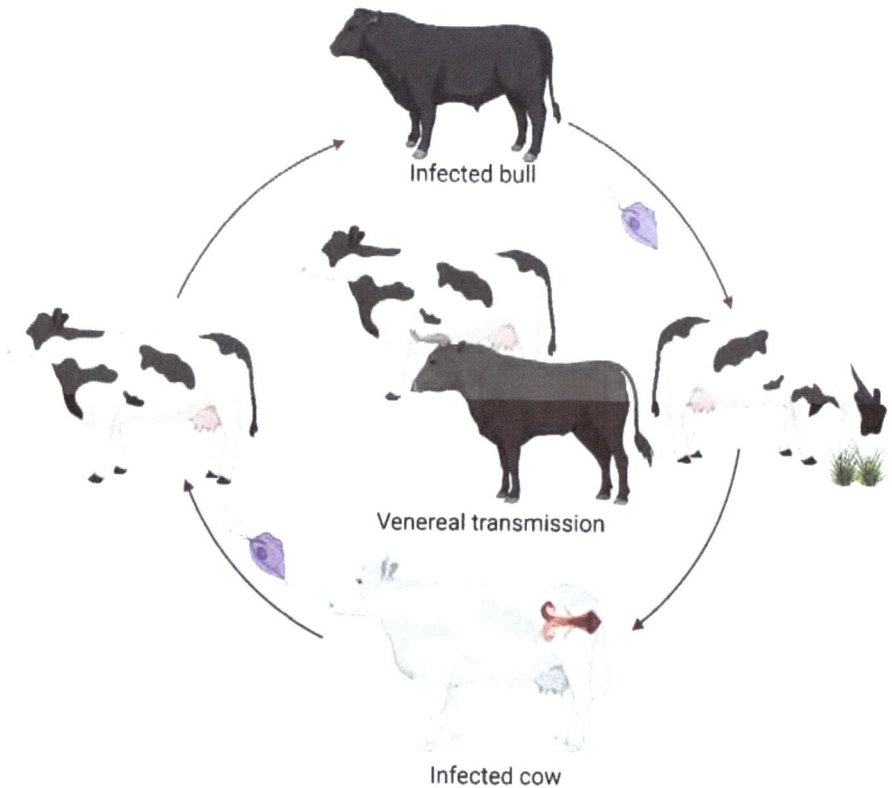

Fig. (2). Life cycle of *Trichomonas* spp.

It has a long life cycle with many stages. It mostly affects the urinary and reproductive systems of cattle, resulting in decreased fertility and reproductive losses [14]. Trophozoites, the parasite's active and mobile form, are the first stage of the life cycle. Both male and female cattle have these trophozoites living in their reproductive and urinary tracts. Bulls that have contracted the parasite host it in their prepuce, sheath, and accessory sex glands, acting as its carriers [15].

During mating, female cattle, especially cows, come into touch with diseased bulls and get infected. The parasite is transferred from the bull to the cow during mating when the prepuce of the bull comes into contact with the cow's vagina and cervix. The trophozoites are introduced into the cow's reproductive system through this transfer. Once inside, the trophozoites carry on growing by engaging in a process known as binary fission. A greater number of trophozoites are produced within the reproductive tract as a result of this replication [16]. The parasite can harm the lining of the reproductive system by causing irritation, inflammation, and damage. Reduced fertility, early fetal mortality, and, in extreme circumstances, abortion can all be consequences of this injury. The characteristic of the infection is its negative effects on fertility and reproductive success. The immune system of the cow elicits an inflammatory response to the infection in order to get rid of the parasite. While some cows are able to effectively fight off the pathogen, others might not [17]. Cows that have a persistent illness may have ongoing reproductive problems that affect both their fertility and overall reproductive performance.

During the breeding season, infected bulls could transmit the parasite to numerous cows since they continue to harbor it. Longer calving intervals and a higher percentage of open (non-pregnant) cows also affect this cycle of transmission. In the end, this has a negative impact on the efficiency of the herd and calf production. Its management demands multifaceted strategies such as routine testing of bulls, enacting biosecurity measures to prevent the introduction of sick animals, and culling infected bulls. Separating animals depending on their reproductive status can also aid in limiting the parasite's ability to spread across the herd [18]. It is transmitted from infected bulls to susceptible cows during mating throughout the life cycle of cattle. Abortion, diminished fertility, and embryonic death are all caused by the parasite's presence in the reproductive and urinary tracts. In order to apply efficient management techniques to prevent and control trichomoniasis and, ultimately, ensure the health and productivity of cattle herds, it is essential to understand its life cycle [19].

It might be difficult to diagnose *Trichomonas* infections in the urinary system. Urinary infection symptoms might be vague and simple to ignore. To further confirm the presence of Trichomonas in the urinary system, specific testing is necessary. Utilizing diagnostic methods like PCR testing enables early identification and prompt intervention. When assessing the health of cattle, veterinarians must take a wider range of diagnostic options into account, particularly when urine signs are present. To relieve discomfort and lessen the effect on general health, infected cattle should get timely treatment and supportive care if identified [20].

The finding of a *T. foetus* in the cattle urinary system emphasizes how active parasite relationships are. To completely comprehend the effects of urinary infections brought on by this parasite, more study is necessary. The prevalence, clinical importance, and potential long-term effects of *Trichomonas* infections in the urinary system can all be clarified through research [21]. In conclusion, the discovery of *T. foetus* in the urinary tract of cattle adds a new perspective to our knowledge of the problems caused by parasites in livestock. Although the main effects of *Trichomonas* on reproduction are well known, their presence in the urinary system emphasizes the need for thorough veterinary treatment and management techniques. Cattle farmers can safeguard the health, productivity, and welfare of their herds in the face of changing parasite problems by being aware of the possibility for urinary infections, putting in place suitable testing and treatment practices, and supporting continuing research.

Stephanurus Dentatus

Pigs and occasionally other animals like cattle are afflicted with the parasitic worm *Stephanurus dentatus* (*S. dentatus*). Due to its propensity to infest the host's kidneys and surrounding tissues, this nematode is also known as the kidney worm [22]. The life cycle of *S. dentatus* is intricate and involves various stages of development both inside the host and outside (Fig. **3**). Usually, the mature worms live in the renal tissues of their host, inflaming and harming these important organs. Through the host's urine, the adult worms release their eggs into the surrounding environment. The eggs are released onto the ground, where they develop and release larvae that earthworms eat. The *S. dentatus* larvae continue to develop inside the earthworms and eventually become contagious to other species [23]. When pigs and cattle consume these earthworms while grazing on contaminated pastures, they become diseased. The life cycle is completed after consumption when the larvae are expelled from the earthworms and move to the kidneys and surrounding tissues. Animals with *S. dentatus* infections may have a range of health problems. Although cattle are not the parasite's main host, they can nevertheless have kidney-related issues. Renal damage and impaired renal function may result from adult worms present in the kidney tissues [24]. Additionally, diseased animals' released eggs add to environmental contamination, continuing the infection cycle.

It takes a mix of clinical observation, diagnostic tests, and veterinary knowledge to find the infection in cattle. Because the parasite prefers pigs to cattle, it can be difficult to identify clinical indications in infected cattle. The suspicion of a kidney-related problem may arise if cattle, however, exhibit symptoms of kidney dysfunction, such as increased thirst, decreased hunger, weight loss, or aberrant posture [25]. A critical step in establishing the presence of a *S. dentatus* infection is diagnostic testing. To find possible parasite presence signs, veterinarians may conduct tests including fecal inspection, urine analysis, or blood tests [26]. These tests can reveal important details about kidney function and general health even if they might not immediately reveal the parasite.

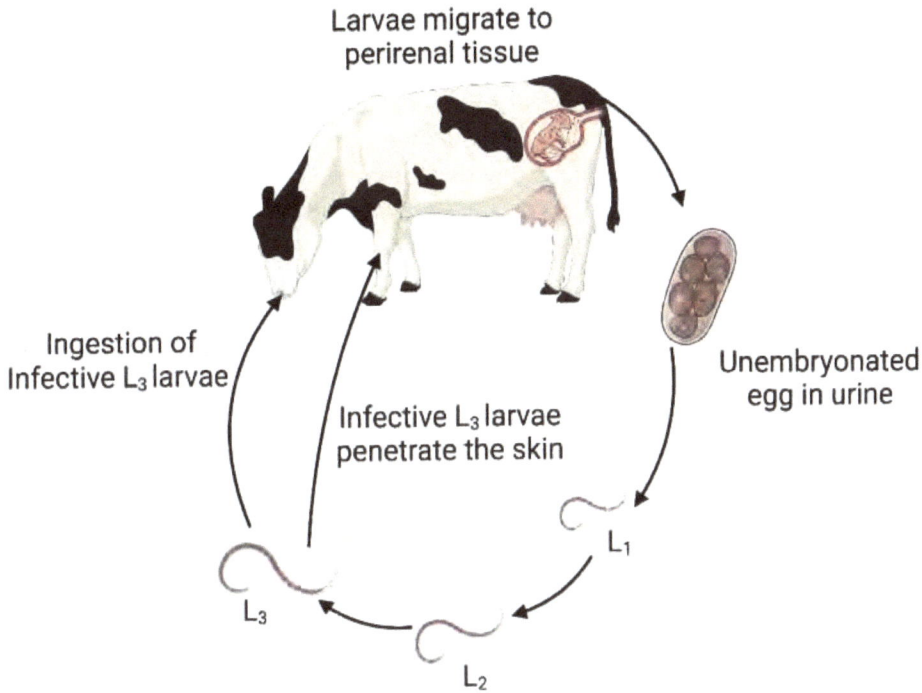

Fig. (3). Life cycle of *Stephanurus dentatus*.

Practices that reduce exposure to polluted settings and consumption of infected earthworms are essential for managing *S. dentatus* infections in cattle effectively. This entails keeping animal housing spaces clean and well-drained and employing tactics like rotational grazing to sabotage the parasite's life cycle. Additionally, targeted deworming and routine health checks on cattle might lessen the effects of this parasite. Livestock management should take proactive steps to lower the risk of infection and protect the health of their cattle by being aware of the life cycle and effects of *S. dentatus* infections.

Neospora Caninum

An internal protozoan parasite called *Neospora caninum* (*N. caninum*) has become a serious problem for the health and reproduction of cattle. It has drawn attention as a significant factor in affecting the productivity and general well-being of cow herds due to its intricate life cycle involving several hosts and potential effects such as abortions and decreased milk output [27]. The life cycle of *N. caninum* is essential to understanding how it affects cattle (Fig. **4**). The definitive host and the intermediate host are the two primary hosts involved in the life cycle. Canids, especially domestic dogs, act as the parasite's primary host and carry out its sexual stage. Sexual reproduction takes place inside the final host, producing oocysts are released into the environment through feces [28]. These oocysts release sporozoites as they sporulate, which can infect intermediate hosts. Other mammals, such as sheep and deer, as well as cattle, serve as intermediate hosts. Cattle become infected when they consume sporulated oocysts from tainted feed, water, or pasture. When sporozoites are consumed, they are released and penetrate host cells, beginning a complicated life cycle in the intermediate host. Particularly in the central nervous system and reproductive tissues, including the placenta, infected host cells produce tissue cysts [29].

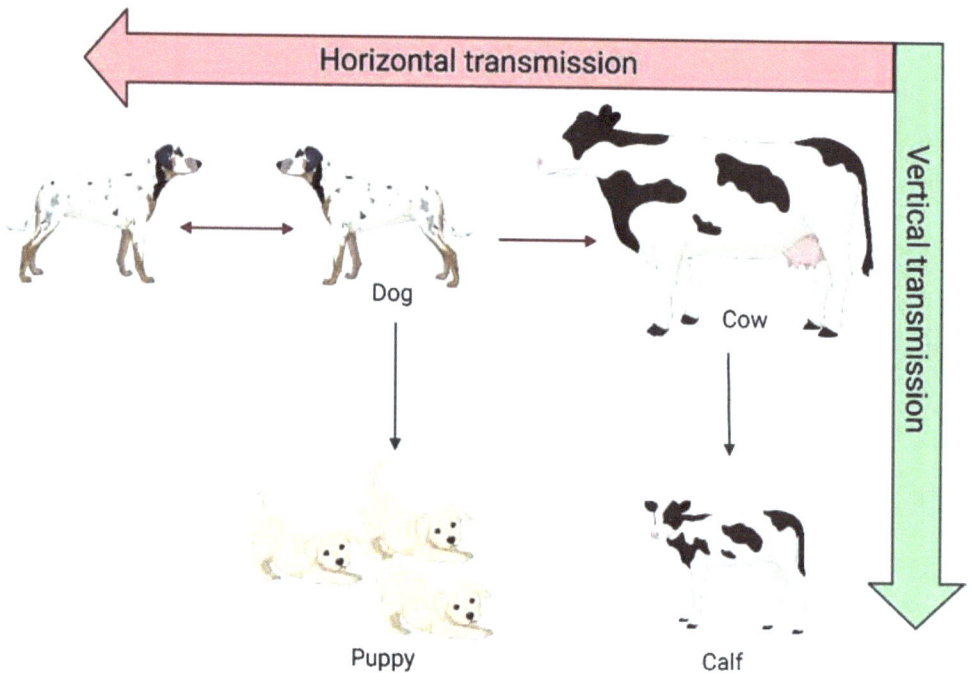

Fig. (4). Transmission of *Neospora caninum* in animals.

Numerous changes in cattle productivity, reproduction, and health may result from the infection. The infection in pregnant cows can result in miscarriages, stillbirths, or even the delivery of weak or congenitally ill calves. The impact is made more severe by the parasite's capacity to penetrate the placental barrier and infect the growing fetus. It can also cause infected cows to produce less milk, which lowers the productivity of the entire herd [30]. *Neospora caninum* infections have significant economic repercussions. Calf losses due to abortions and stillbirths can have a significant impact on the calf crop and earnings. The profitability of cattle operations may be hampered by veterinary costs related to treating diseased animals and decreased milk production [31]. Effective care of the infection depends on accurate diagnosis. PCR (polymerase chain reaction) testing to identify the parasite's DNA, serological tests to identify antibodies in blood samples, and post-mortem examinations to look for recognizable cysts and lesions are some of the diagnostic techniques. While PCR tests offer conclusive proof of the parasite's presence, serological tests, such as ELISA (enzyme-linked immunosorbent assay), can detect exposure to the parasite. The degree of tissue damage and cyst formation is revealed by post-mortem exams [32].

A multifaceted strategy is needed to manage *N. caninum* in order to lessen the negative effects on cattle herds. It is crucial to implement biosecurity procedures to stop diseased canines from being introduced to cattle areas. Dog waste that has been contaminated may contain oocysts that are excreted into the environment. Dogs should not be fed raw meat to avoid the possibility of canine infection and subsequent contamination of the environment. Because the infection can cause abortions and other reproductive losses, managing pregnant cows is essential [33]. During pregnancy, proper diet, stress management, and veterinary care are crucial. To stop further transmission and reduce financial losses, killing affected animals may be an option in cases of confirmed *N. caninum* infection. It poses a significant problem for contemporary cattle ranching, affecting animal reproduction, milk output, and business viability. Its life cycle, impacts, diagnostic techniques, and management techniques must be understood in order to protect cattle health and maximize productivity [34]. Cattle farmers may traverse the complexity of *N. caninum* and protect the health of their herds in the face of this parasite danger by employing strict biosecurity procedures, proactive monitoring, and knowledgeable veterinarian treatment.

Trypanosoma Brucei Brucei

The protozoan parasite *Trypanosoma brucei brucei* is well known for its role in the development of African Animal Trypanosomiasis or Nagana in cattle. However, this parasite, which mostly affects the lymphatic and blood systems, has also shown an unusual capacity to emerge in cows' urinary tracts [35]. It is a parasite that lives mostly in the bloodstream and infects cattle when infected tsetse flies bite them. Once inside the host, the parasite multiplies and produces a variety of symptoms, such as lethargy, anemia, fever, and weight loss. However, this parasite has occasionally been discovered in cows' urinary tracts, straying from its usual location in the circulation and lymphatic system [36].

The urinary system can become infected with the parasite, which can cause a number of issues. Increased frequency of urination, pain during urination, and even blood in the urine are possible signs in infected cattle. The parasite's existence and its interactions with the vulnerable tissues of the urinary system are probably to blame for these symptoms of the urinary tract. Additionally, the parasite in the urinary system has the potential to make pre-existing medical conditions worse [37]. The infection-induced immune response may be a factor in the development of further inflammation and tissue damage. Furthermore, the animal's overall health and well-being may be negatively impacted if the primary bloodstream infection of the parasite and the urinary tract infection coexist.

The mammalian host and the tsetse fly vector engage in intricate interactions throughout the *T. brucei brucei* life cycle in cattle. When tsetse flies eat infected mammalian hosts, they contract *Trypanosoma brucei brucei*. The parasites change into procyclic trypomastigotes in the tsetse fly's midgut, where they multiply and develop into epimastigotes. The salivary glands are where they travel. During a blood meal, infected tsetse flies inject metacyclic trypomastigotes into the host's blood. In the bloodstream of the host, metacyclic trypomastigotes change into blood trypomastigotes [38]. Parasites reproduce within the bloodstream through binary fission. Some change into stout shapes. Blood from the host is consumed by tsetse flies to get infected. In the fly's midgut, stumpy forms separate into procyclic trypomastigotes. In the salivary glands, they develop into epimastigotes and eventually metacyclic trypomastigotes. During a blood meal, infected tsetse flies transfer metacyclic trypomastigotes to a new host. The cycle continues as the parasites change, proliferate, and transfer from cattle to tsetse flies, aiding in the infection's spread [39].

Cattle urinary tract infections caused by *T. brucei brucei* exhibit a special set of diagnostic difficulties. Frequent urination and discomfort, which are typical signs of a urinary tract infection, are generic and readily explained by other conditions. This emphasizes the requirement for sophisticated diagnostic procedures that can reliably detect the parasite's presence in the urinary system. Veterinarians may use a mixture of methods to identify *T. brucei brucei* infection in the urinary system. Urine samples can be examined for the presence of the parasite's distinctive flagellated forms, which can be used to directly demonstrate an infection within the urinary system. Infection may be detected if antibodies to *T. brucei brucei* are found in the bloodstream [40]. This approach, meanwhile, might not be able to pinpoint the involvement of the urinary tract precisely. With the help of PCR testing, the parasite's DNA can be found in urine or tissue samples, providing a sensitive and accurate way to diagnose urinary tract infections. Using methods like ultrasound or other imaging modalities, it may be possible to spot changes or anomalies in the urinary tract that could be a sign that a parasite is involved.

Drugs created particularly to target and get rid of the parasite from the bloodstream are used to treat Trypanosoma brucei brucei infection in cattle. The capacity of the parasite to acquire treatment resistance as well as the possibility of negative host consequences make trypanosome infections very difficult to treat. The severity of the infection, the choice of medication, and the general condition of the cattle must all be taken into account while administering treatment under the direction of a veterinarian [41]. The following medications are frequently used to treat cattle with *Trypanosoma brucei brucei* infection, Suramin, pentamidine, diminazene aceturate, isometamidium, and melarsomine.

The complex character of parasite infections and their tendency to vary from conventional patterns are shown by the unusual expression of *T. brucei brucei* in the urinary system of cattle. Although the parasite is primarily known for its bloodstream infection, its presence in the urinary tract presents special difficulties for diagnosis, therapy, and cattle management in general. Veterinarians and cattle producers can work together to create tactics that protect both animal health and the productivity of cattle herds by comprehending this atypical presentation and its implications.

Dioctophyma Renale

The interesting but uncommon parasitic nematode *Dioctophyma renale* (*D. renale*), also referred to as the big kidney worm, occasionally infects cattle. It offers fascinating insights into the intricate relationships between parasites and their hosts because this particular parasite can live inside the kidneys of its hosts [42]. It has a complex and distinctive life cycle. It usually involves aquatic intermediary hosts, like annelid worms or aquatic insects, that consume the parasite's eggs discharged in the urine of infected hosts, like dogs, wild predators, and, on occasion, cattle. The eggs hatch inside the intermediate host, and the larvae grow into the second-stage larvae, an infectious stage. When the host consumes the intermediate host holding the infectious larvae while grazing or drinking water from polluted sources, the larvae can spread to the final host, such as cattle. The infectious larvae enter the body of the definitive host and move through the circulatory system before settling in the kidneys. Here, they reach adulthood and begin to grow, with females becoming noticeably bigger than males. One of the largest nematode parasites known, adult worms can grow up to 100 centimeters in length [43].

Cattle with *D. renale* in their kidneys may experience a variety of health problems. The size and location of the parasite within the kidney might physically harm renal tissues and perhaps impair kidney function. Clinical symptoms such as abdominal pain, weight loss, decreased appetite, and changes in urine patterns may occasionally be present in infected cattle. It is crucial to remember that many diseased cattle may not display visible signs. It can affect cattle in many ways, depending on the quantity of parasites present and the general health of the animal. The parasites' kidney damage might result in problems and secondary infections that worsen the cattle's health [44].

Due to its rarity and vague symptoms, infection in cattle can be difficult to diagnose. Diagnostic techniques comprise the existence of the parasites and any corresponding structural alterations in the kidneys can be determined with the aid of ultrasonography. Indirect proof of infection can be obtained by testing the urine for the presence of parasite eggs. Large masses within the kidneys can be detected using imaging techniques like X-rays or computed tomography scans. To establish the existence of the parasites, surgical exploration, and kidney biopsy may be required in severe cases.

The infection in cattle can be treated by surgically removing the adult worms from the kidneys. This strategy is often saved for situations where the infection results in serious clinical symptoms or consequences. Because of the size and placement of the worms inside the kidney, surgery can be challenging. The recovery of the cattle depends on post-surgical care and observation. In controlling the infection, preventive measures are essential. The risk of infection can be decreased by making sure that water sources are clean and limiting cattle exposure to aquatic intermediate hosts. Additionally, regular medical exams and diagnostic tests can help identify infections early on and treat them, increasing the likelihood of a full recovery [45].

Although infections with *Dioctophyma renale* in cattle are rather uncommon, they serve as a reminder of the wide variety of parasites that can have an influence on livestock. To keep cattle healthy and avoid the potential repercussions of parasite diseases, vigilance, correct husbandry techniques, and veterinary care are crucial.

The presence of parasites in the kidneys of cattle emphasizes the complex interactions between parasites and their hosts. Although uncommon, this particular parasitic nematode deserves consideration because of the potential harm it could cause to cattle. Cattle farmers and veterinarians can better manage and alleviate the problems caused by *D. renale* infection, enhancing the general health and productivity of their cattle herds, by being aware of its life cycle, consequences, diagnosis, and treatment choices.

FUTURE PERSPECTIVES

The future looks bright for the creation of diagnostic instruments that are more precise and sensitive. Rapid developments in molecular biology, such as PCR and next-generation sequencing (NGS), have the potential to improve our capacity to recognize and distinguish between distinct parasite species and strains. These methods can help with earlier and more precise infection identification, enabling quick responses and stopping the spread of parasites throughout cattle herds. The study of the genetics of cattle urinary system parasites opens up fascinating opportunities in the realm of genomics. Researchers can learn more about the biology, medication resistance mechanisms, and possible weaknesses of various parasite species by mapping their genomes. The creation of innovative medications and focused treatment plans may be made possible by genomic investigations [46].

The evolution of medication resistance poses a serious problem, much like with many infections. Monitoring and comprehending the processes of drug resistance in cattle urinary tract parasites should be the main goals of future studies. Researchers can design alternate treatment plans, combination medicines, and tactics to prevent the emergence of resistance by figuring out these pathways. The management of parasites in cattle will require integrated approaches in the future [47]. The effect of parasites on cattle health can be diminished by a comprehensive strategy that integrates actions including pasture management, selective deworming, genetic selection for resistance, and biosecurity regulations. Implementing integrated programs helps as a preventative step against possible developing problems in addition to addressing present challenges. In the field of parasite research, the idea of "One Health," which acknowledges the interdependence of human, animal, and environmental health, is gaining ground. To fully address zoonotic potential, environmental issues, and the broader ramifications of parasite infections beyond bovine health alone, future perspectives in the study of urinary tract parasites in cattle should embrace a One Health approach. The potential for developing vaccinations against cattle urinary tract parasites is enormous. Antigens and vaccination formulations that might elicit a protective immunological response in cattle are being investigated by researchers. While there are obstacles, such as the intricacy of parasite biology, future developments in vaccine development could fundamentally alter how we treat and prevent these illnesses [48].

Both difficulties and promising prospects lie ahead for the study of and management of parasites in the cattle urinary tract. Diagnostic, genomic, integrated management and holistic health advancements have the power to influence the direction of parasite research and control. The cattle farming community can successfully navigate the changing landscape of urinary tract parasites by adopting innovative strategies, encouraging interdisciplinary collaborations, and staying alert to new trends. This will ensure the health, welfare, and productivity of their herds for future generations.

CONCLUSION

In conclusion, bovine urinary tract parasites pose a challenging, complicated issue that has significant effects on both animal health and agricultural productivity. The complex life cycles, a wide variety of parasites, and different clinical presentations of these infections highlight the necessity for a thorough study of them. Understanding the importance of urinary tract parasites equips us to take proactive steps that advance cow health, avert financial loss, and guarantee sustainable livestock management. A multifaceted strategy is needed to combat parasites of the urinary tract. There is a promise for early detection and accurate parasite identification because of improvements in diagnostic procedures, such as molecular tools and imaging technologies. This makes it possible to create focused treatment plans and timely interventions, thereby reducing the negative effects of diseases on the health of cattle. Furthermore, cooperation among researchers, veterinarians, farmers, and policymakers is essential as we move forward. The secret to lowering parasite burdens and stalling the emergence of drug resistance is to embrace integrated parasite management strategies, which include a variety of tactics from pasture management to deworming protocols. Future times also demand a stronger focus on awareness and education. Better outcomes for the health of livestock can be achieved by arming cattle farmers with information on the dangers, precautions, and financial costs of urinary tract infections. A holistic approach to parasite management is also ensured by advocating a One Health paradigm that acknowledges the interdependence of animal, human, and environmental health. Final thoughts: Cattle urinary tract parasites present a challenge for collaboration, innovation, and adaptation. We can negotiate this complex environment and guarantee the ongoing health and profitability of cattle herds all over the world by being at the forefront of research, embracing technology innovations, and encouraging a group commitment to animal welfare.

REFERENCES

[1]   Almeria S, Robertson L, Santin M. Why foodborne and waterborne parasites are important for veterinarians. Res Vet Sci 2021; 136: 198-9.
[http://dx.doi.org/10.1016/j.rvsc.2021.02.020] [PMID: 33684793]

[2]   Mouritsen KN, Poulin R. Parasitism, community structure and biodiversity in intertidal ecosystems. Parasitology 2002; 124(7) (Suppl.): 101-17.
[http://dx.doi.org/10.1017/S0031182002001476] [PMID: 12396219]

[3]   Schwebke JR, Burgess D. Trichomoniasis. Clin Microbiol Rev 2004; 17(4): 794-803.

[http://dx.doi.org/10.1128/CMR.17.4.794-803.2004]

[4]   Jabbar A, Cotter J, Lyon J, Koehler AV, Gasser RB, Besier B. Unexpected occurrence of Haemonchus placei in cattle in southern Western Australia. Infect Genet Evol 2014; 21: 252-8.
        [http://dx.doi.org/10.1016/j.meegid.2013.10.025] [PMID: 24189197]

[5]   Ploeger HW, Ankum L, Moll L, *et al.* Presence and species identity of rumen flukes in cattle and sheep in the Netherlands. Vet Parasitol 2017; 243: 42-6.
        [http://dx.doi.org/10.1016/j.vetpar.2017.06.009] [PMID: 28807308]

[6]   Klobucher KN, Stahl TC, Islam T, Gray AS, Curreri SI, Erickson PS. Supplementing sodium butyrate to limit-fed heifers: Effects on growth, coccidiosis, urinary purine derivatives and apparent total tract nutrient digestibility. J Dairy Sci 2023; 18: S0022-0302(23)00256-4.
        [http://dx.doi.org/10.3168/jds.2023-23275]

[7]   Kulda J. *Trichomonads*, hydrogenosomes and drug resistance. Int J Parasitol 1999; 29(2): 199-212.
        [http://dx.doi.org/10.1016/S0020-7519(98)00155-6] [PMID: 10221623]

[8]   Yao C. Diagnosis of *Tritrichomonas foetus*-infected bulls, an ultimate approach to eradicate bovine trichomoniasis in US cattle? J Med Microbiol 2013; 62(1): 1-9.
        [http://dx.doi.org/10.1099/jmm.0.047365-0] [PMID: 23082032]

[9]   Ondrak JD. *Tritrichomonas foetus* Prevention and Control in Cattle. Vet Clin North Am Food Anim Pract 2016; 32(2): 411-23.
        [http://dx.doi.org/10.1016/j.cvfa.2016.01.010] [PMID: 27039692]

[10]   Craig TM. Impact of internal parasites on beef cattle. J Anim Sci 1988; 66(6): 1565-9.
        [http://dx.doi.org/10.2527/jas1988.6661565x] [PMID: 3294225]

[11]   Takeuchi-Storm N, Moakes S, Thüer S, *et al.* Parasite control in organic cattle farming: Management and farmers' perspectives from six European countries. Vet Parasitol Reg Stud Rep 2019; 18: 100329.
        [http://dx.doi.org/10.1016/j.vprsr.2019.100329] [PMID: 31796188]

[12]   Barkema HW, von Keyserlingk MAG, Kastelic JP, *et al.* Invited review: Changes in the dairy industry affecting dairy cattle health and welfare. J Dairy Sci 2015; 98(11): 7426-45.
        [http://dx.doi.org/10.3168/jds.2015-9377] [PMID: 26342982]

[13]   McMillen L, Lew AE. Improved detection of *Tritrichomonas foetus* in bovine diagnostic specimens using a novel probe-based real time PCR assay. Vet Parasitol 2006; 141(3-4): 204-15.
        [http://dx.doi.org/10.1016/j.vetpar.2006.06.012] [PMID: 16860481]

[14]   Castro C, Menna-Barreto RFS, Fernandes NDS, *et al.* Iron-modulated pseudocyst formation in *Tritrichomonas foetus*. Parasitology 2016; 143(8): 1034-42.
        [http://dx.doi.org/10.1017/S0031182016000573] [PMID: 27253439]

[15]   Okafor CC, Strickland LG, Jones BM, Kania S, Anderson DE, Whitlock BK. Prevalence of *Tritrichomonas foetus* in tennessee bulls. Vet Parasitol 2017; 243: 169-75.
        [http://dx.doi.org/10.1016/j.vetpar.2017.06.024] [PMID: 28807288]

[16]   Mendoza-Ibarra JA, Pedraza-Díaz S, García-Peña FJ, *et al.* High prevalence of *Tritrichomonas foetus* infection in Asturiana de la Montaña beef cattle kept in extensive conditions in Northern Spain. Vet J 2012; 193(1): 146-51.
        [http://dx.doi.org/10.1016/j.tvjl.2011.09.020] [PMID: 22178360]

[17]   Michi AN, Favetto PH, Kastelic J, Cobo ER. A review of sexually transmitted bovine trichomoniasis and campylobacteriosis affecting cattle reproductive health. Theriogenology 2016; 85(5): 781-91.
        [http://dx.doi.org/10.1016/j.theriogenology.2015.10.037] [PMID: 26679515]

[18]   Hancock AS, Younis PJ, Beggs DS, Mansell PD, Pyman MF. Infectious reproductive disease pathogens in dairy herd bulls. Aust Vet J 2015; 93(10): 349-53.
        [http://dx.doi.org/10.1111/avj.12369] [PMID: 26412115]

[19]   Yao C. Control and eradication of bovine trichomonosis in Wyoming, USA by testing and culling

positive bulls. Vet Res 2021; 52(1): 129.
[http://dx.doi.org/10.1186/s13567-021-00996-w] [PMID: 34620238]

[20]   Waldner CL, Parker S, Gesy KM, Waugh T, Lanigan E, Campbell JR. Application of direct polymerase chain reaction assays for *Campylobacter fetus* subsp. *venerealis* and *Tritrichomonas foetus* to screen preputial samples from breeding bulls in cow-calf herds in western Canada. Can J Vet Res 2017; 81(2): 91-9.
[PMID: 28408776]

[21]   Ortega-Mora LM, Sánchez-Sánchez R, Rojo-Montejo S, *et al.* A new inactivated *Tritrichomonas foetus* vaccine that improves genital clearance of the infection and calving intervals in cattle. Front Vet Sci 2022; 9: 1005556.
[http://dx.doi.org/10.3389/fvets.2022.1005556] [PMID: 36277069]

[22]   Deng YP, Zhang XL, Li LY, Yang T, Liu GH, Fu YT. Characterization of the complete mitochondrial genome of the swine kidney worm *Stephanurus dentatus* (Nematoda: Syngamidae) and phylogenetic implications. Vet Parasitol 2021; 295: 109475.
[http://dx.doi.org/10.1016/j.vetpar.2021.109475] [PMID: 34062343]

[23]   Perin PP, Lapera IM, Arias-Pacheco CA, *et al.* Epidemiology and Integrative Taxonomy of Helminths of Invasive Wild Boars, Brazil. Pathogens 2023; 12(2): 175.
[http://dx.doi.org/10.3390/pathogens12020175] [PMID: 36839447]

[24]   Roepstorff A, Mejer H, Nejsum P, Thamsborg SM. Helminth parasites in pigs: New challenges in pig production and current research highlights. Vet Parasitol 2011; 180(1-2): 72-81.
[http://dx.doi.org/10.1016/j.vetpar.2011.05.029] [PMID: 21684689]

[25]   Bainbridge MH. *Stephanurus dentatus* in an ox in the Northern Territory. Aust Vet J 1970; 46(7): 347.
[http://dx.doi.org/10.1111/j.1751-0813.1970.tb07929.x] [PMID: 5465994]

[26]   Prado RGS, Gardiner CH, Moura MAO, *et al.* Parasitic encephalitis caused by *Stephanurus dentatus* in a pig in Brazil. J Vet Diagn Invest 2021; 33(5): 949-51.
[http://dx.doi.org/10.1177/10406387211021489] [PMID: 34078210]

[27]   da Costa LS, Withoeft JA, Bilicki JV, *et al.* Neospora caninum-associated abortions in cattle from Southern Brazil: Anatomopathological and molecular characterization. Vet Parasitol Reg Stud Rep 2022; 36: 100802.
[http://dx.doi.org/10.1016/j.vprsr.2022.100802] [PMID: 36436886]

[28]   Lindsay DS, Dubey JP. Neosporosis, Toxoplasmosis, and Sarcocystosis in Ruminants. Vet Clin North Am Food Anim Pract 2020; 36(1): 205-22.
[http://dx.doi.org/10.1016/j.cvfa.2019.11.004] [PMID: 32029185]

[29]   Gharekhani J, Yakhchali M. Vertical transmission of Neospora caninum in Iranian dairy cattle. Ann Parasitol 2020; 66(4): 495-500.
[http://dx.doi.org/10.17420/ap6604.290] [PMID: 33646765]

[30]   Haddad JP, Dohoo IR, VanLeewen JA. A review of Neospora caninum in dairy and beef cattle--a Canadian perspective. Can Vet J 2005; 46(3): 230-43.
[PMID: 15884645]

[31]   Hall CA, Reichel MP, Ellis JT. Neospora abortions in dairy cattle: diagnosis, mode of transmission and control. Vet Parasitol 2005; 128(3-4): 231-41.
[http://dx.doi.org/10.1016/j.vetpar.2004.12.012] [PMID: 15740860]

[32]   Jenkins M, Baszler T, Björkman C, Schares G, Williams D. Diagnosis and seroepidemiology of Neospora caninum-associated bovine abortion. Int J Parasitol 2002; 32(5): 631-6.
[http://dx.doi.org/10.1016/S0020-7519(01)00363-0] [PMID: 11943234]

[33]   Cao H, Zheng WB, Wang Y, *et al.* Seroprevalence of *Neospora caninum* infection and associated risk factors in cattle in Shanxi Province, north China. Front Vet Sci 2022; 9: 1053270.
[http://dx.doi.org/10.3389/fvets.2022.1053270] [PMID: 36524222]

[34] Innes EA. The host-parasite relationship in pregnant cattle infected with *Neospora caninum*. Parasitology 2007; 134(13): 1903-10.
[http://dx.doi.org/10.1017/S0031182007000194] [PMID: 17958926]

[35] Van den Bossche P, Ky-Zerbo A, Brandt J, Marcotty T, Geerts S, De Deken R. Transmissibility of *Trypanosoma brucei* during its development in cattle. Trop Med Int Health 2005; 10(9): 833-9.
[http://dx.doi.org/10.1111/j.1365-3156.2005.01467.x] [PMID: 16135189]

[36] Van den Bossche P, De Deken R, Brandt J, Seibou B, Geerts S. Recirculation of *Trypanosoma brucei brucei* in cattle after T. congolense challenge by tsetse flies. Vet Parasitol 2004; 121(1-2): 79-85.
[http://dx.doi.org/10.1016/j.vetpar.2004.02.011] [PMID: 15110405]

[37] Doko A, Verhulst A, Pandey VS, Van der Stuyft P. Artificially induced *Trypanosoma brucei brucei* infection in Lagune and Borgou cattle in Benin. Vet Parasitol 1997; 69(1-2): 151-7.
[http://dx.doi.org/10.1016/S0304-4017(96)01097-7] [PMID: 9187040]

[38] Schuster S, Lisack J, Subota I, *et al.* Unexpected plasticity in the life cycle of *Trypanosoma brucei*. eLife 2021; 10: e66028.
[http://dx.doi.org/10.7554/eLife.66028] [PMID: 34355698]

[39] Guegan F, Figueiredo L. A two-stage solution. eLife 2021; 10: e72980.
[http://dx.doi.org/10.7554/eLife.72980] [PMID: 34534076]

[40] Cunningham LJ, Lingley JK, Tirados I, *et al.* Evidence of the absence of human African trypanosomiasis in two northern districts of Uganda: Analyses of cattle, pigs and tsetse flies for the presence of *Trypanosoma brucei gambiense*. PLoS Negl Trop Dis 2020; 14(4): e0007737.
[http://dx.doi.org/10.1371/journal.pntd.0007737] [PMID: 32255793]

[41] Pereira RM, Greco GMZ, Moreira AM, *et al.* Applicability of plant-based products in the treatment of *Trypanosoma cruzi* and *Trypanosoma brucei* infections: a systematic review of preclinical *in vivo* evidence. Parasitology 2017; 144(10): 1275-87.
[http://dx.doi.org/10.1017/S0031182017000634] [PMID: 28578742]

[42] Bizhani N, Najafi F, Rokni MB, *et al.* Tracking the existence of Dioctophyma renale in Parthian Empire of Iran (247 BC–224 AD). Parasitol Res 2023; 122(2): 413-8.
[http://dx.doi.org/10.1007/s00436-022-07735-w] [PMID: 36416951]

[43] Miyazaki I. An illustrated book of helminthic zoonoses. Tokyo: Internal Foundation of Japan 1991; pp. 459-62.

[44] Measures LN. Dioctophymatosis, parasitic diseases of wild mammals. Iowa State Univ Press 2001; pp. 357-64.
[http://dx.doi.org/10.1002/9780470377000.ch13]

[45] Toshihiro Tokiwa, Tsunehito Harunari, Tsutomu Tanikawa, Nobuaki Akao, Nobuo Ohta. *Dioctophyme renale* (Nematoda: Dioctophymatoidea) in the abdominal cavity of *Rattus norvegicus* in Japan. Parasitology International 60(3): 324-6.
[http://dx.doi.org/10.1016/j.parint.2011.03.003]

[46] Hunt PW, Lello J. How to make DNA count: DNA-based diagnostic tools in veterinary parasitology. Vet Parasitol 2012; 186(1-2): 101-8.
[http://dx.doi.org/10.1016/j.vetpar.2011.11.055] [PMID: 22169224]

[47] Canton C, Canton L, Lifschitz A, *et al.* Monepantel pharmaco-therapeutic evaluation in cattle: Pattern of efficacy against multidrug resistant nematodes. Int J Parasitol Drugs Drug Resist 2021; 15: 162-7.
[http://dx.doi.org/10.1016/j.ijpddr.2021.03.003] [PMID: 33799058]

[48] Sharma N, Singh V, Shyma KP. Role of parasitic vaccines in integrated control of parasitic diseases in livestock. Vet World 2015; 8(5): 590-8.
[http://dx.doi.org/10.14202/vetworld.2015.590-598] [PMID: 27047140]

CHAPTER 4

Parasites in the Circulatory System

Pallabi Pathak[1] and **Joken Bam**[2,*]

[1] *Lakhimpur College of Veterinary Science, Assam Agricultural University, Joyhing, Lakhimpur, Assam, India*

[2] *ICAR-Research Complex for the Northeastern Hill Region, Arunachal Pradesh Centre, Basar, India*

Abstract: Parasitic diseases affecting the circulatory system of cattle are a significant concern in veterinary medicine. The impact of these parasites on cattle health can be significant, resulting in decreased productivity, anaemia, and, in extreme cases, death. Haemoprotozoa like *Trypanosoma, Theileria, Babesia,* and *Anaplasma,* as well as helminths like *Schistosoma* and *Onchocerca,* are among the parasites that impact cattle's circulatory systems. Because the majority of these diseases are transmitted by invertebrate vectors, a comprehensive approach comprising vector control targeted medicine administration, and biosecurity measures is required to ensure cattle health and productivity. Regular monitoring and early action are critical for reducing the parasites' influence on cattle herds.

Keywords: Abortion, Cattle, Circulatory system, Death, Production.

INTRODUCTION

Parasitic diseases of the circulatory system are among the most economically important diseases of cattle. Haemoprotozoan parasites such as *Trypanosoma, Theileria, Babesia,* and *Anaplasma*are among them, as are a few helminths such as *Schistosoma* and *Onchocerca*. The disease manifestation caused by these parasites ranges from anorexia, mild fever, anaemia, and threatening abortion to death in acute cases. These parasites have a significant impact on the health and productivity of cattle.

Schistosoma

Schistosomiasis is common among cattle in Africa and Asia, caused by members of the genus Schistosoma commonly known as blood fluke due to its location in the blood vessel of its host. Six species have been reported in cattle, namely

---

* **Corresponding author Joken Bam:** ICAR-Research Complex for the Northeastern Hill Region, Arunachal Pradesh Centre, Basar, India, E-mail: jode.vet@gmail.com

Tanmoy Rana (Ed.)

Schistosoma bovis, S. mattheei, S. spindale, S. intercalatum, S. indicum and *S. nasalis. Schistosoma* produces severe disease in dairy cattle and work bullocks.

The parasite is slender, elongate, unisexual, and dimorphic trematodes that inhabit the blood vessels of their hosts. The female is thin and usually longer than the male, and the female is usually carried by the latter in a ventral, gutter-like groove, the gynaecophoric canal produced by the body's incurved lateral borders. Adult Schistosomes are blood-feeders that dwell in the portal and mesenteric veins of the host, with the exception of *S. nasalis*, which lives in the nasal mucosa veins [5]. The female lays eggs with a distinctive terminal or lateral spine that is excreted. The eggs are non-operaculate, with a thin shell and a lateral or terminal spine. The *Schistosome* egg morphologies are characteristic, therefore used to differentiate across species. The intermediate hosts include aquatic snails such as *Indoplanorbisexustus* and *Lymnealuteola*, as well as *Biomphalaria, Bulinus*, and *Oncomelania*. The disease transmission is dependent on three major factors:

- Pollution of fresh water with cattle faeces containing *Schistosoma* eggs.
- Presence of intermediate snail host.
- Contact of a definitive host with cercaria-infested water.

Schistosomes are the only trematodes that are transmitted through cercariae skin penetration of their host, although in cattle, the infection can also be acquired orally while drinking water. Cercariae evolve into schistosomula upon penetration and are transferred to their preferred sites *via* lymph and blood. The prepatent period varies between species but typically ranges between 45-70 days.

The disease is manifested in three forms depending on the species involved:

1. Nasal Schistosomiasis: Nasal Schistosomiasis is caused by the eggs of *S. nasalis* irritating the nasal mucosa, resulting in cauliflower-like growths that partially block the nasal cavity causing snoring sounds when breathing. Hemorrhagic and/or mucopurulent nasal discharge is a common feature of the condition. After the abscesses rupture, eggs and pus are released into the nasal cavity, extensive fibrosis develops at the lesion. The clinical presentation of the illness is used to make the diagnosis, and confirmed by the presence of distinctive Boomerang eggs in the faeces of the infected animal. Adult worms could be found on macroscopic examination of mesenteric veins at necropsy.

2. Intestinal syndrome is an acute form of Schistosomiasis that most commonly affects young calves. There have been isolated epidemics of symptomatic intestinal schistosomiasis caused by *S. mattheei, S. bovis*, or *S. spindale*. in endemic areas, occasional incidences of clinical intestinal schistosomiasis caused

by *S. mattheei, S. bovis*, or *S. spindale* occurs. The disease is characterised by diarrhoea, weight loss, anemia, hypoalbuminemia, hyperglobulinemia, and severe eosinophilia that develop after the onset of egg excretion. Symptoms start 7-9 weeks after infection and last depending on the severity of the infection. Health of the animals that are severely infected declines quickly and usually die within a few months of illness, but those that are less severely infected acquire chronic disease with growth retardation. Pathological and histological examination of the intestinal mucosa revealed extensive hemorrhagic lesions. The mucosa of the intestine is oedematous and coated in hemorrhagic foci. Adult parasites induce mesenteric vein phlebitis. Granulomatous lesions in the mucosa and submucosa, as well as infiltration of eosinophils, lymphocytes, macrophages, and plasma cells, may occur surrounding the eggs in the lamina propria.

3. Hepatic syndrome: It is an immunological disease caused by the host's cell-mediated immune response to *Schistosome* eggs in the liver. The immunologically specific host reaction to the eggs leads to extensive damage to the portal vascular system. Soluble antigens escaping through pores in the eggshell sensitise the host, causing lymphocytes, eosinophils, and macrophages to gather near the eggs. The soluble antigens escaping through pores in the eggshell sensitise the host and stimulate the accumulation of lymphocytes, eosinophils and macrophages around the eggs. The inflammatory response becomes persistent, with the presence of epitheloid cells, giant cells, fibroblasts and avascular granuloma can grow to be 100 times the size of the eggs. Large numbers of these egg granulomas grow and heal in heavy infections, causing enormous fibrosis in the portal triads of the liver and the appearance of "Clay Pipe stem" fibrosis.

Diagnosis in the endemic area is based on a clinicopathological picture of diarrhoea, wasting and anaemia, coupled with a history of access to natural water sources in the endemic area. Diarrhoea is persistent and often with blood stains and contains mucous. The detection of characteristic eggs (spindle/ oval shaped with terminal/ lateral spine) in the faeces could be confirmatory of the disease.

Praziquantel at the dose rate of 60 mg/kg body weight is highly effective and is the drug of choice. Other drugs like Oxyclosanide (10 mg/kg thrice at weekly intervals) and Triclabendazole (20 mg/kg) are also effective. For nasal schistosomiasis, intramuscular injection of anthiomaline (15 ml) is effective in reducing the size of the nasal granuloma. Complete recovery could be achieved through two or three injections of Anthiomaline at weekly intervals [5]. Although treatment options are available, in endemic areas, control efforts must be directed towards.

- Preventing contact between the cattle and contaminated water.
- Supply of clean drinking water.
- Control of snail intermediate host.
- Treatment of infected animals.

Onchocerca

Onchocerciasis is a widespread illness in many temperate and tropical areas. In cattle, buffaloes and goats, *Onchocera armillata* is found in the tunica intima of the thoracic aorta. Several reports of the parasite in cattle have been published from Assam [1] and Orissa [2]. Adult worms are thin and long, with malesmeasuring up to 7 cm and females could be as long as 70 cm. The adult worms remain coiled up in the fibrous tissue nodules of the aorta, while the microfilariae, on the other hand, are typically found in the skin of the hump or wither. The life cycle is not well understood. Adult worms are forming convoluted tunnels and aorta nodules. Early infection produces few nodules; later infection produces numerous tortuous tunnels and nodules with yellow caseous or slimy fluid and coiled worms. The parasite causes no clinical symptoms, but nodules are discovered in the aortic wall, and aortic aneurysms can occur. Microfilariae can be detected in skin biopsy materials to aid in diagnosis.

Theileria

Theileriosis is a tick-borne disease of ruminants and captives caused by the parasites of the genus *Theileria*, characterised by high fever, anaemia and enlargement of lymph nodes. The parasite is widely distributed across the globe, from Africa, Asia and Europe. *Theileria parva and T. annulata* are the two major species that afflict cattle, and their intermediate tick hosts are *Rhipicephalus appendiculatus* and *Hyalomma anatolicum anatolicum*, respectively. *T. parva* causes East coast fever, whereas *T. annulata* causes tropical theileriosis [5, 6].

The parasite utilises both lymphocytes and erythrocytes at various phases of development during its life cycle. Non-dividing piroplasm seen in erythrocytes can be ovoid, circular, comma, ring-shaped, rod-like, or irregular in shape and can measure up to 2 μm. The organisms appear with blue cytoplasm and a red chromatin dot at one end blue in Romanowsky stain. The actively reproducing schizont stage is present in the cytoplasm of lymphocytes and, occasionally, endothelial cells. There are two varieties of schizonts based on the size of their chromatic granules: macrochizonts and microschizonts. Macroschizonts create macro merozoites, while microschizonts produce micro merozoites, which penetrate erythrocytes and constitute the parasite's sexual stage. Macroschizonts are 2-16 μm in size and contain approximately 8 nuclei and microschizonts are comparable in size but have about 30-120 nuclei.

The disease is spread by tick saliva harbouring sporozoites while they feed on cattle. Sporozoites enter lymphocytes of regional lymph nodes and multiply *via schizogony*, resulting in the formation of macroschizonts (Koch's blue bodies). Macroschizonts are later discovered in all lymph node lymphocytes, the spleen, liver, and other organs, as well as in circulation. Following macroschizont replication, the creation of microschizonts begins, and the liberated micro merozoites penetrate the RBCs to create piroplasm.

Macroschizonts in lymphocytes and reticuloendothelial cells of parenchymatous organs cause a rise in the infected lymphoblast population, lymphocytolysis, and leucopenia. The piroplasmic stage is responsible for macrophage erythrophagocytosis, which results in the development of anaemia, particularly in high piroplasm parasitemia. High fever (104-107°F), enlargement of superficial lymph nodes, loss of appetite and drop in milk production are the first obvious visible clinical signs of the disease. Other symptoms include cessation of rumination, nasal discharge, dry muzzle, lacrimation, diarrhoea with blood and mucus, tachycardia, and occasionally nervous symptoms. The condition of infected animals goes down rapidly and mortality could reach up to 90%. Mortality is caused by dyspnoea as a result of severe pulmonary oedema. Postmortem lesions include generalised enlargement of lymph nodes. Haemorrhages are seen in lymph nodes, spleen, liver and kidneys and lungs show massive congestion and oedematous. The abomasum mucosa presents punched-out ulcers of 2-12 mm in diameter surrounded by a zone of inflammation.

Diagnosis is made on the basis of clinical signs like fever and enlargement of superficial lymph nodes, and supported by a blood exam confirming the presence of piroplasms in the RBCs (Fig. **1**) and/or Koch's blue bodies in the lymph node biopsy. In case of dead animals, the impression smears of lymph nodes, spleen and liver are stained and examined for the parasite. Antigen-specific ELISAs or PCR on lymph node aspirates can also be used to confirm a definitive diagnosis [5, 6].

Treatment with Buparvaquone started in the early stages of clinical disease is effective but in the latter phases when the disease has already set in with extensive lymphoid and hematopoietic tissue damage, treatment is less effective. Buparvaquone is the drug against *Theileria* and the development of resistance to it is reported in *T. annulata*. Oxytetracycline has also been used in treatment. Control approaches include tick control through the use of acaracide and integrated tick management practices, vaccination of cattle against *T. parva* and *T. annulata* in countries where vaccines are available, and the infection-an--treatment technique, which is becoming more popular in some places.

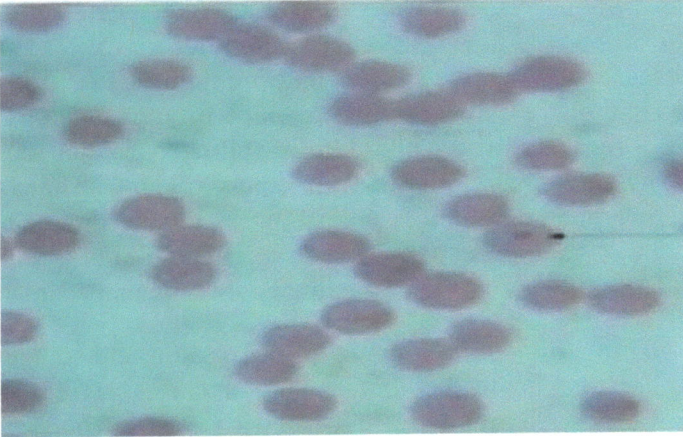

Fig. (1). *Theileria* spp. in Geimsa's stained blood smear of cattle.

Babesia

Babesiosis is an important cattle disease caused by blood protozoa, *Babesia* spp. transmitted by ixodid ticks of the genus *Boophilus* [5]. The disease also known as Redwater fever, Tick fever, Texas fever or piroplasmosis is a serious disease in cattle and is characterised by a very high fever ($\geq 106°F$), anaemia and haemoglobinuria.

Four species of *Babesia* infect cattle across the world, namely, *Babesia bovis, B. bigemina, B. divergens* and *B. major*, the most virulent being *B. bovis* followed by *B. bigemina*. In India, *Babesia bigemina* is an important species infecting cattle, buffalo, Mithun and yaks. *Babesia divergens* and B. major are mostly restricted to temperate zones [5]. It is a large piroplasm occurring singly or in pairs inside the red blood cells of their host. The shape could be pyriform, round, oval or elongated and often lies in pairs forming an acute angle. The size varies from species to species.

An infected tick injects sporozoites into the blood. The sporozoites infect the red blood cells where they divide asexually through binary fission to generate two or, in rare cases, more piroplasms. Infected red blood cells may rupture, allowing piroplasms to enter new red blood cells. When a tick ingests contaminated blood piroplasm is liberated with gamonts in the tick gut, which then undergo sexual reproduction to produce sporozoites. Transovarial or transstadial transmission can occur. In the case of transovarial transfer, sporozoites migrate to the ovary; and in transstadial transmission, they migrate to the salivary glands. These infective sporozoites are thus passed to the next host by transovarian transmission or stage-to-stage transmission.

Pathogenesis is influenced by a variety of factors, like species involved, age and breed of the host. Inverse age resistance is common. Exotic animals are more prone to the diseases than native species and premunity is seen in animals from endemic areas. Pathogenesis occurs due to intravascular haemolysis caused by fast parasite proliferation in red blood cells followed by cell destruction, and extravascular haemolysis primarily in the spleen. There may occur haemoglobinaemia, haemoglobinuria, hilirubinuria, and anaemia, as well as tissue hypoxia, metabolic acidosis, hyperkalemia, hypovolemic shock, and the development of multiple organ failure, all of which can lead to mortality.

Clinical signs include high fever, anorexia, depression and reluctance to move, haemoglobinuria, pale mucous membranes, jaundice, increased pulse, respiratory, and heart rates, and sudden death in untreated cases. Diarrhoea or constipation may also have been seen in a few animals, sudden drop in milk production and abortion in pregnant cows. Nervous signs like ataxia and incoordination are common in *B. bovis* infection along with other symptoms. Diagnosis is made on the basis of clinical presentation of high temperature and haemoglobinuria. The disease needs to be differentiated from other similar diseases through the examination of peripheral blood for *Babesia* organism in the Geimsa's stained blood smear (Fig. **2**). Necropsy reveals splenomegaly, hepatomegaly, subcutaneous and intramuscular oedema with icterus, blackened kidney, urinary bladder filled with dark urine, and organ congestion. There are numerous serological and molecular assays available for the diagnosis of babesiosis in cattle [5]. Polymerase Chain Reaction (PCR) based technologies with extreme sensitivity and specificity are now widely utilised to diagnose subclinical babesiosis.

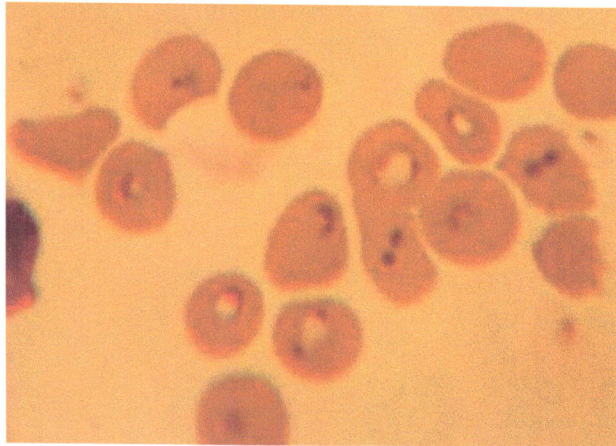

Fig. (2). *Babesia bigemina* in Geimsa's stained blood smear of cattle.

Diminazene aceturate (Berenil) at an intramuscular dose of 3.5 mg/kg and Imidocarb dipropionate at a subcutaneous dose of 1-2 mg/kg are effective in treating clinical infection. Like other tick-borne infections control measures should focus on tick control, which can be achieved with chemotherapy and chemoprophylaxis of the susceptible host population.

Anaplasma

Anaplasma is another obligatory intra-erythrocytic parasite of the order Rickettsiales and family Anaplasmataceae that affects Cattle, buffalo and wild ruminants. It is basically a disease of the tropical and subtropical regions. Diseases are reported from all over the world, Asia, Africa, Asia, Europe and South and Central America. Bovine anaplasmosis is an economically significant disease in the cattle sector. *Anaplasma marginale* and *A. centrale* are the two species that infect cattle. *A. marginal* is located in the erythrocyte's outside perimeter, while *A. centrale* is found in the erythrocyte's centre. Infection is spread by intermediate tick hosts of other important blood parasites such as *Boophilus, Rhipicephalus, Hyalomma etc.*, as well as mechanically by biting insects such as tabanid flies, Stomoxys, and mosquitoes, and even through infected surgical tools. Once in the blood, the organisms enter into the erythrocyte through the invagination of the cytoplasmic membrane resulting in the creation of a vacuole, following which the initial body multiplies by binary fission to produce an inclusion body composed of 4-8 original bodies [5, 6].

A clinical disease is predominantly associated with *A. marginale*. Inverse age resistance is seen in anaplasmosis with severe infection occurring in animals over 2 years of age and milder forms in younger ones. The incubation period ranges from 15-36 days and depends directly on the infective dose after the incubation period, fever and parasitaemia appear and in severe cases, within a week 70% of the erythrocytes are destroyed. The diseases are characterised by febrile reactions along with increasing haemolytic anaemia due to extravascular destruction of both infected and uninfected erythrocytes. The diseases could be peracute, acute or chronic. The clinical signs include a drop in milk production, inappetence, abortion in pregnant animals, loss of coordination, breathlessness when exerted, and a rapid pulse, which are usually evident in the late stages. Anaplasmosis is clinically similar to Babesiosis except there is no hemoglobinuria and fever rarely exceeding 106°F. The disease is more severe in exotic animals. The post-mortem findings are similar to Babesiosis *i.e.*, jaundiced, enlargement of the gall bladder, spleen and lymph nodes and petechial haemorrhages in the heart muscle. Diagnosis of an active infection is based on clinical signs and blood smear examination. Treatment with tetracycline, imidocarb and diminazene aceturate is effective in controlling the diseases since it very often happens in conjunction with babesiosis or theileriosis [5].

Trypanosoma

Trypanosomes are haemoflagellates present in the blood, plasma, lymph, and tissue fluids of mammals and birds. They are members of the Trypanosomatidae family, all of which are parasitic. Bovine trypanosomiasis is a severe health issue worldwide and a substantial cause of economic loss in the cattle industry. The disease is distinguished by gradual emaciation, anaemia, oedema, pyrexia, decreased weight gain, decreased milk and meat yields, abortion, and animal mortality [5]. Table **1** shows the *Trypanosoma* spp. that infects cattle worldwide, as well as their host, vector, and distribution.

Table 1. Cattle *trypanosomes* with their host, vector and distribution.

Sl. No.	Species	Host	Vector	Distribution
a. Salivaria				
1	*T. congolense*	Cattle, sheep, horse, pig	*Glossina*& mechanically by Tabanid	Africa, America
2	*T. vivax*	Ruminants, horses and dog		
3	*T. brucei*	Domestic mammals		
4	*T. simiae*	Pig, cattle, camel and horse	*Glossina*	Africa
5	*T. uniforme*	Antelope and ruminants	*Glossina*	Africa
6	*T. dimorphon*	Cattle, sheep, horse, pig	*Glossina*	Africa
b. Mechanical Transmission				
7	*T. evansi*	Horse, camel, dog, ruminants, elephant	Tabanid&*Stomoxys*	Cosmopolitan
c. Stercoraria#4				
8	*T. theileri*	Cattle	Tabanid	Cosmopolitan

African trypanosomiasis in cattle is caused by three trypanosome species viz. *Trypanosomacongolense*, *T. vivax*, and *T. brucei*, which are transmitted by numerous species of tsetse flies, *Glossina*. The widespread existence of the disease is attributable to the dispersal of tsetse, the wide host range, and the ability of the *trypanosomes* to bypass host defence mechanisms through antigenic variation. Cattle with trypanosomiasis have lower productivity. The disease is characterised by the enlargement of superficial lymph nodes, severe anaemia, and a general loss of body condition. There is intermittent fever with parasitaemic peaks. The condition can last for several months if left untreated, and it usually results in the animal's death. There is no field vaccination for bovine trypanosomiasis, and control approaches include chemotherapeutic and chemoprophylactic medicines, tsetse eradication, or control. Cattle can also serve as carriers for the human trypanosome, *T. Brucei rhodesiense.*

T. evansi is found throughout the Indian subcontinent. Cattle and buffalo primarily act as reservoir hosts for equines; however, epizootic mortality rates ranging from 20% to 90% have been documented in them [3]. *T. evansi* spread mechanically by vectors such as *Tabanus, Stomoxys, Chrysops, Haematopota* flies, and vampire bats. Other methods of transmission include eating infected meat, particularly carnivore meat, transplacental transmission, blood transfusion, and contaminated needles and syringes are also reported [4]. The parasite causes a subclinical illness in cattle and buffalo, but peracute cases with mortality within a few hours can also occur.

The diagnosis is predicated on the presence of a vector in the past, clinical indicators, and microscopical detection of *trypanosomes* in a blood smear (Fig. **3**). The commonly used method of diagnosis is a wet blood smear or thick dehaemoglobinized stained blood smear examination. Haematocrit centrifugation technique (HCT), quantitative buffy coat method (QBC), and anion exchange centrifugation technique are some other sensitive tests. A variety of chemical tests, such as the Mercuric chloride test, Stilbamidine test, Formol gel test, and others, as well as serological assays, such as IFAT, ELISA, and CFT, have been described. Molecular diagnostic tests, such as PCR, have become widely used and extremely specific for diagnosing trypanosomiasis. Diminazeneaceturate, isometamidium and Quinapyramine are the common drugs used for treating trypanosomiasis in cattle [5, 6].

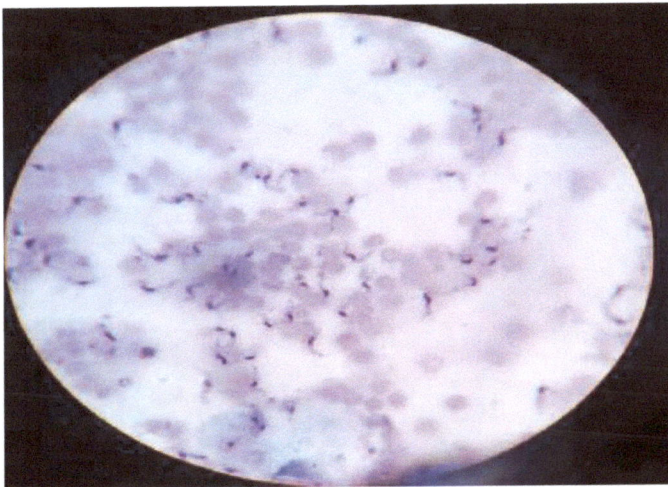

Fig. (3). *Trypanosoma* spp. in Geimsa's stained blood smear of cattle.

CONCLUSION

This chapter covered the parasitic diseases affecting the circulatory system of cattle and examined the vast variety of blood-borne parasites, including *Trypanosoma* spp., *Babesia* spp., *Theileria* spp., *Anaplasma* spp., *Schistosoma* spp., and *Onchocerca* spp. These parasitic diseases cause anaemia, weakness, decreased milk production, and, in severe situations, can be deadly to the animals. Understanding the biology, transmission, and pathophysiology of these parasite organisms is critical for developing effective control and prevention techniques. Vector management, tailored medicine administration, and effective biosecurity measures emerge as critical instruments in combating these parasitic infections. Furthermore, continued research and improvements in veterinary medicine are critical for establishing novel treatment choices, diagnostic tools, and preventive measures.

REFERENCES

[1]   Begam, R. Islam, S., Saikia, M., Kalita, A., Bulbul, K.H., Bam, J. and Pathak, P.. Prevalence of aortic Onchocerciasis in cattle of Assam. Veterinary Practitioner 2015; 16(2): 225-7.

[2]   Patnaik B. Onchocerciasis due to O. armillata in cattle in Orissa. J Helminthol 1962; 36(3): 313-25. [http://dx.doi.org/10.1017/S0022149X00023981] [PMID: 14484347]

[3]   Gill BS. Trypanosomes and trypanosomiases in Indian livestock. New Delhi: Indian Council of Agricultural Research 1991; p. 191.

[4]   Singh V, Singla LD. Trypanosomosis (Surra) in Livestock. In: Katoch R, Godara R, Yadav A, Eds. Veterinary Parasitology in Indian Perspective. Delhi: Satish Serial Publishing House 2013; pp. 305-30.

[5]   Soulsby EJL. Helminths, Arthropods and Protozoa of Domesticated Animals. 7th ed., London: ELBS, BaillierTindall 1982.

[6]   Taylor MA, Coop RL, Wall RL. Veterinary Parasitology. 3rd ed., Blackwell Publishing Ltd. 2007.

CHAPTER 5

Parasites in the Integumentary System

Bhupamani Das[1,*], Niral Patel[1], Dhyanjyoti Sarma[1] and R. M. Patel[1,2]

[1] *Department of Clinics (Veterinary Parasitology), College of Veterinary Science & Animal Husbandry, Kamdhenu University, Sardarkrushinagar, Gujarat, India*

[2] *Department of Veterinary Medicine, College of Veterinary Science & Animal Husbandry, Kamdhenu University, Sardarkrushinagar, Gujarat, India*

Abstract: The integumentary system is the largest organ system in the body and a physical barrier to the external environment. This intricate system maintains the animal's body in a state of homeostasis thanks to its many vital activities and complex structure. Worldwide, a wide range of parasitic diseases significantly increase the morbidity and mortality rate of cattle. Through the various ways that parasitic illnesses infect their host to collect nutrients and complete their lifecycle, as well as the possibility of becoming infection vectors, they have an impact on the health and productivity of cattle. Numerous protozoa, ectoparasites, and helminths mostly affect the integumentary system. A number of diseases have the potential to seriously affect both public and animal health; some are notifiable, while others are zoonotic.

Keywords: Cattle, Health, Homeostasis, Integumentary system, Parasite.

INTRODUCTION

The integumentary system is the largest sophisticated organ that protects the body and controls numerous vital functions [1]. It includes the glands that create sweat and oil as well as the skin, hair, and hoof. Together, these tissues safeguard the body against illness and damage and control physiological functions. The skin acts as the body's first line of defence against the outside world by protecting and maintaining the health of the inside organs. Although, the integumentary system is prone to a number of illnesses, conditions, and wounds.

EFFECT OF PARASITIC DISEASE ON INTEGUMENTARY SYSTEM

Animals' health is impacted by parasitic infections of the skin because they result in tissue loss, blood loss, and discomfort. Pests can make it difficult for an animal to survive quietly, which can lead to weight loss and loss in production. Ectopara-

*** Corresponding author Bhupamani Das:** Department of Clinics (Veterinary Parasitology), College of Veterinary Science & Animal Husbandry, Kamdhenu University, Sardarkrushinagar, Gujarat, India; E-mail: bhupa67@kamdhenuuni.edu.in

Tanmoy Rana (Ed.)

sites including flies, lice, ticks, mites, and leeches are most widely prevalent amongst cattle creating havoc with their infestations [1, 2]. Cattle are also commonly affected by different genera of skin helminths; *Parafilaria, Onchocerca, Stephanofilaria, Strongyloides,* and *Nasal schistosomes.* Protozoan pathogens affecting the skin are less frequent but *Besnoitia* and *Theileria* are capable of causing diseases affecting the skin and integumentary system. The main effect of parasites on the integumentary system has been described in Fig. (1).

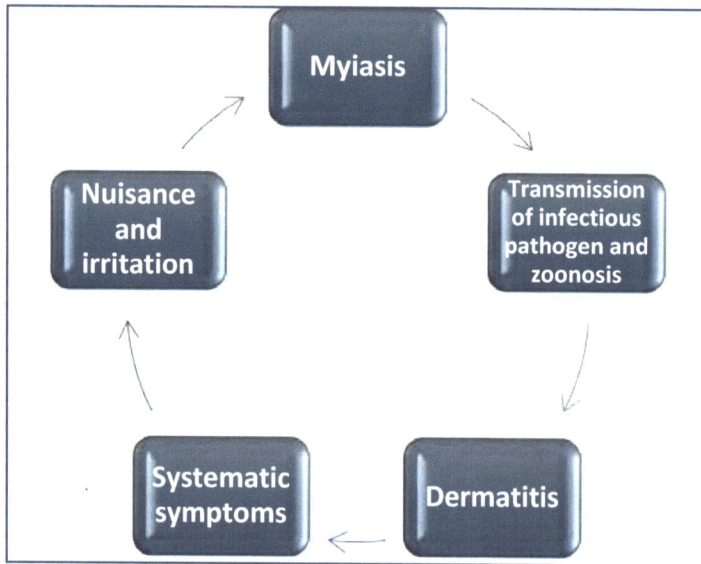

Fig. (1). Effect of parasitic pathogen on skin.

Helminth Parasite Affecting Integumentary System

a. *Parafilaria bovicola:* Cattle parasite, *Parafilaria bovicola* causes subcutaneous lesions that resemble bruises. Additionally, it has been noted in water buffalo (*Bubalus bubalis*). The adult males and females of the worm are 30-35 mm and 50–65 mm long, respectively. It is found in Africa (Morocco, Tunisia, Rwanda, Burundi, South Africa, Namibia, Botswana, Zimbabwe), Europe (Bulgaria, Romania, France, Sweden), and Asia (the Philippines, Japan, Russia, Pakistan, India). It has been determined that *Parafilaria* infection causes the beef industry to suffer significant financial losses. Cattle infected with *Parafilaria* only show outwardly as focused cutaneous haemorrhages (sometimes called "bleeding spots") that leak for a few hours before clotting and drying in the coat's matted hair. The cause of bleeding patches is the female worm, which pierces the skin, develops a tiny nodule, and oviposits in the blood dripping from the core lesion [3, 4]. The parasite's microfilariae first larval stage is present in the small eggs. Bleeding spots are distinctly seasonal, occurring most frequently in the spring and early summer in both the northern and southern hemispheres [5, 6]. The majority of bleeding areas are seen in the animal's dorsum, notably in the forequarters. Face flies of the genus *Musca* (subgenus *Eumusca*) are the invertebrate hosts, and they consume the eggs while eating at the bleeding sites. It takes the fly 10–12 days to develop into infectious third-stage larvae. When the flies feed on wounds, *Parafilaria* bleeding spots, or eye secretions, transmission to cattle most likely happens. However, the main significance of *Parafilaria* in beef-producing countries is damage to the subcutaneous tissues. Severe infections of *P. bovicola* have been found to limit the production of working bullocks in India due to seasonal bleeding and cutaneous nodules [7, 8]. Lesions that resemble bruises are irregular, edematous, greenish-yellow, and present on the carcasses of sick animals. These are often superficial, although on rare occasions, deeper muscles are also heavily implicated. The spring and summer months are when lesions are at their worst. Trimmed carcasses are frequently severely deformed and subsequently devalued. The carcass may be condemned in extreme situations. Bulls experience lesions more frequently and severely than steers, who in turn experience less severe effects than female animals. The diagnosis can be done by examination of blood from dermal lesions for parasitic eggs and microfilariae and also histopathology to identify nematodes or ELISA can be performed. The subcutaneous administration of nitroxynil (20 mg/kg) or ivermectin (200 mcg/kg) reduces the quantity and surface area of *Parafilaria* lesions. Animals should receive therapy for at least 70 to 90 days before death to allow the lesions to heal [9, 10].

b. *Onchocerca* species: *Onchocerca* (Filariidae) is a genus of parasites found in, cattle, sheep, horses, donkeys, and goats. The parasite is responsible for causing dermatitis in ruminants including cattle caused by microfilariae produced by adult *Onchocerca*. The adult worm resides in the nodules, and the fertilised females release microfilariae into the tissue lymph spaces from where an insect vector serves as the intermediate host by ingesting them [11, 12]. Although *Onchocerca* species are generally considered of little veterinary interest due to their low pathogenicity, *O. ochengi* is common in African cattle and is a human vector. For co-infection with onchocerciasis [13, 14] and its potential as a model for *O. volvulus* [15, 16]. The midges of the genus *Culicoides* are the most prevalent vectors. The intermediary hosts can be other biting flies. In these insect vectors, the larvae grow into the infective stage. When these biting flies feed on cattle while carrying the infectious larvae, cattle become infected. The hosts' connective tissue has nodules where the adults reside. Depending on the *Onchocerca* species involved, these nodules may be seen in a particular place. The top dermis is reached by the microfilariae that the adults create after moving through the connective tissues. *O. gibsoni, O. dukei,* and *O. ochengi* in cattle cause intradermal and subcutaneous nodules in the brisket and sporadically elsewhere. Other clinical symptoms are absent in infected animals. The microfilariae migrate to the dermis, and the mature worms reside in numerous ligaments and tendons in horses. Horses with cutaneous onchocercosis exhibit erythema, crusting, depigmentation, pruritis, and baldness [17, 18]. The ventral midline, tail head, face, and neck all have lesions. The microfilariae's pathogenicity remains controversial. Subcutaneous nodules are palpable in the brisket and buttock areas. Once the nodules have been removed, the afflicted carcasses may be passed [19, 20]. Before the carcasses are passed, the tissue and fascia surrounding the stifle and the brisket are peeled off in cases of severe infestations. The condition can be distinguished by cysticercosis, eosinophilic myositis, neurofibromatosis, and abscesses. Beytut *et al.* (2005) found extensive teat lesions associated with microfilariae of the *Onchocerca* spp [3].

c. *Stephanofilaria* species. Infections caused by Stephanofilariae are a prevalent cause of cow skin disease known as "Humpsore" on the Indian subcontinent. Only *Stephanofilaria assamensis* has been identified as the causal agent of tuberous ulcers in East India, despite reports of nine distinct species of *Stephanofilaria* protozoa from various regions of the world [21, 22]. While the term "cusp wound" implies that sores only appear in the cusp region, *Stephanofilaria* dermatitis can affect other body areas as well. The illness is endemic in tropical nations like India and other places, where the house fly is the primary carrier [23]. West Bengal, India, is the disease's endemic region [24]. *Stephanofilaria stilesi* is the most common cause of ventral midline filarial dermatitis in cattle in the United States. The horn-fly Adult worms live in the dermis, while microfilariae are consumed by *Haematobia irritans*. Fly microfilariae develop into infected larvae in two to three weeks, which are injected into the cow's skin during eating. Papules, crusts, and serous exudates are the initial indications and symptoms of ventral midline dermatitis. When it is persistent, it causes baldness, hyperkeratosis, and thickening of the skin. Large lesions usually occur between the navel and sternum, though they might extend deeper to the cranium or tail. Visible breast lesions could also be present. Cows who are irritated will lie down part of the way and scratch their tummies. To ease the itching caused by dermatitis, cows may rock their chests and abdomens while seated on their knees. Combining clinical signs with skin samples is the most effective way to reach a definitive diagnosis. For nursing cattle with stephanofilariasis, there is currently no recognised treatment. However, it is conceivable that this parasite can be controlled by ectoparasiticides belonging to the avermectin and milbemycin families. While doramectin is only useful for female dairy calves under 20 months of age, ivermectin, eprinomectin, and moxidectin can all be administered topically to nursing cattle.

Stephanofilarial otitis or Ear sore: Parasitic otitis caused by *Stefanofilaria zaheeri* occurs most commonly in older cows during wet weather. Infestation is uncomfortable, and biting flies have been linked to the parasite's spread to the auricle. Macroscopic lesions range from congestion to inflammation with haemorrhage to severe crusting (parakeratosis) if chronic, to alopecia with depigmentation, and are particularly noticeable on the concave surface of the auricle. Microscopically, lymphocytes, macrophages, hyperplastic or degenerate sebaceous glands, haemorrhage, and microfilaria are found in the auricular epidermis and dermis. Microfilariae within the dermis are usually dead and present in areas infiltrated by macrophages, eosinophils, and plasma cells. It has been hypothesized that the lesions represent some form of immune-mediated response. Chronic cases of "earache" can lead to dysplasia or neoplastic changes in epidermal cells, possibly related to excessive cellular mitosis and genetic mutations that occur in rapidly dividing somatic cells [17].

Leg sore: Cattle throughout the world are commonly infected with the worm genus *Stephanofilaria*, which causes a range of pathological symptoms. It seems that various species have distinct lesions at different locations. The lesions often referred to as "Krian sore" in Malaysia are always present in the limbs of cattle and are caused by *Stephanofilaria kaeli* [14]. With mononuclear cells and a preponderance of eosinophils, the inflammatory infiltration exhibits the same characteristics as the majority of parasite infections. The cells, however, are not limited to the area around the parasites. They are dispersed evenly throughout the entire lesion. In certain regions, lymphocytes take the lead among eosinophils as the predominant cell type. The idea that there may be a non-specific inflammatory illness that is superimposed upon or even precedes the parasite infection is created by the lesion's widespread nature and mixed look. The latter could account for the lesion's propensity to occur in the limb extremities, which are vulnerable to trauma and general secondary infections.

a. *Strongyloides* species: Otitis externa in cattle is brought on by a free-living, saprophytic rhabditiform worm of the genus *Rhabditis* [15]. Additionally, typical are concurrent infections with the yeast *Malassezia* spp. and the ear mite *Raillietia auris*. *Rhabditis* species are found in some areas of Brazil and tropical and subtropical climate zones of Africa. The external auditory meatus is infected with and overrun by *Rhabditis* species. Cattle that have been exposed to an infestation may not show any symptoms or show depression, otorrhea, otitis media and interna, cranial nerve paralysis, meningitis, circling recumbency, and death. High humidity and a higher ambient temperature are the two main risk factors for this condition. Other risk factors include age, breed, horniness, use of certain insecticide dips, and irritation or damage to the auricular skin. Among the risk factors are the following examples:

1. Purebred and crossbred *Bos indicus* cattle, such as Gir, have long, pendulous auricles that create a more favourable environment for infection;
2. In *Bos indicus* cattle breeds, horns are believed to compress the external acoustic meatus and thereby increase their susceptibility to infection;
3. Cattle "dip treated" with an acaricide have greater infestations with *Rhabditis* spp.

b. *Schistosoma* species: Schistosomiasis frequently affects cattle in Africa and Asia, but it hardly ever affects other domestic animals. Most schistosome infections in endemic areas are asymptomatic, despite the fact that they can occasionally function as important pathogens that encourage intense transmission. However, huge incidence rates of subclinical illnesses cause large losses because of their long-term effects on growth and productivity, as well as their increased susceptibility to other bacterial or parasite diseases. The disease that causes snoring in cattle might result in much reduced market prices. Schistosomes are members of the genus *Schistosoma*, which is part of the family Schistosomatidae. Adult worms are inevitable circulatory system parasites in mammals. The gynecophoric canal, a ventral groove formed by the ventrally flexed lateral outgrowths of the male body, is where the adult female is usually carried. Compared to the male, the adult female is thinner. While an animal may have an oral infection while it is drinking, the most common way that cercariae enter ruminants is through the skin. The lymph and blood transport the schistosomula, which are transformed from cercariae upon penetration, to their predilection sites. Depending on the species, the prepatent period might be anywhere between 45 and 70 days. Nasal schistosomiasis can partially obstruct the nasal cavity and produce snoring due to cauliflower-like growths on the nasal mucosa. It is possible to experience a localised cutaneous hypersensitivity reaction after cercariae skin penetration, which presents as small, itchy maculopapular sores.

Ectoparasites Affecting Integumentary System

The term "ectoparasite" refers to a group of organisms with a wide taxonomic range that live on both human and animal skin. The ability of a solitary organism to cause skin lesions large enough to be seen with the unaided eye makes ectoparasitic arthropods and nematodes comparable. Ectoparasitic infestations frequently have a severe itching sensation that is quite annoying and uncomfortable. These illnesses frequently have a high frequency in disadvantaged families, homes, and neighbourhoods in underdeveloped areas.

Ectoparasite-borne skin diseases and injuries: mechanisms: Arthropod ectoparasites that feed on human blood or tissue juice (such as fleas, lice, mites, and ticks) or that burrow into human skin or orifices and live there can directly endanger people's health. The spread of infectious diseases by the arthropod ectoparasites (fleas, mites, and ticks) can potentially pose a hazard to human health indirectly. The most adaptable ectoparasitic arthropod, ticks may transmit a wide range of infectious illnesses (viral, bacterial, and protozoan), as well as inject paralytic toxins (tick paralysis), all while consuming a protracted blood diet. Ticks, in contrast to other ectoparasites, can transmit disease to both males and females at birth (*via* transovarial pathogen transmission) and at all phases of development through trans stadial pathogen transmission [20].

Ectoparasitic diseases epidemiology: Many of the common traits of developing infectious illnesses are also present in ectoparasitic diseases [5]. The following are characteristics of ectoparasitic infestations and newly developing infectious illnesses that are frequently shared:

1. Infection by endemic agents given selective advantages by changing ecological or socio-economic conditions;
2. Introduction into new, susceptible host populations;
3. The recent migration of endemic human host populations from rural to urban settings in search of improved economic possibilities.

FLIES

a. Old world screw worm fly-*Chrysomya bezziana*: *Chrysomya bezziana*, the old world screw worm fly: Adult screwworms are rarely found in the wild. The bodies of adults are dark metallic green, with a narrow stripe running the length of the abdomen along the tail. The legs have partially brown or black in colour. It has an orange/yellow face. It is quite possible that the first instar larvae, which can grow to a length of 3 mm, will go undetected when they moult into the second instar larvae. The second stage is 4-9 mm long and resembles the third stage. Larvae measure up to 18 mm in size in their third instar. There is a broad ring of thorns encircling the body, which is divided into 12 segments.

Every third instar resembles a maggot and has a tail. Every third instar resembles a maggot and has a distinctive tail coil for this species. At the end of the eighth segment of the abdomen, there is a deep cleft where the larval caudal spiral disc is situated. Large, clearly distinct spiral plates are seen triple breathing slots and a wide rim. The Old World screwworm fly *C. bezziana* produces the incredibly nasty myiasis. Female flies are attracted to open wounds on people and domesticated and wild animals, congregating in masses of 150–500 around body orifices or along the edge of wounds. Larvae enter the third stage of development two days after hatching. Because they have buried themselves so deeply in the wound, only their caudal ends are visible. It takes 5-7 days for the larval stage to fully develop. The pupal stage lasts 7-9 days in warm climates and longer in cooler climates. The adult flies then come out to breed, look for a new host, and repeat the cycle. For prevention and control, it is essential that female flies only spawn once in their lifespan. Under perfect conditions, there may be eight generations per year. Even though they are attracted to open wounds, female flies occasionally lay their eggs on the thin, intact skin of various body parts, especially if such areas have been contaminated by mucus or blood secretions. After hatching, the larvae rip at the host's flesh, severing tissues and severing tiny blood vessels with their hooked mouthparts. Larvae consume a lot of blood. During the bloodsucking phase, only the caudal ends of the maggots with their blackish peritremes remain visible at the surface of the lesion, allowing the larvae to breathe. Up to 300 maggots have been seen in some wounds. When left untreated, the larvae's destructive activity might quickly result in the animal's death. The diagnosis is based on identifying the rarely observed adult flies. Treatment for screwworm infestation involves killing the larvae in the lesions, promoting healing, and preventing secondary reinfestation with larvae of the facultative myiasis-producing flies. To determine the extent of the lesions, the hair coat is clipped and as many larvae as possible are extracted. The removed larvae should be killed in order to prevent them from pupating and developing into adults. Larvae that are firmly entrenched in tissues must be removed. Doses of 50, 100, 200, and 300 mcg/kg of ivermectin prevent cattle from being infested with *C. bezziana*.

a. Face fly-*Musca autumnalis: Musca autumnalis*, often known as face flies, get their name from the way they congregate around the eyes and muzzles of farm animals, notably cattle. They can also be seen on the flank, sternum, withers, and neck. Their mouthpieces are designed for soaking up mucous, tears, and saliva. Due to the fact that face flies have sponging mouthparts rather than piercing or bayonet-like ones like those of *Stomoxys calcitrans*, they are typically not classified as blood eaters. They do, however, pursue blood-feeding flies, agitate them while they are feeding, and then slurp up the blood and other fluids that collect on the host's skin. Face flies are typically only found on outdoor-living animals and do not follow them inside barns. The host is irritated by face flies, which ultimately hinders the host's productivity. Females consume face secretions like saliva, nasal mucus, and tear fluid to get the protein they need for egg formation. The discomfort around the host's eyes causes the host to cry more frequently, which draws more flies. Face flies also consume other liquids, such as milk on the faces of calves and blood from wounds. Face flies can irritate and mechanically harm the host's ocular tissue because of the short, rough spines (prestomal teeth) on their sponging mouthparts. The feeding behaviour of face flies promotes *Moraxella bovis* transmission. *Thelazia* species and *Parafilaria bovicola* can both use face flies as intermediate hosts. From a morphological perspective, adult-face flies resemble house flies. The only real distinctions between these two species are in the colour of the abdomen and the position of the eyes. The abilities of a qualified entomologist are needed for speciation. In general, a medium-sized fly feeding near a cow or horse's eyes and nostrils is most likely a face fly. Different insecticides and application methods, including dust sacks, mist sprays, and wipe-on formulations, have been used extensively. Additionally, feed additives including pesticides and insect growth regulators are employed. Results, however, are typically far from adequate. Even with two tags (one in each ear) per animal, the seasonal face fly population has been reduced by only 70%–80% after the introduction of ear tags filled with pesticides.

b. Horn fly-*Haematobia irritans:* This term refers to the fact that *Haematobia irritans* often congregate in huge groups close to the base of bull horns. This important cattle pest can be found in most of the world's cattle-producing regions. Horn fly adults live their whole lives on their host; females only come off to lay eggs on new cow faeces, which is where the larvae and pupae grow. In warmer climates, the life cycle can take as little as one week, while in the southern US, it might take up to two weeks for development to complete. Male flies are not as aggressive as horn flies, which feed up to 20 times a day by sucking on blood and other bodily fluids. Cattle experience pain, discomfort, and blood loss when feeding. Animals who are disturbed also lose weight because they eat less efficiently. When an infestation is severe, lesions develop along the ventral midline of the animal. In the United States, horn flies commonly cause weaned calves to lose 12–14 pounds, and range cattle to gain 14% less weight. In dairy cows, milk output might drop by 10% to 20%. These flies are also an intermediate host for the parasite *Stephanofilaria stilesi*, which produces plaque-like lesions on the ventral abdomen of cattle. The black hue, small size (3-6 mm, or around half the size of a stable fly), and bayonet-shaped proboscis that extends from the head of horn flies make them immediately distinguishable from other flies. It is usual to find hundreds of them clustered at the base of the cattle horn. Whole-animal chemical sprays and forced-use self-treating devices (such as dust bags or back rubbers) are effective ways to control horn flies. Cattle work best when they have to go under dust bags each day in order to get water or supplements of minerals. Dust bags carry insecticides down the dorsum, where horn flies spend much of their time. Back rubbers allow cattle to reward themselves while they scratch. Herbicide, as recommended by the label, is to be diluted with premium mineral oil.

c. Buffalo fly-*Haematobia irritans exigua*: Similar to horn flies in size, appearance, feeding, and reproductive behaviours is the *Haematobia irritans exigua* (Fig. **2**). Although rarely feeding on horses, sheep, or other animals, the buffalo fly is mostly a pest of cattle and water buffalo. It is prevalent in portions of southern, southeastern, and eastern Asia as well as Oceania, but is absent from New Zealand. Similar to horn flies, it has a life cycle where the adult leaves the host long enough to lay an egg on new dung, where development takes place. Depending on the weather, the life cycle could be completed in as little as 7–10 days. Animals are irritated and annoyed by buffalo flies, which typically bite near the shoulders and withers. Blood is consumed by both sexes 10–40 times per day. Infection with the screwworm *Chrysomya bezziana* may occur in bite wounds. The flies relocate to shady areas of the body in hot weather. Even 100 flies per animal can significantly reduce feed efficiency and production. Affected animals lose blood and become agitated by the flies. The saliva of flies causes allergies in some animals. More flies are drawn to calves with dark coats and animals in poor condition.

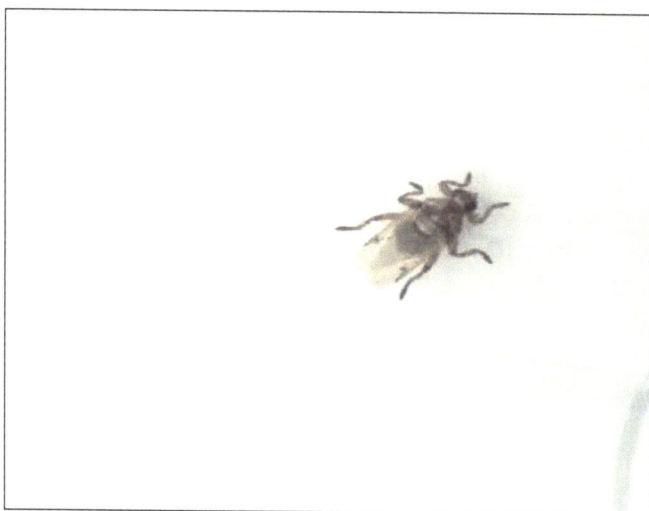

Fig. (2). Buffalo fly collected from cattle.

a. Head flies or plantation flies-*Hydrotaea irritans:* Non-biting flies called *Hydrotaea irritans* are a major problem for cattle, sheep, and other livestock. This insect is between 4 and 7 mm long and resembles the housefly. The wing bases are orange-yellow, the abdomen is olive green, and the thorax is black with grey patches. Head flies are a nuisance to both domestic animals and people because they are drawn to fluids around the mouth, nose, ears, eyes, and wounds. *H irritans* produces one generation each year, with three larval instar stages, in contrast to other *Hydrotaea* spp. Larvae emerge from eggs laid in the late summer within a few days. Before reaching the stage where it preys on other insect larvae, the saprophagous stage is short. Larvae in their late stages overwinter. Adults are most active from early June to late September, and they frequently congregate in thickets or forests where they take refuge between feeding times. When an animal moves, large swarms of flies are drawn to the activity and gather there to feed on the fluids from the eyes and nose as well as the cellular waste near the base of the developed horn. Animals scratch and rub their heads to relieve the ongoing irritation, which causes open wounds or "broken heads," especially on the poll. Flies perch on these self-inflicted sores after being drawn by the blood and spread the edges by feeding them. Humans, deer, horses, cattle, and rabbits are all targets of head flies. Although calves do not have comparable broken head lesions, *Trueperella pyogenes*-caused summer mastitis does occur. The only entirely reliable method of avoiding harm is to remove producing animals from fly-infested areas during the fly season. Once damaged heads have occurred, the only effective way to stop additional fly damage is to stall-feeding the animals.

b. The biting midges, "no-see-ums," or punkies-*Culicoides* spp.: The most prevalent biting midges, *Culicoides* spp., like damp soil or mud near streams, ponds, and marshes, among other aquatic or semiaquatic settings. Biting midges are tiny gnats (1-3 mm long) that, like black flies, bite painfully and draw blood from their hosts, which can include both people and farm animals. The aggressive biting *Culicoides* spp. can be extremely upsetting and inconvenient. They can make production animals anxious and disrupt their feeding schedules if they are present in big numbers. Depending on the species, these biting gnats prefer to feed on the dorsal or ventral regions of the host. They are most active before and during sunset and only fly during the warm months of the year. Animals that are bitten frequently develop allergies to the bites and scratch and rub the affected areas, leading to baldness, excoriations, and skin thickening. It is also known as summer dermatitis because it is frequently observed during the summertime. Onchocerciasis, a nonseasonal dermatosis that affects the head, neck, and abdomen, is comparable to a sweet itch but typically less itchy. The bluetongue virus is also spread by *Culicoides* species in cattle.

c. House fly-*Musca domestica:* House flies, or *M. domestica*, have been a problem for people throughout recorded history and are an important agricultural and public health nuisance [33]. The fly can exploit practically any place that is occupied by people and the animals they live with thanks to its capacity to grow in a wide variety of unevenly distributed and transient organic larval substrates [13]. With the predicted warming of the Earth's temperature, fly populations appear to be increasing [9]. Farmworkers and nearby homeowners have nuisance issues due to the fly population being above the threshold level. More significantly, adult flies' propensity to regurgitate and defecate on both human and animal food allowed for the early identification of their function as carriers of human and animal infections, particularly those responsible for gastrointestinal disorders [13]. In addition to poultry, all farm animals (cattle, camels, and sheep) also experience economic difficulties as a result of houseflies. Houseflies decrease farm worker productivity because they interfere with tasks like feeding and milking. They also increase the frequency of animal disease transmission, increasing the need for veterinary services, medication costs, and the risk of the spread of human diseases [6]. Houseflies reduce milk production because cows must expend extra energy fending off flies. Most insecticides used to combat the medical and veterinary pest *Musca domestica L.* are no longer effective. The quest for new alternative control methods is ongoing as a result [6, 11, 25].

d. The common cattle grub (*H. lineatum*) and the northern cattle grub (*H. bovis*): Both the northern cow grub, *Hypoderma bovis*, and the common cattle grub, *Hypoderma lineatum*, are ubiquitous in the Holarctic and can be found wherever cattle are reared. They are serious cattle pests for commercial use. Larvae of *Hypoderma bovis* move through the epidural spaces of cattle. An infestation usually occurs between July and October. SCI results from the death or destruction of the larvae in the epidural space, which triggers a major immune response. The clinical symptoms usually appear in cattle treated with organophosphate insecticides during the epidural larvae migration. Clinical signs usually appear acutely hours to days after therapy and are caused by injury to the thoracolumbar spinal cord. Notable symptoms include paresis of the pelvic limbs and ataxia of the GP. In the event that the lumbosacral cord is compromised, the pelvic limbs may show LMN signs. The indicators are typically not symmetrical [4]. Ineffective attempts on the part of hosts to escape ovipositing flies lead to losses such as skin damage and self-harm. Adults are therefore commonly referred to as "gad fly." The phrase "heel flies" describes adult members of the *Hypoderma* species and describes the defensive reaction of cattle in which their hooves are lifted [4]. Bovine hypodermiasis has a negative effect on productivity and welfare, which results in significant losses despite the fact that it does not significantly increase mortality and morbidity. These losses include decreased meat and milk production, poor weight gain and growth in calves infected with primovirus, trimming carcasses to remove damaged tissues, severe depreciation of hides due to breathing holes, and increased susceptibility to other diseases. On bright, sunny days, cattle may run away with their tails tucked up while they are being chased by female heel flies, particularly *H. bovis*. Cattle utilise a strategy known as "gadding" to avoid female flies and their attempts to lay eggs. This kind of stampeding or gadding has also been observed in the absence of heel flies, so it is not always a response to their attacks. Cattle gadding can result in decreased productivity, hampered procreation, self-harm, or even fatality. When newly hatched larvae penetrate the skin, it can cause a hypodermal rash. This happens more often in older animals that have already been affected. The puncture sites are usually painful and inflamed, and they often leak a yellowish serum.

Larval secretions are associated with modulatory processes that impact inflammatory and specific immune responses. This immunomodulation aids in the survival of larvae during initial infestations. In otherwise healthy cattle, *H. bovis* larvae and their secretions in the epidural fat of the spinal canal are associated with inflammation, fat necrosis, and disintegrating connective tissue. Sometimes the swelling extends to the periosteum and bone, causing osteomyelitis and periostitis in a particular area. Sometimes the perineurium and epineurium are implicated. In rare instances, severe episodes can lead to neurological disorders such as paralysis. Similar to this, *H. lineatum* in the submucosa of the oesophagus may cause enough inflammation and tissue edema to impede swallowing or eructation. Clinical parasitism signs, however, are not usually evident throughout the migratory season. From the topline to approximately one-third of the way down the sides and from the tailhead to the shoulders, the diseased animal's back may exhibit warbles. The warbles are frequently raised and firm, protruding well beyond the skin's natural contours. Every warble may have a breathing hole, which can range in size from a microscopic slit to a circular aperture (3–4 mm in diameter) for more mature larvae. Usually, secondary infection is inhibited; however, large, purulent abscesses can occasionally develop warbles. As soon as the third-stage larvae appear, are expelled, or die inside the cysts, the lesions often heal without any issues. The carcasses and hides of infected animals exhibit obvious signs of animal grub infestation, and their value has decreased. Most afflicted animals have less than 100 warbles, while they can have up to 300.

The presence of individual animals without larvae is common in infected herds. Young animals are most commonly affected since older animals develop some resistance to the condition. When animals come into contact with migrant *Hypoderma* spp. larvae that die in the oesophagus (*H. lineatum*) or near the spinal canal (*H. bovis*), they may react severely and sometimes even die. These reactions appear to be connected with the number of larvae, but they are infrequent regardless of the number of larvae present. The mortality of *H. lineatum* L1 larvae in the submucosal connective tissue of the oesophagus causes dysphagia, drooling, and bloating. Again, recovery occurs rapidly and entirely (48–72 hours following therapy); nevertheless, in severe cases, the bloat may be lethal. If a stomach tube is tried to be placed into an affected animal, the animal may explode from its oesophagus. Cattle experienced stiffness, ataxia, muscle weakness, and paralysis of the hind limbs as a result of the death of *H. bovis* L1 larvae in the spinal canal following systemic pesticide treatment. Most of the time, recovery is swift and total; extremely sometimes, paralysis may be irreversible. These parasites' clinical significance has decreased in North America due in part to the widespread usage of macrocyclic lactones; concurrently, the prevalences of *H. lineatum* and *H. bovis* in cattle have decreased. Nonetheless, serologic investigations have demonstrated that cattle continue to be exposed to *Hypoderma* spp. If treatment programmes are discontinued, or if effective therapies for *Hypoderma* spp. are no longer used, clinical signs of infestation will most likely reappear.

Effect of fly larvae on skin: Myiasis

The infestation of living vertebrates with fly larvae, whose species change depending on where they are in the world, is known as myiasis. The term "myiasis" is typically used to describe those genera of flies that occasionally infiltrate deeper tissues in addition to the skin and subcutaneous tissues of humans, domestic animals, and wildlife. Despite migrating through the tissues of the host, the larvae of warble and bot flies (such as *Hypoderma* in cattle) are typically not linked to skin lesions. The myiasis-causing larvae must consume the tissues of the affected animals, which can occasionally result in major clinical complications and even death. When adult female flies are drawn to a wound or to macerated skin that is contaminated with urine and/or faeces, they lay eggs (or larvae - *Wohlfahrtia* species), which causes myiasis in the affected animals. The eggs hatch and go through three phases of larval development on the animals. The third-stage larvae fall to the ground, where they form pupae which the immature adult flies develop before hatching. These larvae's feeding activities can badly harm the host. Animals who are neglected or immobile are more prone to myiasis because they can't ward off adult flies or get rid of the eggs and larvae. The flies connected to myiasis can be divided into two categories:

1. Obligatory flies, which must develop on living hosts (such as *Wohlfahrtia vigil*, a type of meat fly); and
2. Facultative flies, which can develop on living or dead hosts as well as organic debris.

Genera that cause facultative myiasis are further divided into primary and secondary genera. Primary genera, such as *Lucilia* species, *Calliphora* species,

Phormia species, and *Wohlfahrtia* species, can initiate myiasis while primary and secondary genera, such as Lucilia species, *Calliphora* species, *Phormia* species, and *Wohlfahrtia* species, require obligate or primary genera to do so. These genera are all found in Canada. According to a study done by Singh & Singh, 2016, dairy animals in the State of Punjab, India, are frequently affected by screwworm flies, house flies, and flesh flies.

TICK

The bodies of dairy cattle are covered in a variety of external parasites including ticks. By virtue of their name, it is clear that they stick to the bodies of animals and draw blood from them. They survive by sucking blood from these animals [19]. Ticks are typically located inside and outside of an animal's external ears, under its tail's inner and exterior surface, on its neck, and in the spaces between its hooves, where they stick and cling securely to draw blood (Fig. **3**). Ticks on animals can be found in 106 different species, with scientific names like *Ixodes, Amblyomma, Boophilus, Hyalomma, Rhipicephalus*, and *Dermacenter*.

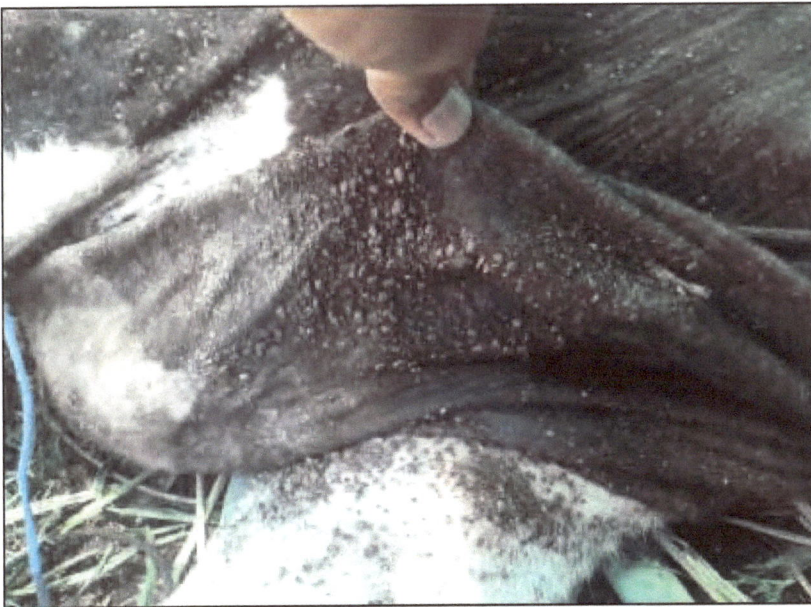

Fig. (3). Heavy infestation of tick in crossbred cattle.

The most significant external parasite typically seen in cattle, ticks cause significant economic losses both directly through blood sucking and indirectly through their role as carriers of infections that promote disease. Ticks are the most important external parasite. Ticks consume animal blood. As a result, animals experience blood loss and anaemia, which cause them animal to gradually get weaker. One tick consumes 0.5 to 2.0 milliliters of animal blood in a single day. Animals lose their hunger, which causes them to become dull. Skin irritation is present. Animals who are scratched are mentally agitated and occasionally enraged. Animal skin deteriorates over time. Skin hair begins to come out (alopecia). The milk supply has drastically decreased. Animals with a heavy tick population have lower fertility and reproductive ability. Bullocks' ability to labour is diminished, and their capacity for work is gone. Ticks' indirect effects on performance and production include skin rashes, anaemia, weight loss, decreased milk supply, and disease transmission. There are some tick species that significantly reduce the value of cattle by spreading disease (most commonly the protozoan Rickettsia) from one animal to another. Ticks are therefore considered to be important disease vectors. Ticks can cause a variety of infectious diseases in animals, including spirochetosis (Tick fever), encephalitis (viral), theileriosis, babesiosis, and anaplasmosis (protozoon diseases). On the one hand, ticks sucking the blood of animals reduces their productivity. On the other hand, they can indirectly transmit different types of bacteria, viruses, and protozoon parasites. Typically, "Acaricides"—chemical insecticides—are used to control tick infestations in cattle. For this, synthesized organophosphorus chemicals are specifically used. The majority of adult ticks on an animal's body are almost fully eliminated (killed) by these substances, but the ticks' eggs are not eliminated since they hide in the cracks and crevices of the flooring and walls of the stables.

LICE

Cattle are agitated by lice, which makes them bite, scratch, and rub. This persistent annoyance could develop into a welfare problem. Fences, yards, and trees that the cattle use as rubbing posts may sustain damage from unruly animals. A rough, scruffy appearance develops on the coats of bad animals, and sometimes the skin is scraped raw. In addition to potentially being in conflict with on-farm quality assurance programmes, this will lower hide value at slaughter. There is ongoing discussion over the impact of lice on the growth and productivity of cattle. Numerous research works with conflicting findings suggest that a combination of factors influences how much lice affect cattle. When cattle are not in good health or if infestations are severe, lice can be a significant source of financial loss. Always seek an underlying cause if a mob's lice infestation is limited to a few numbers of severely infected animals. Animals that are unwell or under nutritional stress will experience more severe infestations of lice than healthy animals.

a. Bitting Lice: Lice that bite feed on dead skin cells and can be extremely irritating. The reddish-brown, 2 mm long cattle biting louse (*Bovicola bovis*) has a brown head. It primarily affects the back, rump, shoulders, and neck. Lice-sucking blood is drawn from skin piercings by sucking lice. If a lot of them are present, anaemia may result.

b. *Haematopinus eurysternus*, the short-nosed cattle louse: It is a dark grey shade. Length of the female: 3.5–5 mm. The man is not as big. Although it can appear anywhere in the hair coat in cases of severe infestation, it is primarily found in the long hair surrounding the cattle's neck and tail and around their eyes. It is located under the tail and in and around the ears in the summer.

c. The long-nosed cattle louse (*Linognathus vituli*): Bluish-black and about 2.5 mm long. Like the short-nosed cattle louse, it may be found anywhere in the hair coat including the neck, dewlap, inner thigh, and scrotum.

d. The tubercle-bearing louse (*Solenoptes capillatus*): Smallest louse, only 1.2 mm long. It has a brown head and a bluish abdomen. It is usually found around the head and neck in distinct dark clusters.

Winter is when lice numbers are highest, and summer is when they are lowest. Lice infestations are known to be more severe in cooler skin temperatures. Lice thrive in colder climates with thicker winter coats. It seems that healthy, well-fed cattle are not heavily infested with lice, and when they are, their performance is not negatively impacted by the lice. When the cattle's nutrition declines, the number of lice tends to rise. In the winter, significant infestations of lice typically occur when cold weather is combined with inadequate nourishment. Sick cattle typically have more extensive lice infestations, especially if they are dealing with another issue like a chronic illness. Nonetheless, certain cattle are referred to as "louse carriers" since they seem to be very susceptible to lice. It has been proposed that variations in the greasiness of the hair coat among different breeds of cattle could account for observed variations in lice susceptibility. Nonetheless, it is more likely that variations in lice burdens between people are a reflection of variations in an animal's immune system, nutrition, or general health.

Scratching, hair loss brought on by rubbing the rump, shoulders, and neck tearing and scratching. Fences, yards, and trees that the cattle use as rubbing posts may sustain damage from unruly animals. A rough, scruffy appearance develops on the coats of bad animals, and sometimes the skin is scraped raw. There is ongoing discussion over the impact of lice on the growth and productivity of cattle. Numerous researches with conflicting findings suggest that a combination of factors influences how much lice affect cattle. When cattle are in poor health or have extensive infestations, lice can be a significant source of financial loss. Seek an underlying cause whenever a small number of animals within a mob exhibit severe lice infestations. More severe lice infestations will occur in diseased or nutritionally challenged animals than in healthy ones.

Insecticides can be used to treat infected cattle. However, they may not be as effective on louse eggs. This means that after treatment, eggs can still hatch and continue the infestation. With some insecticides, a follow-up treatment 2–3 weeks later is necessary. This time interval is critical to achieve control, as it allows time for the eggs to hatch but not to mature into adults which will lay eggs themselves. It can be important to know whether you have sucking or biting lice because the different method of feeding means that they have different susceptibilities to treatments. This is particularly important if you are going to use an avermectin injection (such as ivermectin) as these are much more effective against sucking than biting lice. Different treatments are available including pour-ons, sprays, ear tags or injections. There are some concerns about resistance to treatments.

MITE

Several mite species afflict cattle and cause the skin ailment known as mange. Mites are little ectoparasites, or arachnids, that belong to the same class as spiders and ticks. Adult mites have two body parts and eight legs, compared to three body parts and six legs for adult insects.

a. *Sarcoptes scabiei* var *bovis*: The extremely contagious disease, *Sarcoptes scabiei bovis*, commonly referred to as sarcoptic mange, is transmitted by contaminated feed or direct contact between infected and uninfected animals. Lesions from this burrowing mite can start on the shoulders, neck, and head and subsequently spread to other parts of the body. The complete body may be impacted in six weeks. The skin gets thick and wrinkled, the pustules harden into crusts, and there is excruciating itching. The diagnosis is made using deep skin scrapings, skin biopsies, or therapy results. *S. scabiei bovis* can infect humans and result in transient, self-limiting dermatitis. The materials doramectin, eprinomectin, and ivermectin have been approved for use against sarcoptic mange mites in cattle.

b. *Psoroptes ovis:* Psoroptic mange in cattle is caused by *Psoroptes ovis*, a non-burrowing mite that resides on the skin's surface. The sides and backs of afflicted animals are home to the majority of these mites. *P. ovis* mites penetrate the host tissue in order to feed on the serum and other fluid discharges from the biting wound. A week after infestation, clinical signs may manifest. Congealed exudates form thick, scabby crusts. Alopecia is often a part of exudative dermatitis. The occurrence of papules, crusts, excoriation, and lichenification on the shoulders and rump initially occurs before almost the whole body is covered in extremely itchy infestations. Secondary bacterial infections are common in harsh environments. If left untreated, calves may lose weight, produce less milk, and become more prone to infections. Since *P.*

ovis may survive for up to two weeks without the host under the right conditions, it can also spread through contaminated environments and fomites. Direct contact between infected and vulnerable hosts is the main way that *P. ovis* spreads. Treatment options include the topical use of nonsystemic acaricides, spray dipping, vat dipping, systemic drug formulations, and oral, topical, or injectable formulations. Most cattle are infected with *C. bovis* subclinically. The mites may, however, cause an allergic, exudative, somewhat itchy, flaky dermatitis. Lesions that typically begin at the pastern and progress up the legs to the udder, scrotum, tail, and perineum include nodules, papules, crusts, and ulcers. There may be signs of self-trauma and alopecia. Lesions and clinical signs emerge in late winter and gradually go away in the summer. Sarcoptic or psoroptic mange is more pathogenic than chorioptic mange in cattle. Treatments like pour-on doramectin, eprinomectin, and moxidectin have been approved for use against *C. bovis* at the dosages indicated on the label.

c. *Chorioptes bovis: Chorioptes bovis* or *C. texanus* infestation is the primary cause of chorioptic mange in cattle. Domestic ruminants and horses globally serve as hosts for *C. bovis* since *Chorioptes* species are not host-specific. *C. bovis* is a surface-dwelling, non-burrowing organism. Direct contact between infected people and unreliable hosts is how the virus spreads. Since the mites can survive for up to three weeks without a host, cattle can become infected through contaminated housing and food. *C. bovis* most likely consumes dead skin cells and other surface detritus. The excrement and secretions of the mites contaminate the abrasions that *C. bovis* causes in the host's skin when it feeds.

d. *Demodex bovis*: Three species of *Demodex* are known to infect cattle and produce demodectic mange in those animals. *D. bovis* is the most common kind of infection in cow hair follicles. *D. ghanensis* has invaded the meibomian glands of Ghanaian cattle. The sebaceous glands and hair follicles of cattle from former Czechoslovakia have been found to harbour *D. tauri*. Certain species of *Demodex* are host-specific and not zoonotic. Among parasitic mites, *Demodex* spp. (Fig. **4**) are unique due to their elongated body and short, stumpy legs. It is believed that their distinct shape is an adaptation that allows them to reside in their hosts' hair follicles and sebaceous glands. These mites consume protoplasm, sebum, and epidermal debris as food. *D. bovis* is spread by close contact between infected and naive hosts; the primary pathway for mite transmission is from infected dams to neonates. Lesions consisting of follicular papules and nodules are most commonly seen across the neck, back, and flanks. Persistent inflammation, follicular rupture, secondary staphylococcal infection, and the formation of ulcers, abscesses, and fistulae are all brought on by *D. bovis* invasion. There isn't any itching. An infestation of *D. bovis* can seriously damage hides. Demodectic mange can afflict cattle of any age, however it is more apparent in younger animals. Most occurrences involving dairy cows occur in the late winter or early spring. Infestations with *D. bovis* are usually asymptomatic and can extend for several months. Recovery usually happens on its own; treatment is seldom used. If treatment for *Sarcoptes scabiei bovis* or *Chorioptes ovis* is initiated, consideration should be given to the macrocyclic lactones that are advised for this condition.

e. *Psorobia bos*: Psorergatic mange is caused by a microscopic mite called *Psorobia* (previously *Psorergates*) *bos*, which lives in the upper layers of cattle skin. Generally speaking, *P. bos* is not pathogenic, and very few cattle exhibit clinical signs of infection. Rarely, baldness, increased licking and rubbing, and moderate pruritus have all been related to this mite infection. *P. bos* have been detected in cattle in the US, Canada, the UK, and South Africa. Not zoonotic at all. Because the illness does not cause large financial losses, animals are typically not treated for it. Most likely, the macrocyclic lactone drugs that are authorised for use on sarcoptic, chorioptic, and psoroptic mange effectively control this infestation [26].

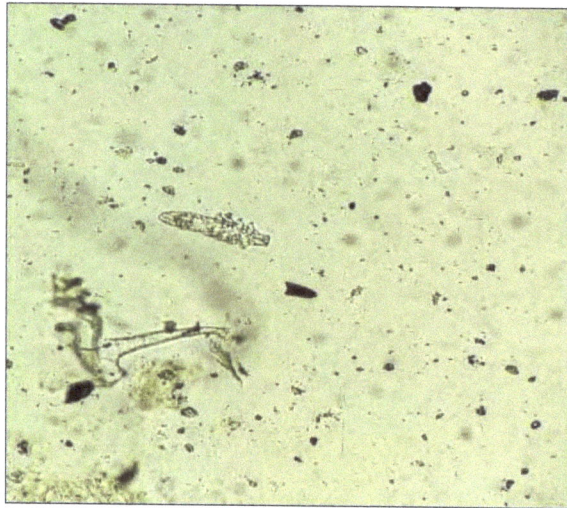

Fig. (4). *Demodex* species collected from skin scrapping of cattle.

FLEA

Pathogens of several diseases that affect both humans and domestic animals are spread by fleas. The majority of fleas temporarily infest one host before moving on to another of the same sort, although some fleas switch to different host species. According to Rust and Dryden [22], flea infestations and the resulting hypersensitivity reactions are major clinical and parasite issues for animals kept as pets [22]. They are typically restricted to hosts with nests or lairs as this can provide circumstances for the conclusion of their life cycle [27]. In some regions, they comprise over 50% of all the dermatological cases brought to small animal clinics. As a result, they are typically not considered to be serious pests of large domesticated animals. However, there have been instances of flea infestations on cattle and other livestock [2]. Less frequently reported fleas in cattle are *C. felis*, which has been found in Brazil, Japan, the United States, and Iran [2, 7, 18, 21]. Animals can be treated by being dipped in pyrethroids or sprayed with them, together with an insect growth regulator within the animal house.

LEACH

a. Paddy field leech or buffalo leech, *Hirudinaria manillensis*: Leeches are segmented, hermaphroditic worms under the phylum annelida and order hirudinea. Sanguinivorous leeches suck the blood of various vertebrate animals, including cattle, and buffalo. *Hirudinaria manillensis* is the most common leech found in India especially in the wetlands of Assam [12]. The leech bite causes annoyance, discomfort, and severe blood loss to the affected animal. Besides sucking blood, it can also transmit pathogenic bacteria, virus and also that protozoan parasites can survive up to 1-2 years in ingested blood. Chemical control by DEET is effective for controlling this parasite [16]. The application of a concentrated solution of salt is also effective for the removal of leeches from infested animals.

Miscellaneous

A range of insect pests affect dairy farm pastures all over the world. These pests include (Fig. **5**).

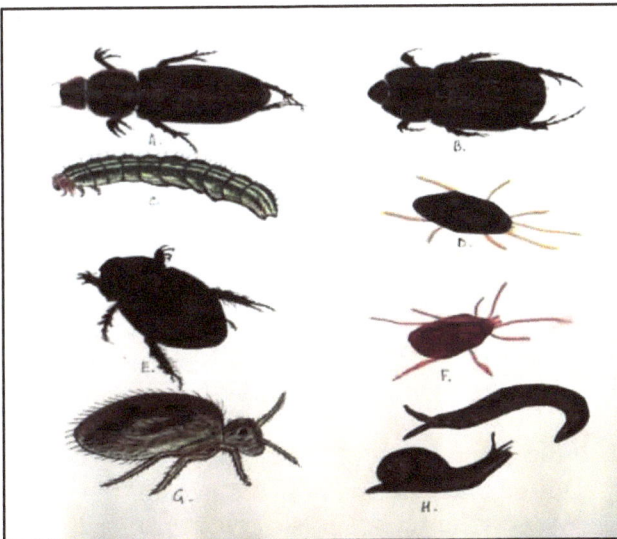

Fig. (5). A. Black headed cockroaches. **B**. Red headed cockroaches. **C**. Army worm. **D**. Red legged earth mite. **E**. African black beetle. **F**. *Bryobia* mite. **G**. Lucerne flea. **H**. Slung and snail. (*Picture by Jayesh purohit).*

A. Black-headed cockroaches.
B. Red-headed cockroaches.
C. Armyworm.
D. Red legged earth mite.
E. African black beetle.
F. Bryobia mite.
G. Lucerne flea.
H. Slung and snail.

Protozoa Affecting Integumentary System

a. *Besnoitia besnoiti*: Bovine besnoitiosis is exudative dermatitis that is distinguished by skin thickening, folding, hair loss, fissures, scabs, edema, and enlargement of the superficial lymph nodes. It is brought on by the apicomplexan *Besnoitia besnoiti*, an obligate intracellular protozoan parasite [28, 29]. Worldwide, it affects horses, donkeys, and cattle older than six months. Though the virus may start in cats, the disease is spread by biting flies. Once cattle have contracted *B. besnoiti*, the incubation period could last anywhere from two weeks to two months. Next, the two stages of bovine besnoitiosis develop sequentially: febrile acute (anasarca) and chronic (scleroderma). Fever is the first symptom of the disease's acute stage, which may go unnoticed when tachyzoites invade blood vessel endothelia. The following edema causes an increase in vascular permeability. Vasculitis, thrombosis, and degenerative and fibrinoid necrotic vascular lesions also appear, primarily in the skin and testes. In this stage, symptoms like lameness, orchitis, hyperemia of the skin, and enlargement of the superficial lymph nodes may appear. Severe respiratory diseases may also result from edema in the lungs' interstitial and alveolar tissues, which is often accompanied by pneumonitis and emphysema. The slow replication of bradyzoites inside tissue cysts with a preference for connective tissue, particularly the superficial layers of skin, mucous membranes of the upper respiratory tract, the vestibulum vaginae, and in males, the testes and epididymis, is what causes chronic infection. Pathognomonic tissue cysts can be seen in the scleral conjunctiva. Other common clinical indicators of the chronic stage include cutaneous abnormalities, such as thickening and folding of the skin in the scrotum and neck, loss of necrotic epidermis, and atrophy and induration of the bull testes. Vascular diseases in the scrotal skin and pampiniform plexus are likely to blame for male infertility. Both the acute and chronic stages of the illness might result in death. In severe cases, convalescence is sluggish despite low mortality. During acute and chronic infections, severely damaged bulls may become sterile.

Animals who are affected by the condition are always carriers [1]. Most animals in endemically infected herds continue to be subclinically diseased, but a minority develop the typical acute and chronic disease. Animals under a year of age only sometimes develop clinical instances, and as they get older, more animals become seropositive and develop clinical symptoms. Bradyzoite-containing intradermal cysts with inflammatory infiltrates in skin sections can be seen during diagnosis. The most effective and difficult forms of treatment are wound dressing and secondary infection management. Sulfanilamide, antimony, or oxytetracycline produce effective results. Culling or separating sick from healthy animals are two methods of prevention. South Africa has access to vaccination [10].

b. *Theileria annulata:* *Theileria annulata* infection, also known as bovine tropical theileriosis, is a protozoan illness that is spread by numerous tick species that are all members of the genus *Hyalomma*. It is a significant disease spread by ticks in many nations. The protozoan is found throughout the world, including North Africa, southern Europe, and a sizable portion of Asia [30, 31]. The detection of clinical cases of tropical theileriosis by field veterinarians constitutes a cornerstone in controlling this disease and lessening its economic burden because the condition is linked to large economic losses and some mortality. This calls for an excellent and thorough understanding of all potential clinical symptoms [32, 33]. The symptoms of tropical theileriosis are polymorphic and manifest at various frequencies, which could result in a false positive and worsen the disease's effects. Several writers have described skin lesions caused by *T. annulata* Among these symptoms, Nodular, hemorrhagic, and/or necrotic lesions are examples of infections. Cattle and buffaloes have been observed to develop skin lesions in many parts of the world [30]. Two clinical instances of tropical theileriosis with the unusual symptom of skin nodules were described by Gharbi *et al.* [8] in northern Tunisia [8].

CONCLUSION

The skin and subcutaneous tissues are infected by a variety of arthropods, protozoa, and helminths, all of which can be recognised by parasitologists using conventional and advanced diagnostic methods. Arthropods, helminths, and protozoa are the most frequent parasites found in the skin and subcutaneous tissues. Understanding these diseases is becoming more crucial because of how easily animals can spread to different parts of the world causing transboundary diseases. Vector control, medications, insecticides, and enhanced management practices are all examples of control measures (Fig. **6**). When taken in concert, these steps can greatly lessen the global toll that parasitic illnesses are taking on both human and animal health as well as agricultural output.

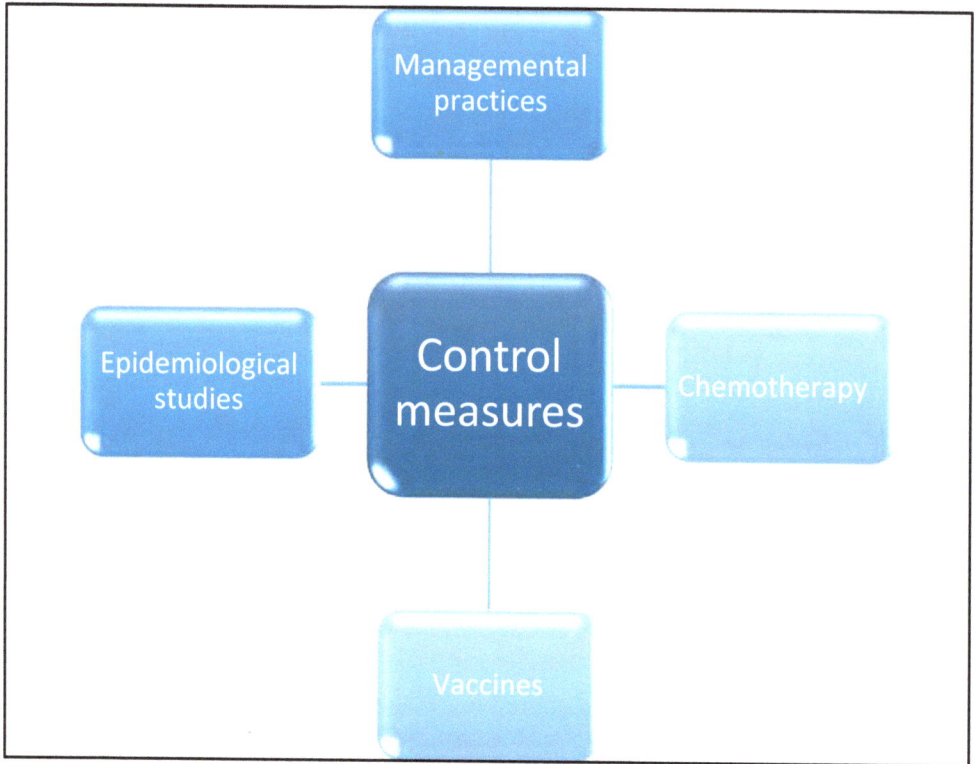

Fig. (6). Control measures of parasites.

REFERENCES

[1]   Álvarez-García G, Frey CF, Mora LMO, Schares G. A century of bovine besnoitiosis: an unknown disease re-emerging in Europe. Trends Parasitol 2013; 29(8): 407-15.
       [http://dx.doi.org/10.1016/j.pt.2013.06.002] [PMID: 23830145]

[2]   Araújo FR, Silva MP, Lopes AA, *et al.* Severe cat flea infestation of dairy calves in Brazil. Vet Parasitol 1998; 80(1): 83-6.
       [http://dx.doi.org/10.1016/S0304-4017(98)00181-2] [PMID: 9877075]

[3]   Beytut E, Akca A, Bain O. Teat onchocercosis in cows with reference to prevalence, species involved and pathology. Res Vet Sci 2005; 78(1): 45-51.
       [http://dx.doi.org/10.1016/j.rvsc.2004.05.007] [PMID: 15500839]

[4]   Catts EP, Mullen GR. Myiasis (Muscoidea, Oestroidea). In Medical and Veterinary Entomology. Academic Press 2002; pp. 317-48.
       [http://dx.doi.org/10.1016/B978-012510451-7/50018-9]

[5]   Diaz JH. Introduction to ectoparasitic diseases. Eighth Edition In Mandell, Douglas, and Bennett's Principles and Practice of Infectious Diseases. WB Saunders 2015; 2: pp. 3243-5.
       [http://dx.doi.org/10.1016/B978-1-4557-4801-3.00293-9]

[6]   Douglass ES, Jesse C. Integrated pest management for fly control in Maine dairy farms. Texas Agricultural Extension Service. 2002; 4: p. 6.

[7]   Dryden MW, Broce AB, Moore WE. Severe flea infestation in dairy calves. J Am Vet Med Assoc

1993; 203(10): 1448-52.
[http://dx.doi.org/10.2460/javma.1993.203.10.1448] [PMID: 8276708]

[8]   Gharbi M, Souidi K, Boussaadoun M A, *et al.* Dermatological signs in bovine tropical theileriosis (Theileria annulata infection), a review. Scientific and Technical Review - Office international des epizooties 2017; 36(3): 807-16.

[9]   Goulson D, Derwent LC, Hanley M, Dunn DW, Abolins SR. Predicting calyptrate fly populations from the weather, and probable consequences of climate change. J Appl Ecol 2005; 42(5): 795-804.
[http://dx.doi.org/10.1111/j.1365-2664.2005.01078.x]

[10]   Hamid ME. Skin Diseases of Cattle in the Tropics: A Guide to Diagnosis and Treatment. Academic Press 2016.

[11]   Huang JG, Zhou LJ, Xu HH, Li WO. Insecticidal and cytotoxic activities of extracts of *Cacalia tangutica* and its two active ingredients against Musca domestica and Aedes albopictus. J Econ Entomol 2009; 102(4): 1444-7.
[http://dx.doi.org/10.1603/029.102.0407] [PMID: 19736755]

[12]   Joken B, Pallabi P, Bhattacharya D, Islam S. Leeches affecting livestock and man in northeast India. North-East Vet 2014; 14(1): 3-5.

[13]   Lietze VU, Abd-Alla AMM, Vreysen MJB, Geden CJ, Boucias DG. Salivary gland hypertrophy viruses: a novel group of insect pathogenic viruses. Annu Rev Entomol 2011; 56(1): 63-80.
[http://dx.doi.org/10.1146/annurev-ento-120709-144841] [PMID: 20662722]

[14]   Loke Y W, Ramachandran CP. The Pathology of Lesions in Cattle caused by Stephanofilaria kaeli Buckley, 1937. Journal of Helminthology 1967; 41(2- 3): 161-6.

[15]   McGavin MD, Zachary JF. Pathologic basis of veterinary disease. Elsevier Health Sciences 2006.

[16]   Nath DR, Das NG, Das SC. Bio-repellents for land leeches. Def Sci J 2002; 52(1): 73-6.
[http://dx.doi.org/10.14429/dsj.52.2151]

[17]   Njaa BL. Chapter 20- The Ear. Pathologic Basis of Veterinary Disease. 2017; pp. 1223-64.

[18]   Otake O, Maehara K, Imai S. Massive infestation of fleas in dairy rearing calves. Journal of the Japan Veterinary Medical Association (Japan) 1997; 50: 92-4.

[19]   Pathak KML. 2020. Tick Infestation in Dairy Cattle and its Control. Indian; 2020 https://indiancattle.com/

[20]   Pollack RJ, Engelman D, Steer AC, Norton SA. Ectoparasites. International Encyclopedia of Public Health, 2nd edition. 2017; pp. 417-28.
[http://dx.doi.org/10.1016/B978-0-12-803678-5.00123-5]

[21]   Rahbari S, Nabian S, Nourolahi F, Arabkhazaeli F, Ebrahimzadeh E. Flea infestation in farm animals and its health implication. Iran J Parasitol 2008; 3(2): 43-7.

[22]   Rust MK, Dryden MW. The biology, ecology, and management of the cat flea. Annu Rev Entomol 1997; 42(1): 451-73.
[http://dx.doi.org/10.1146/annurev.ento.42.1.451] [PMID: 9017899]

[23]   Singh A, Singh D. A study on the incidence of myiasis among dairy animals in the State of Punjab, India. IOSR Journal of Agriculture and Veterinary Science (IOSR-JAVS) 2016; 9: 30-4.

[24]   Subha G. Biological and scientific opinion on study on the various aspects of "humpsore" in cattle population of India. A Review of Journal Biological Science Opinion 2013; 1: 98-100.

[25]   Tarelli G, Zerba EN, Alzogaray RA. Toxicity to vapor exposure and topical application of essential oils and monoterpenes on Musca domestica (Diptera: Muscidae). J Econ Entomol 2009; 102(3): 1383-8.
[http://dx.doi.org/10.1603/029.102.0367] [PMID: 19610461]

[26]   Tiwari A, Udainiya S, Dubey A, Agrawal V. Parasites in the integumentary system. Organ-Specific

Parasitic Diseases of Dogs and Cats. Academic Press 2023; pp. 89-111.
[http://dx.doi.org/10.1016/B978-0-323-95352-8.00007-2]

[27] Traub R. Co-evolution of Fleas and Mammals. Co-Evolution of Parasitic. Kim, KC (Ed.). Arthropods and mammals. Wily, New York,. 1985; pp. 93-8.

[28] Trees AJ, Graham SP, Renz A, Bianco AE, Tanya V. *Onchocerca ochengi* infections in cattle as a model for human onchocerciasis: recent developments. Parasitology 2000; 120(7) (Suppl.): 133-42.
[http://dx.doi.org/10.1017/S0031182099005788] [PMID: 10874716]

[29] Trees AJ, Wahl G, Kläger S, Renz A. Age-related differences in parasitosis may indicate acquired immunity against microfilariae in cattle naturally infected with *Onchocerca ochengi*. Parasitology 1992; 104(2): 247-52.
[http://dx.doi.org/10.1017/S0031182000061680] [PMID: 1594291]

[30] Uilenberg G, Zwart D. Skin nodules in East Coast fever. Res Vet Sci 1979; 26(2): 243-5.
[http://dx.doi.org/10.1016/S0034-5288(18)32925-4] [PMID: 122267]

[31] Vuong PN, Wanji S, Prod'Hon J, Bain O. Subcutaneous nodules and skin lesions caused by several Onchocerca spp. in African cattle. Revue Elev Medical and Veterinarie Pays Tropica 1994; 47: 47-51.
[http://dx.doi.org/10.19182/remvt.9131] [PMID: 7991898]

[32] Wahl G, Achu-Kwi MD, Mbah D, Dawa O, Renz A. Bovine onchocercosis in North Cameroon. Vet Parasitol 1994; 52(3-4): 297-311.
[http://dx.doi.org/10.1016/0304-4017(94)90121-X] [PMID: 8073613]

[33] West LS. The Housefly Its natural history, medical importance, and control. The Housefly. Its Natural History, Medical Importance, and Control 1951.

CHAPTER 6

Parasites in the Nervous System

Muhammad Mohsin[1], Muhammad Tahir Aleem[2,3,*], Muhammad Zahid Farooq[4], Muhammad Asmat Ullah Saleem[5] and Furqan Munir[6]

[1] *Shantou University Medical College, Shantou, Guangdong, 515045,China*

[2] *MOE Joint International Research Laboratory of Animal Health and Food Safety, College of Veterinary Medicine, Nanjing Agricultural University, Nanjing 210095, China*

[3] *Center for Gene Regulation in Health and Disease, Department of Biological, Geological, and Environmental Sciences, College of Sciences and Health Professions, Cleveland State University, Cleveland, OH 44115, USA*

[4] *Department of Animal Science, University of Veterinary and Animal Sciences (Jhang Campus), Lahore 54000, Pakistan*

[5] *College of Veterinary Medicine, Northeast Agricultural University, Harbin 150030, P.R. China*

[6] *Department of Parasitology, Faculty of Veterinary Science, University of Agriculture, Faisalabad 38040, Pakistan*

Abstract: Parasitic disease of the nervous system of cattle is generally caused by migrating nematodes, cestode cysts, or protozoa in the central nervous system. The parasites namely Hypoderma larvae cause neurological diseases. The toxins liberated by *Dermacentor* ticks, and metabolic changes associated with intestinal coccidiosis are the key factors for neurological complications.

Keywords: Aanthelmintics, Cattle, Control, Economic impact, Mmanagement, Nervous system, Parasites.

INTRODUCTION

The management of parasitic diseases in cattle continues to be a substantial concern with significant effects on animal health, productivity, and financial stability. Due to their complicated interactions with the neurological architecture of the host, neurotropic parasites that target the cow nervous system have drawn the most interest among these illnesses [1]. In order to cross the blood-brain barrier and establish themselves within the central and peripheral nervous sys-

* **Corresponding author Muhammad Tahir Aleem:** MOE Joint International Research Laboratory of Animal Health and Food Safety, College of Veterinary Medicine, Nanjing Agricultural University, Nanjing 210095, China Center for Gene Regulation in Health and Disease, Department of Biological, Geological, and Environmental Sciences, College of Sciences and Health Professions, Cleveland State University, Cleveland, OH 44115, USA;
E-mail: dr.tahir1990@gmail.com

Tanmoy Rana (Ed.)

tems, these parasites have evolved sophisticated tactics, which have resulted in a variety of neurological symptoms. The investigation of these interactions throws light on the basic tenets of neuroimmunology and neuropathology as well as the complex coevolution of parasites and their bovine hosts. A critical hub for an organism's physiological and behavioral functions, the central nervous system coordinates intricate reactions to both internal and external inputs [2]. This complex network is not immune to the influence of parasitic invaders. A wide variety of taxonomic groups of neurotropic parasites have developed varied adaptations to enter and take advantage of the host's brain environment. These parasites, which range in form from protozoans like *Trypanosoma* spp. and *Neospora caninum* to metazoans like *Taenia saginata* and *Setaria digitata*, have developed unique adaptations that let them move through the complex environment of the nervous system (Fig. **1**) [3].

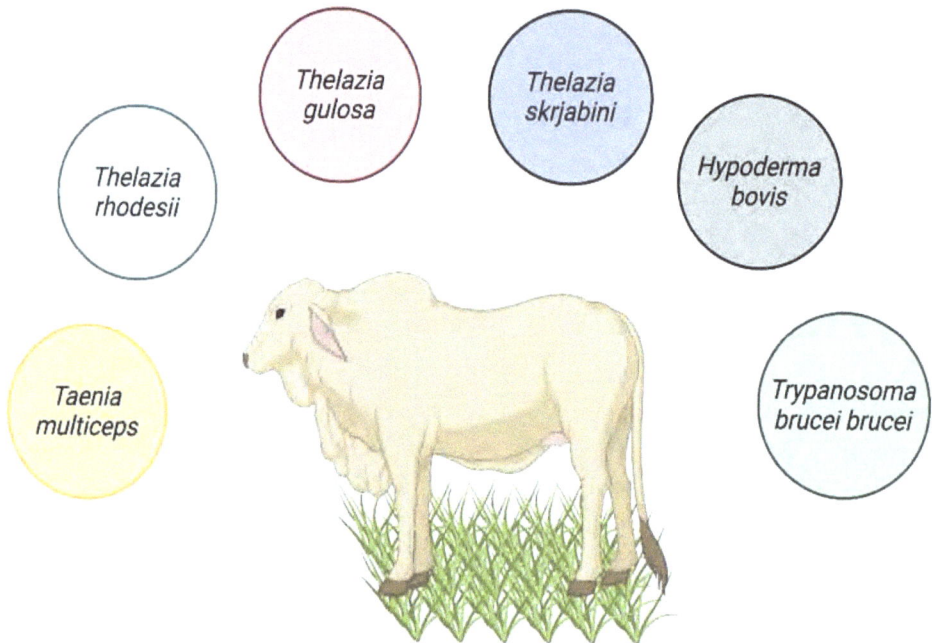

Fig. (1). Parasites affecting the nervous system of cattle.

Infections with neurotropic parasites in cattle can have a variety of negative effects, including neurological dysfunction, changed behavior, impaired motor skills, and even death (Table **1**). The dynamics of infection-induced neuroinflammation, neuronal injury, and subsequent repair processes can be better understood by understanding the complex interactions between the parasites and the host's immune responses in the context of neuroinvasion. These interactions also highlight the complex balancing act between immunological privilege in the

CNS and the requirement to establish strong defenses against invasive infections [4]. Promising paths for therapeutic approaches can be found by investigating the molecular and cellular mechanisms underlying host-parasite interactions in the neurotropic setting. The development of focused antiparasitic drugs is made possible by the identification of critical chemicals and signaling pathways that promote parasite entry and establishment within brain tissues. Deciphering the immunological responses that are brought on by these parasites may also help in the development of immunomodulatory techniques that will strengthen the host's defenses while reducing damage to crucial neurological regions [5].

Table 1. Parasites in the nervous system, site of predilection, symptom, diagnosis, and treatment.

Parasite	Predilection site	Symptoms	Diagnosis	Treatment	References
Taenia multiceps	Muscle, subcutaneous tissue, CNS	Decreased coordination, bizarre behavior, convulsions, and paralysis	Biopsy, autopsy, microscopy	Surgery, anthelmintic drugs	[13 - 16]
Thelazia rhodesii	Eye, conjunctival sac, lacrimal duct	Conjunctivitis, lacrimation, photophobia	Clinical examination, microscopy	Manual removal of larvae, and anthelmintics such as levamisole.	[23 - 26]
Thelazia gulosa	Eye, conjunctival sac, lacrimal duct	Conjunctivitis, lacrimation, photophobia	Clinical examination, microscopy	Manual removal of larvae, and anthelmintics such as levamisole.	[32 - 37]
Thelazia skrjabini	Eye, conjunctival sac, lacrimal duct	Conjunctivitis, lacrimation, photophobia	Clinical examination, microscopy	Manual removal of larvae, and anthelmintics such as levamisole.	[43 - 45]
Hypoderma bovis	Larvae: Epidural fat of spinal cord	Decreased milk production, fluid filled swelling on the back	Presence of larvae under the skin, eggs on hair, immunodiagnostic tests	Organophosphate insecticide, macrocyclic lactone	[47 - 51]
Trypanosoma brucei brucei	Blood, central nervous system, reproductive tract, or myocardium	Intermittent fever, anemia, abortion, edema, decreased fertility	Clinical history, microscopy, ELISA, PCR	Isometamidium and diminazene aceturate.	[52 - 57]

African animal trypanosomiasis, also called Nagana, is brought on by the protozoan *Trypanosoma brucei*. Cattle's central nervous system may become infected, which could result in neurological symptoms and behavioral changes [6]. Another protozoan parasite linked to bovine neosporosis is *Neospora caninum*. Cattle's CNS may be impacted, leading to stillbirth, abortion, or neurological issues in calf calves [7]. Neurocysticercosis is a disorder caused by the larval stage of the *Taenia saginata* tapeworm in which cysts develop in the central nervous system. Cattle may get seizures and other neurological issues as a result of this [8]. Cerebrospinal setariasis is a disorder brought on by the filarial nematode *Setaria digitata*, which can move through the CNS tissues. In cattle, it can cause inflammation of the spinal cord and neurological problems [9]. *Hypoderma* spp. (bot fly) larvae can move inside the spinal cord and other CNS tissues, irritating cattle and resulting in neurological symptoms. This problem is sometimes known as "grub in the head" [10]. Some tick species, such *Rhipicephalus microplus*, can spread pathogens like *Theileria* and *Babesia*, which can cause diseases in cattle that are transmitted by ticks and impact a variety of systems, including the nervous system. Each parasite has unique adaptations and tactics for interacting with the host's nervous system [11]. Since the effects of various infections can range from minor neurological abnormalities to serious clinical problems, it is crucial to understand how they interact in order to develop management and control strategies that are effective.

A fascinating nexus of parasitology, neurology, and immunology is represented by neurotropic parasites that attack the neurological system of cattle. The complexity of host-parasite coevolution is highlighted by their capacity to modify neuronal settings and affect host behavior. In addition to advancing our knowledge of parasite biology, the search to comprehend the molecular subtleties of these relationships opens exciting possibilities for the creation of cutting-edge methods to lessen the negative effects of parasitic infections on the health and welfare of cattle [12]. This in-depth examination into the world of neurotropic parasites promises to reveal not only the factors that contribute to their success but also brand-new directions for boosting productivity and animal welfare in the agricultural sector.

Taenia Multiceps

Parasitic illnesses represent a serious threat to the health and productivity of cattle, having an effect on agricultural economies all over the world. The ability of *Taenia multiceps* to infect the neurological system of cattle makes it stand out among the wide group of parasites as a particularly intriguing and alarming parasite [13]. The central nervous system (CNS) of the intermediate hosts of this tapeworm, sometimes known as the "brain worm," develops cysts as a result of the tapeworm's unusual lifecycle, which involves both definitive and intermediate hosts. This article explores the complexities of *T. multiceps* infection in cattle, focusing on its lifecycle, clinical manifestations, diagnostic techniques, treatment plans, and preventative and control measures. The complex life cycle of the parasite involves two primary hosts: the definitive host, which is frequently a carnivore like a dog, and the intermediate host, which includes cattle [14]. Within the cow CNS, the tapeworm's lifecycle progresses through the stages of egg release, ingestion, migration, and cyst development. The environment is contaminated by the eggs that adult tapeworms in the definitive host's intestines release, eventually making their way into the grass that cattle eat. The oncosphere larvae emerge from the eggs after being consumed, travel through the bloodstream, and eventually arrive at the nervous system (Fig. **2**) [15].

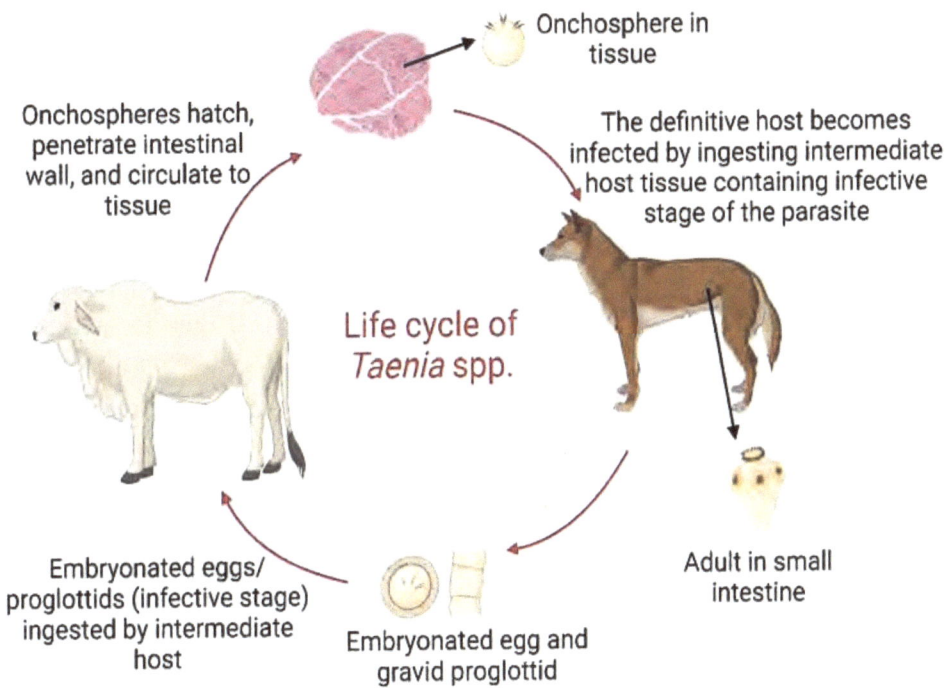

Onchosphere in tissue

Onchospheres hatch, penetrate intestinal wall, and circulate to tissue

The definitive host becomes infected by ingesting intermediate host tissue containing infective stage of the parasite

Life cycle of *Taenia* spp.

Embryonated eggs/ proglottids (infective stage) ingested by intermediate host

Embryonated egg and gravid proglottid

Adult in small intestine

Fig. (2). The life cycle of *Taenia* species.

Taenia multiceps infection in cattle develops as a result of a complicated interaction between the parasite and the host. Once ingested, the parasite eggs or larvae make their way into the brain and spinal cord, as well as other central nervous system organs, causing coenurosis. When the larvae turn into cysts, they start a localized immune reaction and cause inflammation in the brain structures nearby. This inflammatory response may compress nearby structures, resulting in neurological symptoms such as ataxia, seizures, and behavioral changes. In severe situations, the cysts can put pressure on the brain's critical regions, leading to fatal neurological abnormalities and severe neurological deficits [16]. Damage to tissue results from the immunological response to an infection that is being controlled, and cysts interfere with the regular operation of the nervous system.

In an effort to contain the infection, the existence of these cysts can also trigger the development of granulomas, which are immune cells that enclose the parasites. These granulomas, however, have the potential to harm tissue even more. The pressure from the cysts and the inflammatory reaction may cause structural abnormalities in the brain as the infection worsens, which may result in long-term neurological damage [17]. The *T. multiceps* infection's pathogenesis emphasizes how seriously it affects cattle's neurological health, emphasizing the importance of prompt identification and treatment to stop the progression of neurological symptoms and lessen the long-term impacts on the affected animals [18].

The development of coenurus cysts within the CNS is a sign of *T. multiceps* infection in cattle. The development of these fluid-filled cysts in the brain and other neural tissues results in mechanical compression of the nearby structures and a range of neurological symptoms. These symptoms, which include decreased coordination, bizarre behavior, convulsions, and paralysis, can have a serious negative impact on the welfare and general production of the affected animals. Due to the intricacy of the clinical indications and the placement of the cysts inside the CNS, diagnosing the infection in cattle can be difficult [19]. Cysts can be seen and their effects on neurological structures can be evaluated using imaging techniques like MRI and CT scans. When possible, surgical surgery to remove cysts is a common treatment option; however, due to the fragile nature of nerve tissues, this method may pose hazards. Anthelmintic drugs may be used, but because of the CNS's protected environment, their effectiveness may be constrained [20].

A multifaceted strategy is required for the effective management of the infection. The risk of infection can be decreased by limiting contact with definitive hosts, such as dogs, and preventing access to contaminated areas. The lifecycle of the tapeworm must be stopped by implementing sensible deworming programs and ensuring good sanitation and hygiene measures for dogs. For early detection and prompt action, surveillance and monitoring of animal health are essential. In conclusion, the infection of cattle with *T. multiceps* is a potent example of the complex interactions between parasites and their hosts [21]. The peculiar life cycle of the tapeworm and its tendency to attack the neurological system highlights the significance of comprehending its effects on cow health and the requirement for efficient control methods.

Thelazia rhodesi

A type of parasitic nematode worm called *Thelazia rhodesi* frequently infects the eyes of several animal species, including domestic animals and people. It belongs to the family Thelaziidae's genus *Thelazia*. Due to their propensity to reside in the conjunctival sac and other eye structures, these parasites are known as eyeworms [22]. These are typically found in warm areas and are frequently connected to rural and agricultural settings. There have been reports of it in several parts of Africa, especially in East and South Africa, where it can harm livestock including cattle, sheep, and goats. Additionally, *Thelazia rhodesi* infections in humans have been reported in these areas [23].

It goes through numerous significant stages in its life cycle (Fig. **3**). Cattle eyes are where adult worms live and lay their eggs. The host's ocular secretions are used to release these eggs. The first-stage larvae (L1) grow inside the eggs after hatching. Face flies or stable flies, which feed on the secretions in the cattle's eyes, unintentionally consume L1 larvae. These larvae develop into the infectious third stage (L3) inside the fly's mouthparts [24]. The L3 larvae are transmitted to the host when the infected flies subsequently feed on the secretions from the cattle's eyes. The cycle is completed when these larvae move into the tissues of the cattle's eyes and develop into adult worms. The life cycle is continued by adult worms reproducing and laying new eggs. In order to effectively eradicate this parasite, fly populations must be managed and veterinary assistance is required. Cattle with this infection may experience discomfort and damage to their eyes [25].

These adult worms cause the host's immune system to react right away, causing inflammation and discomfort as a result. Mechanical damage is caused as the worms migrate through the ocular tissues, and this leads to an inflammatory response that is defined by the production of immune signaling molecules. In addition, the worms may cause holes in the tissues of the eyes, making them vulnerable to secondary bacterial or fungal infections [26]. This series of events causes increased inflammation and discomfort. The immune system gets more involved, trying to fight off the invaders but unintentionally causing more inflammation and harm overall.

The parasitic worm mainly affects cattle's eyes and does not directly attack the neurological system. Its symptoms are mostly characterized by eye inflammation and discomfort. *Thelazia rhodesi* infected cattle may experience symptoms such as excessive weeping, conjunctivitis, and the emergence of ocular lesions or ulcers. Symptoms of this discomfort include frequent blinking and rubbing the eyes against things [27]. Although it has little effect on the neural system, the irritation brought on by eye infections may lead to behavioral abnormalities because of the discomfort felt. Although the parasites rarely directly damage the neurological system, the stress and discomfort brought on by eye-related problems may have an indirect impact on cattle behavior [28].

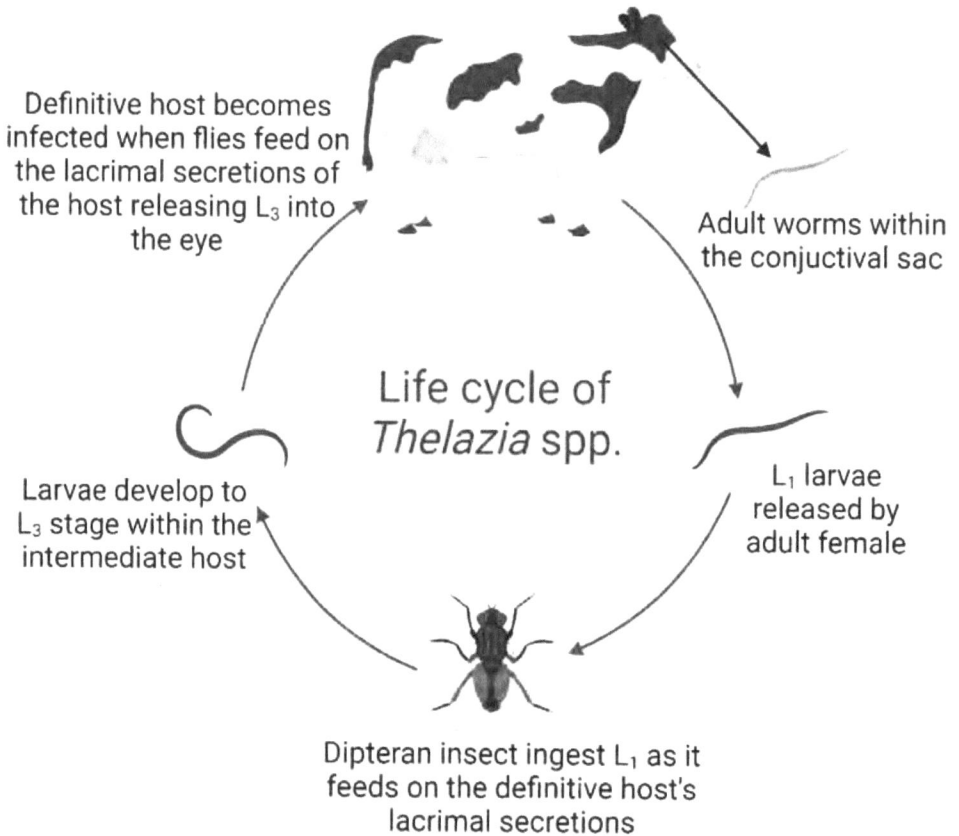

Fig. (3). Life cycle of *Thelazia* species.

To reduce the discomfort these parasitic worms cause, *T. rhodesi* infections in cattle require a multimodal strategy. Veterinary doctors frequently recommend anthelmintic drugs, which are created especially to target and get rid of internal parasites like *Thelazia* worms. The severity of the infection, the age and health of the cattle, and any potential resistance issues all play a role in the choice of the best anthelmintic and how it should be administered. Supportive care is crucial to speed up the healing process in addition to medication [29]. The use of topical medications, such as eye ointments or solutions, can reduce the risk of secondary infections brought on by *Thelazia* worms and ease eye irritation. Additionally, it is essential to keep the area clean and control fly populations around cattle as preventive measures to lessen the possibility of new infestations [30].

The infections in cattle must be prevented and managed using a multifaceted strategy that addresses both the parasites and their vectors. Controlling the fly population is essential because these insects act as intermediate hosts for the parasites. Cattle can be exposed to possible vectors to a lesser extent by implementing fly control measures, such as good waste management and sanitation procedures. Fly breeding and feeding grounds can be disturbed by routinely cleaning livestock housing spaces and removing dung [31]. Additionally, treating cattle with insecticides and using fly repellents can provide protection from flies and thereby reduce the likelihood of *Thelazia* transmission. Flytrap location should be considered to further reduce fly populations. It is possible to prevent the buildup of flies and create an environment that is less favorable to their development by ensuring proper ventilation in locations where cattle are housed.

Thelazia gulosa

A parasitic worm called *Thelazia gulosa* can infect cattle's eyes, causing pain and perhaps even harm to the ocular tissues. *Thelazia* is a genus of worms that comprise multiple species known to parasitize the eyes of a variety of animals, including humans and domesticated animals like cattle. This particular worm is a member of that genus. Cattle's eyes are specifically the target of *T. gulosa*, where it can live, proliferate, and cause a variety of eye-related problems [32].

It has a particular rhythm to its life cycle. Cattle eyes, specifically the conjunctival sac and other ocular tissues, become home to adult worms. These mature worms lay eggs, which are then expelled into the environment through the tears and secretions of the cattle's eyes. Larvae are produced from the eggs once they hatch. These intermediate hosts, which include particular species of flies, are where these larvae go through a vital stage of development [33]. These flies' larvae develop into infectious stages there. The larvae are then returned to the cattle when the infected flies feed on the eye secretions of the cattle. The life cycle of these larvae is completed once they reach the cattle's eyes and develop into adult worms. Cattle may have a variety of symptoms, including conjunctivitis, excessive weeping, and eye discomfort when *T. gulosa* worms are present in the eyes. Worm infestations can seriously harm the cornea [34]. Controlling fly populations and preserving hygienic living conditions for cattle are preventive strategies. For the early detection and prompt treatment of any infections, routine veterinarian exams are crucial. Cattle owners and veterinarians can make well-informed decisions to protect the ocular health and general welfare of the animals by understanding the life cycle of *T. gulosa* [35].

Thelazia gulosa in cattle causes disease by a series of complex interactions between the parasite and its host. Adult worms settle in cattle eyes after infestation, especially in the conjunctival sac and adjacent ocular tissues. These worms cause mechanical damage to the sensitive ocular structures as they travel and eat, which causes an inflammatory reaction in the host. Numerous signaling molecules are released as a result of this immune-driven reaction in an effort to fight off the invaders. In addition, the worms' presence might cause holes in the tissues of the eyes, leaving them prone to secondary bacterial or fungal infections. The interaction of injury, inflammation, and infection intensifies the cattle's suffering [36]. The immune system of the host becomes more active, unintentionally fueling the continuous inflammation and tissue damage. Observable behavioral changes, such as frequent blinking, wiping of the eyes, and light aversion, highlight the animals' efforts to lessen the discomfort the parasites are causing. Severe cases of the infestation might eventually result in serious eye issues such as corneal ulcers and conjunctival scarring if left untreated. *T. gulosa* infections have a complex pathophysiology, which emphasizes the significance of early detection and veterinary intervention in order to reduce inflammation, get rid of the parasites, and diminish the effect on cattle's ocular health [37].

The parasitic infestation in cattle manifests clinically as symptoms that mostly impact the neurological system as a result of the parasite's presence in the eyes. *T. gulosa* predominantly affects the ocular region, but in severe situations, the tension and discomfort brought on by the eye-related symptoms can have an indirect impact on the nervous system [38]. As a result of the discomfort brought on by the parasites present in the eyes, cattle may display symptoms of ocular irritation such as excessive tears, conjunctival inflammation, and eye rubbing. These eye-related problems may result in uncomfortable behaviors such as excessive blinking, head shaking, and aversion to bright light. Despite the fact that worm infections predominantly affect the eyes, the discomfort and irritation they cause might cause behavioral changes that may in turn have an indirect impact on the nervous system [39]. The continuous anguish and agitation brought on by the eye-related symptoms may be a factor in the affected cattle's changed behavior and general restlessness. It is vital to understand that the effects on the nervous system are secondary to the primary ocular symptoms and that infections rarely directly affect the neurological system. To effectively evaluate and treat these eye-related problems, a veterinarian's help is required. This will help to minimize any potential effects on the affected cattle's ocular health and subsequent behavioral responses [40].

An all-encompassing strategy is utilized to treat *T. gulosa* infestations in cattle in order to reduce the discomfort and potential harm these parasitic worms might cause. The main objective is to get rid of the adult worms that are present in the cattle's eyes and control any side effects that may have resulted from the infestation. Veterinary doctors frequently recommend anthelmintic drugs to treat parasites. The severity of the infection, the age and health of the cattle, and any potential resistance issues all play a role in the choice of the best anthelmintic and how it should be administered [41]. Supportive care is also essential to promote recovery and lessen suffering. Topical medications, such as eye ointments or solutions, can ease eye discomfort and reduce any potential secondary infections. Given that some fly species act as *T. gulosa*'s intermediate hosts, effective fly control tactics are crucial to preventing re-infestation.

Infestations of worms in cattle necessitate a thorough strategy that treats both the parasites and their vectors. Managing the fly populations that act as intermediate hosts for the parasite is the first step in taking effective measures. Cattle can be exposed to potential vectors to a great extent, but it can be greatly reduced by putting fly control measures in place, such as good waste management, keeping clean places where cattle are housed, and applying fly repellents. For the early detection and rapid treatment of any infections, routine veterinarian examinations are crucial. Veterinarians can do routine eye exams to look for any indications of discomfort or irritability brought on by the worms. If an infection is verified, the parasites can be removed by administering the proper anthelmintic drugs under a veterinarian's care [42]. The entire prevention strategy can be improved by informing cattle owners and handlers of the value of fly control, upholding proper cleanliness, and routine veterinarian care. Increasing people's knowledge of the symptoms of infection and the possible dangers posed by the parasites can inspire proactive action and prompt intervention. Cattle owners can successfully reduce the occurrence of *T. gulosa* infestations, enhancing the health and well-being of their animals, by taking a proactive approach that incorporates vector control, regular veterinarian treatment, and awareness-raising initiatives.

Thelazia skrjabini

An important role is played by the parasitic worm *Thelazia skrjabini* in the field of veterinary ophthalmology, particularly with regard to cattle. This nematode belongs to the parasitic family Thelaziidae, which is known for producing ocular infestations. It belongs to the Spirurida order, which includes a wide variety of parasitic worms that affect different hosts. *Thelazia skrjabini* is morphologically unique and displays an elongated, thread-like appearance that distinguishes its structural structure. It is distinguished as a relatively small parasite by its adult length, which ranges from 10 to 20 millimeters. Its undetectable existence within the host's eye is aided by the coloring, which frequently ranges from white to pale yellow [43].

Its life cycle in cattle contains several stages that happen within the intermediate host species as well as the parasite worm. The mature female worms settle in cattle eye tissues, namely in the conjunctival sac, to begin the life cycle. Eggs are released into the ocular environment while they reproduce here. Once laid, these eggs can be discovered in the secretions from the cattle's eyes. A crucial stage of the life cycle is when these eggs are found in the secretions of the eyes. These eggs are accidentally consumed by flies while they feed on the secretions of cattle's eyes, particularly those of the *Musca* genus [44]. The ingested *T. skrjabini* eggs hatch inside the flies' bodies, resulting in the appearance of infectious larvae. The larvae then continue to develop while still within the fly. They are flying into contact with livestock while carrying the infectious larvae, infected flies. These flies deposit the larvae after landing on the cattle's eyes, face, or other suitable regions. The larvae begin their migration into the eye tissues after being implanted in the cattle, preferring the conjunctival sac in particular. Within these tissues, these larvae eventually evolve into adult worms.

Thelazia skrjabini infestations in cattle are responsible for inflammation, eye discomfort, and possibly even damage to ocular structures. Cattle's conjunctival sac and other eye tissues harbor adult *T. skrjabini* worms. The delicate ocular structures are mechanically irritated by their presence and mobility within the eye tissues. The conjunctiva, the cornea, and other regions become infected when the worms attach to them, causing localized discomfort and irritation. The host's immune system mounts an inflammatory response in response to the irritation that the worms' presence causes [38]. Neutrophils and eosinophils are drawn to the afflicted areas by the immune cells. Cattle infected with *T. skrjabini* frequently develop conjunctivitis, an infection of the conjunctival tissues bordering the eye, as the immune response worsens. The conjunctiva turns red, swells, and is more prone to produce too many tears. The buildup of tears may make the environment more conducive for the worms and make the irritation worse. Severe parasitic infestations occasionally cause problems with the cornea. The corneal epithelium may be harmed by the cattle's continual scratching of their eyes in an effort to relieve discomfort, which could result in corneal ulcers. In addition to causing discomfort, these ulcers run the danger of developing secondary bacterial infections. *T. skrjabini* affected cattle frequently exhibit photophobia, a dislike of light, as a result of the inflamed eyes' increased sensitivity. This discomfort causes the eyes to rub against things more frequently, which can make them feel even more irritated and help the infection develop. The worm infestations can develop into chronic conditions that last for a long time and cause irritation and inflammation. This tissue scarring from chronicity could affect the cattle's vision.

Additionally, the ongoing presence of the worms can harm the affected animals' general health and well-being [35].

Thelazia skrjabini infestations in cattle can induce a variety of clinical symptoms, with some animals displaying uneasiness due to the discomfort of these parasitic worms in their eyes. Nervous behavior might appear as increased restlessness and agitation in addition to the typical signs of *T. skrjabini* infestations, such as excessive weeping, conjunctivitis, and photophobia. Increased eye rubbing and head shaking may result from the worms' motions within the ocular tissues, which cause continual irritation. Cattle may become more wary and perceptive of their surroundings, reacting exaggeratedly to even small stimuli. This tense attitude is an indirect reaction to the pain and misery the parasite infestation causes them. Cattle's behavior may be affected by the severe itchiness and inflammation that *Thelazia skrjabini* causes, leading them to avoid direct sunlight and seek refuge in the shade [23]. Due to their nervousness, animals frequently rub their eyes against things, which can worsen the discomfort and possibly harm the eye structures. As the discomfort and changing behavior influence the animals' general well-being, the general uneasiness can contribute to a decrease in feed intake.

Clinical observation along with veterinary examination is used to identify worms infestations in cattle. The conjunctival sac or other ocular tissues may be found to contain adult worms or larvae upon close inspection of the eyes. To establish the existence of the parasites, veterinarians frequently perform procedures like conjunctival scraping, in which an eye sample is collected for microscopic analysis. The worms infestations must be treated effectively by removing the adult worms from the eye and administering the necessary drugs. It takes experienced hands to carefully extricate the worms without further harming the eye because the removal procedure is delicate. After that, anthelmintic drugs are given to get rid of any worms and larvae that could still be present. Addressing any secondary diseases brought on by the infestation is also essential [45]. To treat bacterial issues brought on by the ongoing inflammation, doctors may give antibiotics or other treatments.

Preventative measures are also very important. To disrupt the life cycle of the parasite, fly control measures are put in place, such as maintaining good hygiene, eliminating fly habitats, and using insecticides as necessary. To identify and treat infestations early, regular veterinary checkups and eye exams are advised, especially in regions where these parasites are common.

Hypoderma bovis

The parasitic fly *Hypoderma bovis*, sometimes known as the "cattle grub" or "warble fly," infests cattle and other bovines. If not appropriately controlled, this parasite poses a serious threat to cattle production and may result in a number of health problems. During the summer, adult *H. bovis* flies deposit their eggs on the hair of cattle, typically on the legs, neck, and back. The eggs are attached to the hairs with cement, and they soon hatch. The larvae sometimes referred to as neonates, tunnel through the host cattle's skin after hatching [46]. They frequently enter through hair follicles. As the larvae progress through the host's subcutaneous tissues, they dig tunnels. As they move, they trigger an inflammatory reaction that results in swelling and the development of cysts, also referred to as "warbles." The back, shoulders, and neck of cattle are frequently affected by these cysts. The larvae migrate through a variety of body tissues along the way, including muscles, connective tissue, and occasionally even important organs. The developed larvae exit the host's body through a skin hole after several weeks of migration. This may cause an open wound or sore to appear when the larvae first emerge. Mature larvae drop to the ground and bury themselves in the ground to pupate. They undergo a pupal stage before becoming adult flies. After some time, adult flies emerge from the pupae, and the cycle repeats. The primary function of these adult flies is to mate and lay eggs on cattle; they do not feed on the host [47].

Initial localized discomfort caused by the larvae penetrating the skin leads to inflammation and excruciating itching. The cattle then start acting in ways like excessively rubbing against things or licking the entry points as a result. Warbles, which are lumps and palpable swelling that develop as the larvae migrate beneath the skin, cause swelling and discomfort to varied degrees. Further clinical signs are brought on by the larvae moving in the direction of the respiratory tract. In response to the larvae, cattle may undergo episodes of coughing, which shows inflammation along the respiratory passages. Additionally, the feeling of alien objects inside the cattle's bodies may damage their general comfort. The presence of the larvae in the stomach may cause further symptoms [48]. Reduced hunger and weight loss may result from the irritation the larvae's attachment to the stomach lining causes, especially while the animal expends energy defending itself from the parasitic invasion. It is possible for breastfeeding cows to produce less milk, which emphasizes the influence on their productivity and health. The skin is vulnerable to subsequent bacterial infections as a result of the initial sores the larvae leave behind. These infections can worsen discomfort and add to the animal's general condition decrease. The clinical signs and symptoms of a bovine infestation with *H. bovis* include skin irritation, the development of warbles, respiratory discomfort, stomach-related difficulties, a probable reduction in milk output, and the possibility of secondary infections [49].

Clinical assessment, management plans, and focused interventions are used in combination for the diagnosis and treatment of *H. bovis* infestation in cattle. Recognition of the distinctive clinical symptoms, such as the presence of warbles, palpable lumps under the skin, and indications of skin irritation or respiratory discomfort, is frequently essential for making a diagnosis. Veterinarians carry out extensive physical examinations while taking into account the history of the animal and the regional parasite frequency [50]. Timely therapy is essential for success. Typically, veterinarians advise catching the larvae at particular times in their life cycle. To destroy the larvae inside the host, chemical treatments are used, such as insecticides either topically or intravenously. To get rid of the larvae before they finish their migration, these treatments are frequently used in the late winter or early spring. Management procedures can also help reduce infestations of Hypoderma bovis. During the fly season, routine grooming and inspection of cattle allow for the detection and removal of eggs before they hatch. Sanitation practices can stop the parasite's life cycle, for as by removing pupae-containing manure from pastures [51]. The use of methods to reduce fly exposure and effective pasture rotation can also help prevent this.

Trypanosoma brucei brucei

African Animal Trypanosomiasis, or Nagana, is a parasitic disease that affects cattle and other livestock and is brought on by the protozoan parasite *Trypanosoma brucei brucei*. In regions of Central America and Sub-Saharan Africa, nagana is a serious illness. Cattle are exposed to *Trypanosoma brucei brucei* by the biting of infected tsetse flies of the *Glossina* genus, which serve as the parasite's vectors. Cattle become hosts for the parasites after being bitten by an infected tsetse fly [52]. Depending on the parasite strain, the host's immune response, and other variables, these parasites can produce a variety of clinical signs. It displays a distinct and one-of-a-kind morphology. The unicellular organism appears streamlined and spindle-like when viewed under a microscope. The parasites enter the bloodstream of a mammalian host when an infected tsetse fly feeds on the blood of the animal. The trypanosomes replicate within the mammalian host through binary fission, resulting in bloodstream forms. As these forms multiply, the host's bloodstream becomes heavily parasitized. The bloodstream forms of the parasite are consumed by an uninfected tsetse fly when it feeds on the blood of an infected host. The parasites undergo a procyclic trypomastigote transformation inside the midgut of the tsetse fly. They spread out and move to the fly's salivary glands, where they undergo epimastigote differentiation. Then, these epimastigotes go through additional development to become metacyclic trypomastigotes [53]. When the tsetse fly feeds once more, these parasites can infect a fresh mammalian host. The metacyclic trypomastigotes are introduced into the host's bloodstream by the tsetse fly as it feeds on a mammalian host through its saliva. The cycle is soon restarted when the parasites penetrate the host's red blood cells. *Trypanosoma brucei brucei* can spread and spread among susceptible animals thanks to this intricate life cycle that involves both the mammalian host and the tsetse fly vector [54]. This keeps the cycle of infection and sickness going.

The parasites immediately infiltrate red blood cells after entering the bloodstream, where they reproduce by binary fission. Increased parasitemia, or a significant number of parasites in the bloodstream, results from parasites' rapid multiplication. The host's immune system reacts when *T. brucei brucei* is present in the bloodstream. The immune system produces antibodies and activates immune cells in an effort to control the illness. The parasites multiply and reproduce within the host's red blood cells, causing harm to them [55]. Anemia is the outcome of hemolysis, or the breakdown of red blood cells, which happens as a result. Fatigue, weakness, and other clinical indications of anemia can result. Fever and widespread inflammation in the host can be brought on by the immunological reaction to the parasites and the loss of red blood cells. To avoid the host's immunological reaction, the parasite uses many methods. The frequent swapping of variable surface glycoproteins (VSGs) on its cell surface is one of the most important adaptations. The parasite can alter its surface coat and elude detection by the host's immune system thanks to this antigenic diversity. The parasites may occasionally penetrate the blood-brain barrier and enter the central nervous system [56]. This may result in neurological symptoms like paralysis, behavioral abnormalities, and lack of coordination. Weight loss, decreased appetite, and general debilitation in infected cattle can result from the interactions between anemia, the immune system, and the energy requirements of the parasites.

To guarantee accurate detection and efficient care of the disease, infection in cattle requires a thorough strategy. Clinical observation is the first step in diagnosis as vets look for symptoms like anemia, fever, weight loss, and neurological problems. Serological procedures, such as ELISAs, confirm infection by detecting particular antibodies, whereas microscopic inspection of stained blood smears enables direct visualization of the parasites. The genetic makeup of the parasite can be identified with great sensitivity and precision using molecular techniques like PCR tests [57]. Trypanocidal medications, such as diminazene aceturate and isometamidium chloride, are used to treat parasites by either killing them or stifling their growth. The severity of the infection and the overall health of the cattle are among the factors that influence the medication choice, dose, and length of therapy. Monitoring the therapy response entails keeping tabs on changes in clinical symptoms and general health. In addition to pharmaceutical intervention, implementing management practices to reduce tsetse fly exposure is essential, including insecticide-treated ear tags, strategic cattle placement, and regular grooming [58]. In order to negotiate potential drug resistance and customize treatment approaches for specific situations, collaboration with veterinarians is essential.

FUTURE PERSPECTIVE

Future research on parasites that influence cattle's neurological systems offers promising opportunities to deepen our understanding of these intricate connections and enhance disease management. Rapid developments in diagnostic technology, such as more sensitive molecular tests and sophisticated imaging methods, should make it possible to identify brain parasites earlier and with more accuracy. Research into the complex ways through which these parasites interact with neuronal tissues may reveal new targets for therapeutic approaches. In order to maximize the potential of immunization to prevent these illnesses, research may concentrate on creating vaccines specifically suited to parasites that damage the brain system. Additionally, the investigation of novel drug-delivery strategies to reach parasites inside the central nervous system may revolutionize therapeutic modalities [59]. A "One Health" strategy that takes into account animals, people, and the environment could result in all-encompassing disease control techniques as the interconnectivity of health systems becomes more widely recognized. The impact of climate change on the distribution of parasites may spur study into how changing conditions affect the prevalence of parasitic illnesses. The discovery of key parasite factors and pathways could open the door to targeted therapies as genomics and proteomics develop. The future holds the promise of more efficient diagnostics, treatments, and prevention strategies for parasites affecting the nervous system of cattle through collaborative efforts across disciplines, including veterinary medicine, parasitology, and technology, contributing to improved animal welfare and overall agricultural sustainability [60].

CONCLUSION

In conclusion, the study of parasites that impact cattle's neurological systems is an active, quickly developing topic with important repercussions for both veterinary and public health. The complicated interactions among these parasites, their hosts, and the vectors that spread them highlight how difficult a task these problems are. As our knowledge grows, it is evident that these parasite infections can cause cattle to exhibit crippling neurological symptoms, resulting in financial losses and diminished animal welfare. However, novel approaches to diagnosis, treatment, and prevention show promise for the future.

REFERENCES

[1]   van Veen TWS. Parasitic disease of the bovine nervous system. Vet Clin North Am Food Anim Pract 1987; 3(1): 99-105.
[http://dx.doi.org/10.1016/S0749-0720(15)31182-8] [PMID: 3552153]

[2]   Batista JS, Riet-Correa F, Teixeira MMG, Madruga CR, Simões SDV, Maia TF. Trypanosomiasis by *Trypanosoma vivax* in cattle in the Brazilian semiarid: Description of an outbreak and lesions in the nervous system. Vet Parasitol 2007; 143(2): 174-81.
[http://dx.doi.org/10.1016/j.vetpar.2006.08.017] [PMID: 16965857]

[3]   Galiza GJN, Garcia HA, Assis ACO, *et al.* High mortality and lesions of the central nervous system in Trypanosomosis by *Trypanosoma vivax* in Brazilian hair sheep. Vet Parasitol 2011; 182(2-4): 359-63.
[http://dx.doi.org/10.1016/j.vetpar.2011.05.016] [PMID: 21664764]

[4]   Morrison LJ, Steketee PC, Tettey MD, Matthews KR. Pathogenicity and virulence of African trypanosomes: From laboratory models to clinically relevant hosts. Virulence 2023; 14(1): 2150445.
[http://dx.doi.org/10.1080/21505594.2022.2150445] [PMID: 36419235]

[5]   Balemba OB, Mbassa GK, Assey RJ, *et al.* Lesions of the enteric nervous system and the possible role of mast cells in the pathogenic mechanisms of migration of schistosome eggs in the small intestine of cattle during Schistosoma bovis infection. Vet Parasitol 2000; 90(1-2): 57-71.
[http://dx.doi.org/10.1016/S0304-4017(00)00214-4] [PMID: 10828512]

[6]   Latif AA, Ntantiso L, de Beer C. African animal trypanosomosis (nagana) in northern KwaZulu-Natal, South Africa: Strategic treatment of cattle on a farm in endemic area. Onderstepoort J Vet Res 2019; 86(1): e1-6.
[http://dx.doi.org/10.4102/ojvr.v86i1.1639] [PMID: 31170783]

[7]   da Costa LS, Withoeft JA, Bilicki JV, *et al.* Neospora caninum-associated abortions in cattle from Southern Brazil: Anatomopathological and molecular characterization. Vet Parasitol Reg Stud Rep 2022; 36: 100802.
[http://dx.doi.org/10.1016/j.vprsr.2022.100802] [PMID: 36436886]

[8]   Nguyen MTT, Gabriël S, Abatih EN, Dorny P. A systematic review on the global occurrence of Taenia hydatigena in pigs and cattle. Vet Parasitol 2016; 226: 97-103.
[http://dx.doi.org/10.1016/j.vetpar.2016.06.034] [PMID: 27514893]

[9]   Mohanty MC, Sahoo PK, Satapathy AK, Ravindran B. *Setaria digitata* infections in cattle: parasite load, microfilaraemia status and relationship to immune response. J Helminthol 2000; 74(4): 343-7.
[http://dx.doi.org/10.1017/S0022149X0070112X] [PMID: 11138024]

[10]   Ahmed H, Sousa SR, Simsek S, Anastácio S, Kilinc SG. First Molecular Characterization of Hypoderma actaeon in Cattle and Red Deer (Cervus elaphus) in Portugal. Korean J Parasitol 2017; 55(6): 653-8.
[http://dx.doi.org/10.3347/kjp.2017.55.6.653] [PMID: 29320820]

[11]   Almazán C, Scimeca RC, Reichard MV, Mosqueda J. Babesiosis and Theileriosis in North America. Pathogens 2022; 11(2): 168.
[http://dx.doi.org/10.3390/pathogens11020168] [PMID: 35215111]

[12]   Innes EA. The host-parasite relationship in pregnant cattle infected with *Neospora caninum.* Parasitology 2007; 134(13): 1903-10.
[http://dx.doi.org/10.1017/S0031182007000194] [PMID: 17958926]

[13]   Al-Riyami S, Ioannidou E, Koehler AV, *et al.* Genetic characterisation of *Taenia multiceps* cysts from ruminants in Greece. Infect Genet Evol 2016; 38: 110-6.
[http://dx.doi.org/10.1016/j.meegid.2015.12.008] [PMID: 26688203]

[14]   Varcasia A, Tamponi C, Ahmed F, *et al. Taenia multiceps* coenurosis: a review. Parasit Vectors 2022; 15(1): 84.
[http://dx.doi.org/10.1186/s13071-022-05210-0] [PMID: 35279199]

[15]   Oryan A, Akbari M, Moazeni M, Amrabadi OR. Cerebral and non-cerebral coenurosis in small ruminants. Trop Biomed 2014; 31(1): 1-16.
[PMID: 24862039]

[16]   Zhang XY, Jian YN, Duo H, *et al.* Coenurosis of Yak, Bos grunniens, caused by *Taenia multiceps*: A

Case Report with Molecular Identification in Qinghai Tibetan Plateau Area, China. Korean J Parasitol 2019; 57(4): 423-7.
[http://dx.doi.org/10.3347/kjp.2019.57.4.423] [PMID: 31533410]

[17]   Tan L, Wang AB, Zheng SQ, Zhang XL, Huang CJ, Liu W. Molecular characterization and phylogenetic analysis of *Taenia multiceps* from China. Acta Parasitol 2018; 63(4): 721-7.
[http://dx.doi.org/10.1515/ap-2018-0085] [PMID: 30367774]

[18]   Varcasia A, Pipia AP, Dessì G, *et al.* Morphology and genetic variability within *Taenia multiceps* in ruminants from Italy. Vet Parasitol 2016; 223: 181-5.
[http://dx.doi.org/10.1016/j.vetpar.2016.04.039] [PMID: 27198798]

[19]   Hughes EC, Kibona TK, de Glanville WA, *et al. Taenia multiceps* coenurosis in Tanzania: a major and under-recognised livestock disease problem in pastoral communities. Vet Rec 2019; 184(6): 191.
[http://dx.doi.org/10.1136/vr.105186] [PMID: 30683735]

[20]   Afonso SMS, Neves L, Pondja A, *et al.* Efficacy of albendazole against *Taenia multiceps* larvae in experimentally infected goats. Vet Parasitol 2014; 206(3-4): 304-7.
[http://dx.doi.org/10.1016/j.vetpar.2014.09.020] [PMID: 25450723]

[21]   Lescano AG, Zunt J. Other cestodes. Handb Clin Neurol 2013; 114: 335-45.
[http://dx.doi.org/10.1016/B978-0-444-53490-3.00027-3] [PMID: 23829923]

[22]   Deak G, Ionică AM, Oros NV, Gherman CM, Mihalca AD. *Thelazia rhodesi* in a dairy farm in Romania and successful treatment using eprinomectin. Parasitol Int 2021; 80: 102183.
[http://dx.doi.org/10.1016/j.parint.2020.102183] [PMID: 32891881]

[23]   Giangaspero A, Traversa D, Otranto D. Ecologia di *Thelazia* spp. e dei vettori in Italia (Ecology of *Thelazia* spp. in cattle and their vectors in Italy). Parassitologia 2004; 46(1-2): 257-9.

[24]   Naem S. *Thelazia rhodesi* (Spirurida, Thelaziidae), bovine eyeworm: morphological study by scanning electron microscopy. Parasitol Res 2007; 100(4): 855-60.
[http://dx.doi.org/10.1007/s00436-006-0346-1] [PMID: 17096145]

[25]   Otranto D, Traversa D. eyeworm: an original endo- and ecto-parasitic nematode. Trends Parasitol 2005; 21(1): 1-4.
[http://dx.doi.org/10.1016/j.pt.2004.10.008] [PMID: 15639731]

[26]   Ikeme MM. Kerato-conjunctivitis in cattle in the plateau area of Northern Nigeria. A study of *Thelazia rhodesi* as a possible aetiological agent. Bull Epizoot Dis Afr 1967; 15(4): 363-7.
[PMID: 5629276]

[27]   Smeal MG. Observations on the occurrence of *Thelazia* or eyeworm infection of cattle in northern New South Wales. Aust Vet J 1968; 44(11): 516-21.
[http://dx.doi.org/10.1111/j.1751-0813.1968.tb09004.x] [PMID: 5749410]

[28]   Otranto D, Tarsitano E, Traversa D, De Luca F, Giangaspero A. Molecular epidemiological survey on the vectors of *Thelazia gulosa*, *Thelazia rhodesi* and *Thelazia skrjabini* (Spirurida: Thelaziidae). Parasitology 2003; 127(4): 365-73.
[http://dx.doi.org/10.1017/S0031182003003913] [PMID: 14636023]

[29]   Khedri J, Radfar MH, Borji H, Azizzadeh M. Epidemiological Survey of Bovine Thelaziosis in Southeastern of Iran. Iran J Parasitol 2016; 11(2): 221-5.
[PMID: 28096856]

[30]   Anderson RC. Nematode parasites of vertebrates: their development and transmission. 2000.
[http://dx.doi.org/10.1079/9780851994215.0000]

[31]   Soulsby EJL. Helminths, arthropods and protozoa of domesticated animals. 7th ed. Bailliere Tindall, London, UK. 1982.

[32]   Demiaszkiewicz AW, Moskwa B, Gralak A, *et al.* The Nematodes *Thelazia gulosa* Railiet and Henry, 1910 and *Thelazia skrjabini* Erschov, 1928 as a Cause of Blindness in European Bison (Bison

bonasus) in Poland. Acta Parasitol 2020; 65(4): 963-8.
[http://dx.doi.org/10.1007/s11686-020-00243-w] [PMID: 32613456]

[33] Moolenbeek WJ, Surgeoner GA. Southern Ontario survey of eyeworms, *Thelazia gulosa* and *Thelazia lacrymalis* in cattle and larvae of *Thelazia* spp. in the face fly, *Musca autumnalis*. Can Vet J 1980; 21(2): 50-2.
[PMID: 7189135]

[34] Geden CJ, Stoffolano JG Jr. Development of the bovine eyeworm, *Thelazia gulosa* (Railliet and Henry), in experimentally infected, female *Musca* autumnalis de Geer. J Parasitol 1982; 68(2): 287-92.
[http://dx.doi.org/10.2307/3281188] [PMID: 7200515]

[35] Bradbury RS, Gustafson DT, Sapp SGH, *et al.* A Second Case of Human Conjunctival Infestation With *Thelazia gulosa* and a Review of *T. gulosa* in North America. Clin Infect Dis 2019; 70(3): ciz469.
[http://dx.doi.org/10.1093/cid/ciz469] [PMID: 31638142]

[36] Bradbury RS, Breen KV, Bonura EM, Hoyt JW, Bishop HS. Case Report: Conjunctival Infestation with *Thelazia gulosa*: A Novel Agent of Human Thelaziasis in the United States. Am J Trop Med Hyg 2018; 98(4): 1171-4.
[http://dx.doi.org/10.4269/ajtmh.17-0870] [PMID: 29436343]

[37] Miller PE, Campbell BG. Subconjunctival cyst associated with *Thelazia gulosa* in a calf. J Am Vet Med Assoc 1992; 201(7): 1058-60.
[http://dx.doi.org/10.2460/javma.1992.201.07.1058] [PMID: 1429135]

[38] Giangaspero A, Otranto D, Vovlas N, Puccini V. *Thelazia gulosa* Railliet & Henry, 1910 and *T. skrjabini* Erschow, 1928 infection in southern Europe (Italy). Parasite 2000; 7(4): 327-9.
[http://dx.doi.org/10.1051/parasite/2000074327] [PMID: 11147042]

[39] Bani Hassan E, Moshaverinia A, Sheedfar F, *et al.* A report of the unusual lesions caused by *Thelazia gulosa* in cattle. Vet Parasitol Reg Stud Rep 2017; 7: 62-5.
[http://dx.doi.org/10.1016/j.vprsr.2016.12.006] [PMID: 31014660]

[40] Geden CJ, Stoffolano JG Jr. Bovine thelaziasis in Massachusetts. Cornell Vet 1980; 70(4): 344-59.
[PMID: 7193108]

[41] Kennedy MJ, Holste JE, Jacobsen JA. The efficacy of ivermectin (pour-on) against the eyeworms, *Thelazia gulosa* and *Thelazia skrjabini* in naturally infected cattle. Vet Parasitol 1994; 55(3): 263-6.
[http://dx.doi.org/10.1016/0304-4017(93)00644-E] [PMID: 7879384]

[42] Kennedy MJ, Phillips FE. Efficacy of doramectin against eyeworms (*Thelazia* spp.) in naturally and experimentally infected cattle. Vet Parasitol 1993; 49(1): 61-6.
[http://dx.doi.org/10.1016/0304-4017(93)90224-B] [PMID: 8236740]

[43] Kennedy MJ, MacKinnon JD. Site segregation of *Thelazia skrjabini* and *Thelazia gulosa* (Nematoda: Thelazioidea) in the eyes of cattle. J Parasitol 1994; 80(4): 501-4.
[http://dx.doi.org/10.2307/3283182] [PMID: 8064515]

[44] Kennedy MJ, Moraiko DT, Goonewardene L. A study on the prevalence and intensity of occurrence of *Thelazia skrjabini* (Nematoda: Thelazioidea) in cattle in central Alberta, Canada. J Parasitol 1990; 76(2): 196-200.
[http://dx.doi.org/10.2307/3283015] [PMID: 2319419]

[45] Kennedy MJ. Prevalence of eyeworms (Nematoda: Thelazioidea) in beef cattle grazing different range pasture zones in Alberta, Canada. J Parasitol 1993; 79(6): 866-9.
[http://dx.doi.org/10.2307/3283723] [PMID: 8277378]

[46] Bagherzadeh NM, Behniafar H, Rahbari S, Valizadeh S. Prevalence of hypodermosis in cattle slaughtered in industrial slaughtered-house of Ardebil, Iran. J Parasit Dis 2016; 40(4): 1579-82.
[http://dx.doi.org/10.1007/s12639-015-0733-6] [PMID: 27876987]

[47] Hassan M, Khan MN, Abubakar M, Waheed HM, Iqbal Z, Hussain M. Bovine hypodermosis—a

global aspect. Trop Anim Health Prod 2010; 42(8): 1615-25.
[http://dx.doi.org/10.1007/s11250-010-9634-y] [PMID: 20607401]

[48]   Ahmed H, Afzal MS, Mobeen M, Simsek S. An overview on different aspects of hypodermosis: Current status and future prospects. Acta Trop 2016; 162: 35-45.
[http://dx.doi.org/10.1016/j.actatropica.2016.05.016] [PMID: 27260666]

[49]   Reina D, Martínez-Moreno FJ, Gutierrez-Palomino P, Scholl PJ, Hernández-Rodríguez S, Navarrete I. Experimental bovine hypodermosis in Spain. J Med Entomol 2000; 37(2): 210-5.
[http://dx.doi.org/10.1603/0022-2585-37.2.210] [PMID: 10730489]

[50]   Otranto D, Zalla P, Testini G, Zanaj S. Cattle grub infestation by Hypoderma sp. in Albania and risks for European countries. Vet Parasitol 2005; 128(1-2): 157-62.
[http://dx.doi.org/10.1016/j.vetpar.2004.11.016] [PMID: 15725546]

[51]   Boulard C. Durably controlling bovine hypodermosis. Vet Res 2002; 33(5): 455-64.
[http://dx.doi.org/10.1051/vetres:2002032] [PMID: 12387483]

[52]   Latif AA, Ntantiso L, de Beer C. African animal trypanosomosis (nagana) in northern KwaZulu-Natal, South Africa: Strategic treatment of cattle on a farm in endemic area. Onderstepoort J Vet Res 2019; 86(1): e1-6.
[http://dx.doi.org/10.4102/ojvr.v86i1.1639] [PMID: 31170783]

[53]   De Beer CJ, Venter GJ, Kappmeier Green K, *et al.* An update of the tsetse fly (Diptera: Glossinidae) distribution and African animal trypanosomosis prevalence in north-eastern KwaZulu-Natal, South Africa. Onderstepoort J Vet Res 2016; 83(1): a1172.
[http://dx.doi.org/10.4102/ojvr.v83i1.1172] [PMID: 27380653]

[54]   Motloang M, Masumu J, Mans B, Van den Bossche P, Latif A. Vector competence of *Glossina austeni* and *Glossina brevipalpis* for *Trypanosoma congolense* in KwaZulu-Natal, South Africa. Onderstepoort J Vet Res 2012; 79(1): E1-6.
[http://dx.doi.org/10.4102/ojvr.v79i1.353] [PMID: 23327306]

[55]   Kappmeier K, Nevill EM, Bagnall RJ. Review of tsetse flies and trypanosomosis in South Africa. Onderstepoort J Vet Res 1998; 65(3): 195-203.
[PMID: 9809324]

[56]   Oluoch EA, Magnuson NS, McGuire TC, Barbet AF. *Trypanosoma brucei*: Peptide mapping of partially homologous variable surface glycoproteins. Int J Parasitol 1991; 21(5): 573-8.
[http://dx.doi.org/10.1016/0020-7519(91)90062-C] [PMID: 1743853]

[57]   Kayang BB, Bosompem KM, Assoku RKG, Awumbila B. Detection of *Trypanosoma brucei*, *T. congolense* and *T. vivax* infections in cattle, sheep and goats using latex agglutination. Int J Parasitol 1997; 27(1): 83-7.
[http://dx.doi.org/10.1016/S0020-7519(96)00160-9] [PMID: 9076533]

[58]   Nantulya VM, Lindqvist KJ. Antigen-detection enzyme immunoassays for the diagnosis of *Trypanosoma vivax*, *T. congolense* and *T. brucei* infections in cattle. Trop Med Parasitol 1989; 40(3): 267-72.
[PMID: 2617031]

[59]   Jaimes-Dueñez J, Zapata-Zapata C, Triana-Chávez O, Mejía-Jaramillo AM. Evaluation of an alternative indirect-ELISA test using *in vitro*-propagated *Trypanosoma brucei brucei* whole cell lysate as antigen for the detection of anti-Trypanosoma evansi IgG in Colombian livestock. Prev Vet Med 2019; 169: 104712.
[http://dx.doi.org/10.1016/j.prevetmed.2019.104712] [PMID: 31311647]

[60]   Zhang XX, Liu JS, Han LF, *et al.* Towards a global One Health index: a potential assessment tool for One Health performance. Infect Dis Poverty 2022; 11(1): 57.
[http://dx.doi.org/10.1186/s40249-022-00979-9] [PMID: 35599310]

CHAPTER 7

Parasites in the Eye and Ear

Muhammad Mohsin[1]**, Muhammad Tahir Aleem**[2,3,*]**, Muhammad Zahid Farooq**[4]**, Muhammad Asmat Ullah Saleem**[5] **and Furqan Munir**[6]

[1] *Shantou University Medical College, Shantou, Guangdong, 515045,China*

[2] *MOE Joint International Research Laboratory of Animal Health and Food Safety, College of Veterinary Medicine, Nanjing Agricultural University, Nanjing 210095, China*

[3] *Center for Gene Regulation in Health and Disease, Department of Biological, Geological, and Environmental Sciences, College of Sciences and Health Professions, Cleveland State University, Cleveland, OH 44115, USA*

[4] *Department of Animal Science, University of Veterinary and Animal Sciences (Jhang Campus), Lahore 54000, Pakistan*

[5] *College of Veterinary Medicine, Northeast Agricultural University, Harbin, 150030, P.R. China*

[6] *Department of Parasitology, Faculty of Veterinary Science, University of Agriculture, Faisalabad 38040, Pakistan*

Abstract: The eye and earworms are responsible for ocular infections and ear infections in cattle. Larva can migrate the anterior chamber of the eye and can cause severe ocular inflammation in cattle. The antigen present on the surface of the parasite can cause an immune-mediated response with uveitis and keratoconjunctivitis. The transmission occurs through a housefly which feeds on the excretions/ lacrimal/ear discharge and the larva develops in the fly and lodges in mouthparts and when the same fly feeds another animal, the infestation is established. Proper anthelmintic treatment with correct management protocol is needed to combat the parasitic diseases of the eye and the ear.

Keywords: Anthelmintics, Cattle, Control, Economic impact, Eye and ear, Management, Parasites.

INTRODUCTION

The term "parasite" refers to a creature that inhabits or lives on another organism, often known as the "host," from which it derives its nutrition and frequently infl-

* **Corresponding author Muhammad Tahir Aleem:** MOE Joint International Research Laboratory of Animal Health and Food Safety, College of Veterinary Medicine, Nanjing Agricultural University, Nanjing 210095, China Center for Gene Regulation in Health and Disease, Department of Biological, Geological, and Environmental Sciences, College of Sciences and Health Professions, Cleveland State University, Cleveland, OH 44115, USA;
E-mail: dr.tahir1990@gmail.com

icts harm. Different tactics have been developed by these creatures to take advantage of their hosts in order to survive and reproduce [1]. Various health problems for the host might result from interactions between parasites and their hosts. They might vary from minor annoyance and discomfort to more serious illnesses and even death. While some parasites are more specialized, others have complex life cycles involving various host species. Due to lower productivity, increased veterinary expenses, and compromised animal welfare, parasitic infections in cattle can result in large financial losses for the livestock industry [2]. Cattle's eyes and ears are particularly susceptible to parasite infestations among the different organs impacted. These illnesses affect the animals' general health and well-being in addition to causing them anguish and pain. Conjunctivitis, keratitis, and more serious disorders that can result in partial or total blindness are just a few of the parasite infections that cattle's eyes are vulnerable to [3]. *Thelazia* worm, a nematode that infests the conjunctival sac and other ocular tissues, is one of the most frequent offenders. Conjunctival egg-laying by adult worms causes discomfort, severe tearing, and corneal injury. Additionally, Musca flies can spread these parasites, aggravating the issue, particularly in areas with large fly populations [4]. Cattle with parasitic infestations in their ears may experience anything from minor discomfort to excruciating pain. The surrounding tissues, the eardrum, and the ear canal can all be impacted. The ear tick, *Otobius megnini*, is one of the main parasites that afflict cattle's ears. This soft tick enters the ear canal and attaches, causing swelling, itching, and a waxy discharge. Constant irritability may impair an animal's ability to hear because it may result in secondary infections or even eardrum damage [5].

Vectors including flies, ticks, and mites are frequently used in the transmission of parasites that harm cattle's eyes and ears. For instance, flies have been known to transmit infectious larvae or eggs to the ears and eyes, beginning the parasitic life cycle inside the host. Ticks find that direct attachment to the ears offers the best conditions for feeding and reproduction [6]. These parasites can result in secondary illnesses that further jeopardize the health of the animal in addition to doing physical harm. Cattle eye and ear parasites have a complicated life cycle that involves several stages and frequently requires intermediate hosts or vectors. Consider the *Thelazia* worm, a typical parasite that affects cattle's eyes. Adult worms that are living in the host cattle's eyes usually start the life cycle. Through the host's tears, these mature worms generate eggs that are released into the environment. By consuming the eye fluids that contain the eggs, flies of the genus Musca serve as intermediary hosts [7]. The eggs are consumed by the fly, and once inside, they hatch into infectious larvae. These larvae eventually reach an infection-causing stage. These larvae are spread onto the surface of the eyes of cattle by the infected fly as it feeds or looks for moisture. The cycle is subsequently completed when the larvae enter the eye and mature into worms [8].

Otobius megnini, an ear tick, is a parasite that affects the ears. When female ticks lay their eggs in the host's ears or adjacent locations, the parasite's life cycle begins. Larvae developed from the eggs cling to the host's ears after they have hatched. The larvae feed during this period and go through a number of molts before becoming nymphs. The nymphs keep eating and molting until they reach adulthood [9]. When a tick reaches adulthood, it separates from the host's ear and looks for a place where it can lay eggs. As the eggs are laid and the cycle starts over again, this completes the life cycle. In all instances, the host's general health and well-being are impacted by the parasites' pain, irritability, and potential harm to their eyes and ears. To reduce the effects of parasite infections on cattle, it is essential to employ effective preventative and control techniques [10].

Infections with parasites in cattle's eyes and ears have significant negative economic effects. The stress and suffering brought on by these infections may lead to reduced milk production, weight loss, and poor reproduction. Cattle producers may also be severely burdened by the expenses related to veterinary care, drugs, and preventative measures. Prompt resolution of these problems is essential to preventing financial losses and protecting the general welfare of the cattle. To effectively manage parasite diseases in cattle, preventive measures must be put in place [11]. The availability of good hygiene and routine cleaning of cow living facilities might lessen the number of parasite breeding sites. By reducing the number of flies, ticks, and mite populations, insecticides and acaricides can reduce the spread of these parasites. The introduction of new cattle to a herd under quarantine conditions can also aid in halting the spread of parasites from carrier animals [12].

Parasite infections in cattle's eyes and ears pose a serious problem for livestock farmers (Table **1**). These illnesses not only endanger the health and welfare of the animals but also cost the industry money. Implementing efficient management measures requires a thorough understanding of the parasite life cycles, their routes of transmission, and the possible effects of infestations. The impact of parasitic diseases on cattle can be reduced by good cleanliness, routine veterinary care, and the use of preventive measures, enhancing the general success and sustainability of the livestock business. The parasites affecting the eyes and ears of the cattle are discussed below.

Raillietia auris

A parasite mite called *Raillietia auris*, also referred to as "aural ear mites," can infest the ears of many different animals, including cattle. The Raillietiidae family includes these mites. The arachnids that live in the ear canals and feed on skin fragments and wax, irritate and torment the hosts. These mites are distinguished by their small size, elongated shape, and flattened body, which enables them to move around and live in the microscopic areas of the ear [13]. They have a segmented body and a hard exoskeleton that shields them from the host's defenses and aids in keeping them in the ear canal. *Raillietia auris* mites have specialized mouthparts that enable them to feed on skin debris, wax, and other ear canal secretions, contributing to the irritation and inflammation experienced by the host. They frequently cause an ear canal discharge that is dark brown or black [14]. According to microscopic analysis, these mites have features and appendages that are tailored to their parasitic existence, which makes it easier for them to attach to the surfaces of the ear [15]. Direct contact with infected animals frequently results in *R. auris* infections in cattle. Additionally, the mites can be transferred by contact with fomites (inanimate items that might harbor diseases), contaminated bedding, or equipment. Infestations are more likely to affect cattle kept in close quarters, such as herds or small areas [16].

Table 1. Parasites of eye and ear, site of predilection, symptom, diagnosis, and treatment.

Parasite	Predilection site	Symptoms	Diagnosis	Treatment	References
Thelazia rhodesii	Eye, conjunctival sac, lacrimal duct	Conjunctivitis, lacrimation, photophobia	Clinical examination, microscopy	Manual removal of larvae, and anthelmintics such as levamisole.	[26 - 31]
Thelazia gulosa	Eye, conjunctival sac, lacrimal duct	Conjunctivitis, lacrimation, photophobia	Clinical examination, microscopy	Manual removal of larvae, and anthelmintics such as levamisole.	[33 - 37]
Thelazia skrjabini	Eye, conjunctival sac, lacrimal duct	Conjunctivitis, lacrimation, photophobia	Clinical examination, microscopy	Manual removal of larvae, and anthelmintics such as levamisole.	[38 - 42]
Otobius megnini	Ear	Irritation, inflammation, decreased weight gain	Visual examination	Acaricide	[44 - 48]
Rhabditis species	Ear	Agitation, head shaking, ear rubbing, drooping ears, itching, swelling, and pain	Visual examination	Anthelmintic drugs	[22 - 25]
Raillietia auris	Ear canal	Otitis media, otitis interna, head shaking, circling, head rotation	Microscopy, visual examination	Miticidal	[13 - 20]

There are various stages in the life cycle that are perfectly suited to the host and ecosystem. Adult female mites lay eggs in the ear canal environment to start the mite's life cycle. The larvae which emerge from these eggs are incredibly tiny and have just six legs at this stage. The larvae subsequently mature into nymphs, going through molting as they grow and getting eight legs. The nymphs keep consuming the fluids from the ear canal as they develop into adult mites. The nymphs are prepared to procreate once they reach adulthood, continuing the cycle. Cattle's ear canals serve as the final stop in the life cycle of adult female mites, who lay eggs there [17].

The clinical signs and symptoms seen in infected animals are a result of a series of events that are involved in the pathogenesis of mite infestation in cattle. The presence of the mites in the ear canals causes irritation, swelling, and discomfort, which causes a variety of physiological and behavioral reactions. The delicate ear tissues get mechanically irritated as a result of the mites' movement and physical presence inside the ear canal [18]. They can harm the ear canal's epithelial lining while moving and feeding, which causes the host's immune system to react inflammatorily. The infected ear canal becomes inflamed as a result of the mites' discomfort. Various immune cells, cytokines, and inflammatory mediators are released during this immunological response, causing the region to enlarge, become red, and have increased blood flow. To stop the infestation and fix any tissue damage, the inflammatory process is elicited. The clinical signs and symptoms seen in cattle with *R. auris* infestations are caused by a combination of mechanical irritation, mite feeding, and the host's inflammatory reaction. These include trembling, head swaying, head tilting, ear rubbing or itching, restlessness, and discomfort [19].

A thorough clinical examination of the infected animal's ears is necessary for the diagnosis of parasite ear infection in cattle. Otoscopes can be used by veterinarians to view the ear canal and spot mites, debris, and inflammatory symptoms. Additionally, ear swab samples can be examined under a microscope to confirm the presence of *R. auris* mites or their eggs. Acaricidal (mite-killing) drugs are frequently used to treat ear infections caused by mites [20]. These mites are frequently susceptible to the antiparasitic medicine ivermectin. Depending on the infection's severity and the veterinarian's recommendation, it can be given topically or intravenously. Cleaning the ear canal thoroughly to get rid of dirt and mites might also help the healing process. Antibiotics may be used to treat the bacterial component of the infection in more severe situations where secondary bacterial infections are present. To ensure the complete eradication of both mites and any accompanying infections, it is imperative to adhere to the recommended treatment regimen and finish the entire term of drugs [21].

Additionally, keeping their living space clean and inspecting and cleaning their ears frequently can be helpful in preventing re-infestation and lowering the risk of ear infections in cattle. For a precise diagnosis and a customized treatment plan for cattle *R. auris* ear infections, consultation with a veterinarian is essential.

Rhabditis species

Rhabditis species, notably *Rhabditis bovis,* can induce ear infections in cattle which can result in "summer ear syndrome" or "gadfly larvae infestation." The adult gadflies, also known as heel flies or warble flies, lay their eggs on the lower legs of cattle during the warmer months, which is when these parasites generally arise. The newly formed larvae then break through the skin and move within, frequently ending up in tissues in the head and neck area, including the ears [22].

Cattle with ear infections caused by *Rhabditis* species may exhibit agitation, head shaking, ear rubbing, and drooping ears. Itching, swelling, and pain in the ears can result from larvae present. Due to the harm the larvae have done, secondary bacterial infections may occasionally also happen. Clinical observation and physical examination are required for diagnosis [23]. The presence of *Rhabditis* larvae can be further confirmed by microscopic inspection of ear swab samples and identification of the larvae by veterinarians during an ear examination. The removal of the larvae from the ears is often the first step in treating ear infections brought on by *Rhabditis* species. Under the supervision of a veterinarian, this can be accomplished by carefully and delicately retrieving the larvae using forceps or other specialized tools [24]. Acaricidal (mite-killing) drugs may also be utilized to get rid of any lingering larvae in cases of severe infestation. To reduce the possibility of *Rhabditis* species ear infections in cattle, preventive measures are crucial. This may involve putting fly control measures in place to lower gadfly populations and stop egg-laying on livestock. Fly traps, chemical repellents, and keeping cattle in places with shade during fly activity peak seasons can all help with prevention [25].

Thelazia rhodesii

A parasitic nematode (worm) called *Thelazia rhodesii* can infect the eyes of cattle and other animals. It is frequently called an eyeworm. The parasite vector that spreads the larvae of *T. rhodesii,* which are frequently flies of the genus *Musca,* is most common in particular regions of Africa [4]. Adult worms are slender and thread-like in appearance, and they range in length from 10 to 20 millimeters. They have a recognizable anterior end with three lips encircling a mouth. The worms' bodies are translucent, making it possible to see within the body. The male worm has a bursa, a special structure utilized for reproduction, on its curved rear end. On the other hand, female worms are larger and have a straighter posterior end than males [26]. There are multiple stages of the parasite life cycle, and they all lead to eye infections. The worms which live in the eyes of infected cattle lay eggs to start the cycle. Through the host's tears, these eggs are discharged into the environment. The intermediate hosts are flies of the species Musca, also called eye flies. These flies are drawn to the wetness surrounding the eyes and eat the host's tears, unintentionally eating the eggs in the process. *Thelazia* eggs hatch inside the Musca fly's body, and the larvae grow into the infective stage. The larvae are dropped onto the host's eyes while the fly is feeding when it comes into contact with another cattle host [27]. The eye tissues, notably the conjunctival sac and its surroundings, are then penetrated by the larvae. The larvae continue to grow while they are inside the host's eye, eventually becoming adult worms. The life cycle of these worms is finished when they reproduce and release eggs [28].

There are several stages in the pathogenesis of *T. rhodesii* infection in cattle that result in the development of clinical symptoms and pain connected to the eyes in the infected animals. The larvae enter the ocular tissues, especially the conjunctiva and surrounding areas, after depositing onto the host's eyes. This penetration has the potential to cause inflammation and mechanical damage to the eye tissues. The larvae cause an immunological and inflammatory reaction in the tissues of the eyes. This response leads to irritation, redness, and swelling, causing discomfort for the animal [29]. Additionally, inflammation may be a factor in corneal injury and other ocular problems. The larvae can irritate and inflame the eye, causing symptoms such as excessive weeping, conjunctivitis, photophobia (sensitivity to light), and corneal ulcers. In severe circumstances, the worms can cause more serious eye issues as well as possible harm to the cornea and other ocular components [30].

Combining clinical evaluation, preventive measures, and targeted treatments is necessary for the diagnosis and management of infection in cattle. The diagnosis is usually made after a comprehensive ocular examination by a veterinarian, during which the existence of adult eyeworms or any accompanying clinical symptoms is evaluated. The worms may occasionally be visible inside the conjunctiva or the eye. Eye swab samples can be examined under a microscope to further confirm the presence of *Thelazia* larvae [31]. Effective fly control measures must be put in place in order to stop the illness. This includes controlling the number of mosquitoes that carry the parasite's larvae, frequently members of the genus Musca. Insecticides, fly repellents, and maintaining good hygiene in locations where cattle are housed are possible tactics. In order to detect and treat infections early, routine health checkups should also include regular eye exams. Eyeworms are often removed manually from the eye as part of treatment, frequently while the animal is sedated or under anesthetic to reduce discomfort [32]. To relieve pain and reduce inflammation, supportive care and anti-inflammatory drugs may also be recommended. The effects of *T. rhodesii* infections in cattle can be reduced, improving eye health and general welfare, by combining accurate diagnosis, watchful fly control techniques, and quick treatment.

Thelazia gulosa

A parasitic worm called *Thelazia gulosa* infects humans, cattle, and other animals. Due to its propensity for infesting cow's eyes, it is popularly referred to as the "cattle eyeworm". *Thelazia* is a genus of nematode worms that parasitize animals' eyes, and *T. gulosa* is one of these species [33]. It has a complex life cycle that requires both temporary hosts and permanent hosts. The adult worms are found in the ocular tissues of cattle, including the conjunctival sacs. Face flies (*Musca autumnalis*), which act as intermediary hosts, eat the larvae that the female worms deposit into the host's eye. The larvae mature into the infectious stage inside the fly. The larvae are deposited when the infected fly comes into touch with the mucous membranes or eyes of cattle. The larvae then travel to the conjunctival sac, where they mature into adults. The cycle then continues when the mature worms procreate [34].

In cattle, *T. gulosa* causes a dual-pronged pathogenesis: first, the worms alter the ocular environment, causing irritation and inflammation; second, the host's immune system activates to fight foreign invaders. It is known that the immune system tries to eliminate the worms and repair the tissue damage they cause, even if the precise processes underpinning the host's immunological response to these parasites are not fully understood. *T. gulosa* infected cattle may display a variety of discomfort and irritability symptoms. Conjunctivitis, corneal opacity, excessive tearing, and occasionally even corneal ulcers are some of these. Serious eye damage can result from severe infestations, which can harm the cattle's general health and productivity [35].

The eyes of the infected animal are normally thoroughly examined by a veterinarian in cases of *T. gulosa* infestations. The diagnosis can be confirmed by the worms' distinctive presence in the conjunctival sacs or other ocular tissues. The adult worms are typically extracted from the animal's eyes as part of the treatment. A veterinarian can perform this manually while utilizing forceps or other specialized instruments. To get rid of the worms and stop new infestations, doctors may also prescribe medications such as anti-parasitic drugs [36].

The infestations can be avoided by reducing the number of face flies, which serve as intermediate hosts. This can be accomplished in a number of ways, including the use of pesticides, the upkeep of clean and sanitary conditions for cattle, and the use of techniques that lower fly populations near livestock facilities. It should be noted that Human Thelaziasis, a disorder caused by *T. gulosa*, can also harm humans. The worms can make people feel uncomfortable and irritated, and develop conjunctivitis [37]. The same preventative techniques used to manage face flies can aid in lowering the danger of human infections. *T. gulosa* infestations can affect the health and productivity of cattle and provide a possible zoonotic danger to people who come into contact with infected animals or settings. In order to prevent and control these infestations, regular veterinary treatment, sound management techniques, and efficient fly control can all be very helpful.

Thelazia skrjabini

A parasitic worm called *Thelazia skrjabini* affects cattle and other animals. It belongs to the *Thelazia* genus, which contains several worm species well recognized for infesting animals' eyes, including human eyes. *T. skrjabini* is sometimes referred to as the "cattle eyeworm" because of its propensity to reside in its hosts' ocular tissues [38]. It has a multi-stage life cycle that depends on both intermediate and permanent hosts. Cattle conjunctival sacs and the tissues around their eyes are home to adult worms. Face flies (*Musca autumnalis*), which serve as intermediate hosts, consume the larvae that the female worms release. The larvae transition into infectious stages inside the flies. The larvae are shed when infected face flies come into contact with cattle's eyes or mucous membranes. After migrating to the conjunctival sac, the larvae develop into adult worms. The presence of adult *T. skrjabini* worms in cattle's eyes can cause a variety of uncomfortable ocular symptoms [39].

When infected face flies feed close to eyes or mucous membranes, they accidentally spread the larvae to cattle, starting the pathogenesis. The larvae then move to the conjunctival sacs and begin to develop into adult worms, starting a chain of events that have an impact on the host. *T. skrjabini* worms in the eyes cause a variety of physiological reactions and symptoms. Symptoms of discomfort and irritability in infected cattle include excessive tearing, conjunctivitis, and inflammation of the ocular structures [40]. The worms' movement inside the eye may result in mechanical harm, which could cause corneal opacity, ulcers, and potentially more serious ocular conditions. As the body of the host detects the presence of these foreign invaders, the immune system of the cattle is also triggered. Immune cells and inflammation are directed to the area of the infestation, which adds to the cattle's general discomfort and annoyance. A variety of clinical indications pertaining to eye health may manifest in cattle infected with *T. skrjabini*. Excessive tearing, conjunctivitis, irritation, and even corneal damage including opacity and ulceration can be among these symptoms [41]. Strong infestations may be detrimental to the health and production of cattle.

A comprehensive veterinary examination of the eyes is required to identify *T. skrjabini* infestations in cattle. The diagnosis is confirmed by the visual detection of the worms in the conjunctival sacs or other ocular tissues. Adult worms are often manually removed by a veterinarian using specialized tools as part of treatment. Anti-parasitic drugs may also be recommended to get rid of the worms and stop additional infestations. The prevention of parasitic infestations centers on reducing the number of face flies, which act as intermediate hosts. Utilizing insecticides, keeping cattle facilities clean, and putting measures in place that lessen fly prevalence around livestock are some methods to do this [42]. It is crucial to remember that *T. skrjabini* can infect humans as well, leading to a disorder called human thelaziasis. These worms can cause pain, conjunctivitis, and other eye-related problems in people. The same strategies used to manage face flies can also reduce the danger of human infections. Its infestations can affect the health and productivity of cattle and perhaps constitute a zoonotic danger to humans [43]. For the prevention and management of these infestations and the maintenance of both cattle and human welfare, regular veterinarian care, efficient fly control, and appropriate management methods are necessary.

Otobius megnini

The parasitic arachnid *Otobius megnini*, often called the Texas cattle tick or the spinose ear tick is a member of the Argasidae family. It is not a member of the Ixodidae family like many other ticks; rather, it is a member of the Argasidae family of soft ticks [44]. With a body that is leathery and flattened, as well as lengthy spines covering its dorsal side, the spinose ear tick has a striking appearance. Its characteristically prickly or spiky appearance is due to these spines. Its hue might be anything from gray to reddish-brown. Although it can also be found in other livestock species like horses, goats, and sheep, this tick typically infests the ears of cattle [45].

The warmer parts of North and South America are the usual locations for *O. megnini*. It prefers places with a lot of humidity, and the habitats of its host species are frequently linked to where it lives. The tick is sensitive to cold temperatures and has a life cycle that is adapted to warmer climates. It has a unique life cycle compared to many other tick species. Prior to becoming an adult, it goes through a number of nymphal and larval phases [46]. The host's blood is what the larvae and nymphs eat. Soft ticks like *O. megnini*, in contrast to hard ticks, do not adhere securely to their hosts and typically detach after feeding. Their many parasitic behaviors are influenced by this behavior as well as their affinity for protected locations like the ears [47].

While they normally pose less of a health risk to people than some other ticks do, they can irritate and distress cattle and other livestock. Ticks that feed on the blood of the host can irritate and inflame the surrounding area. The presence of these ticks in the ears can cause discomfort, decreased weight gain, and even secondary bacterial infections in cases of severe infestations [48]. Maintaining appropriate hygiene standards in livestock facilities, as well as routine inspection and control actions to limit tick presence, are necessary for managing *O. megnini* infestations. It is possible to apply insecticides, and veterinarian advice should be obtained for the best course of action.

Significance of Parasites of Eye and Ear on Cattle

Cattle's health, well-being, and general productivity can all be significantly impacted by parasites that live in their eyes and ears. These parasites, which include various worms and insects, can damage cattle in a number of different ways. Cattle with infected eyes and ears may experience pain, discomfort, and distress. These animals frequently display signs of discomfort, such as excessive head shaking, rubbing, and increased tear production. The discomfort and inflammation that parasites generate can lower the cattle's quality of life. Conjunctivitis, corneal ulcers, corneal damage, and other issues with the eye's structures can all be brought on by parasite infestations [49]. In addition to impairing the animal's vision, these problems can, if addressed, result in long-term eye diseases. In the case of ear parasites, infestations can lead to secondary infections that impair hearing and balance as well as ear canal inflammation, irritation, and more.

The productivity of cattle with eye and ear parasites may be decreased. In addition to causing discomfort and anguish, parasites can also cause dairy calves to consume less feed, lose weight, and produce less milk. The animals' behavior could alter, which would have an impact on how they interacted with other herd members and how actively they participated in daily activities. The integrity of the mucous membranes and other protective barriers in the eyes and ears may be compromised by parasite infections in these locations [50]. Cattle may become more vulnerable to bacterial and viral illnesses as a result of this weakened immune system. The animal's health may be further impacted by secondary illnesses, which can make the primary issue worse. Certain parasites that infest cattle's eyes and ears can also put humans at risk for zoonotic diseases. For instance, *Thelazia* species can harm both cattle and people, irritating and inflaming human eyes. The chance of transmission to humans can be decreased with proper management and treatment of these parasites in cattle. Producers may suffer financial losses as a result of parasite infections in cattle [51]. Financial strains on livestock enterprises can be caused by decreased productivity, veterinary treatment expenses, and the probable culling of seriously harmed animals.

FUTURE PERSPECTIVES

Progress in a number of areas, including veterinary medicine, parasitology, technology, and animal management, is anticipated to have an impact on future perspectives on parasites of the eyes and ears in cattle. Early and more precise diagnoses might result from improvements in diagnostic methods, such as more sensitive and focused testing for finding parasite infestations. This will enhance the health and welfare of cattle by allowing vets to spot and treat eye and ear parasite problems before they result in significant harm. In the future, eye and ear parasites may be treated with more specialized and effective methods [52]. This could entail the creation of brand-new anti-parasitic medications or formulations that target these parasites directly, minimizing the effects on unintended organisms and preventing the emergence of treatment resistance. Precision cattle farming techniques might become increasingly popular as technology develops. To do so, sensors, data analytics, and monitoring systems might be used to spot the first indications of parasite infestations in cattle. Better management of parasites might result from timely interventions based on real-time data. Future solutions for treating parasites of the ears and eyes might integrate a variety of techniques. This could incorporate both conventional chemical treatments and biological parasite control strategies, such as the use of beneficial insects or nematodes, in addition to these methods. It may become more frequent to breed cattle selectively to increase their genetic resistance to ocular and ear parasites. The development of more resistant cow breeds that are less vulnerable to these parasites may be facilitated by the identification of genetic markers linked to resistance [53]. The possibilities for developing vaccinations or immunomodulatory techniques against certain eye and ear parasites are high. These methods may aid in preventing or lessening the severity of infestations by boosting the cattle's immunological response. The "One Health" idea, which acknowledges the connection between the health of people, animals, and the environment, will probably continue to impact parasite management tactics. This involves designing thorough strategies that benefit both animal and human populations as well as taking into account the zoonotic potential of specific parasites [54]. Campaigns to raise knowledge and awareness among cattle owners, vets, and agricultural experts may be of utmost importance in the future. Campaigns to raise knowledge and awareness among cattle owners, vets, and agricultural experts may be of utmost importance in the future. Greater procedures and results might result from a greater understanding of the effects of eye and ear parasites and the significance of proactive care [55]. In conclusion, the management of eye and ear parasites in cattle is expected to include a combination of technical developments, novel therapeutic approaches, and a holistic approach to animal health and management in the future. The objective will be to reduce the effect of these parasites on cow welfare, production, and human health as our knowledge and techniques continue to advance.

CONCLUSION

In conclusion, parasites that damage cattle's eyes and ears represent serious threats to their health and well-being as well as to the productivity of the livestock business. Conjunctivitis, keratitis, otitis, and in severe cases, blindness or deafness can all be brought on by these parasites, which include different kinds of mites, flies, and worms. The economic ramifications are significant since affected cattle frequently experience decreased milk production, slower weight gain, and higher susceptibility to various illnesses. The management of eye and ear parasites in cattle requires a complex strategy. Regular veterinarian surveillance and early detection, the application of suitable deworming and antiparasitic treatments, the development of hygiene and sanitation in cow housing and feeding facilities, and the adoption of preventative measures like fly control methods are all part of this. It is also critical to inform cattle owners and livestock handlers of the need to maintain good herd health practices and act quickly on any indicators of parasite infections.

REFERENCES

[1] Almeria S, Robertson L, Santin M. Why foodborne and waterborne parasites are important for veterinarians. Res Vet Sci 2021; 136: 198-9.
[http://dx.doi.org/10.1016/j.rvsc.2021.02.020] [PMID: 33684793]

[2] Innes EA. The host-parasite relationship in pregnant cattle infected with *Neospora caninum*. Parasitology 2007; 134(13): 1903-10.
[http://dx.doi.org/10.1017/S0031182007000194] [PMID: 17958926]

[3] Morris CA. A review of genetic resistance to disease in Bos taurus cattle. Vet J 2007; 174(3): 481-91.
[http://dx.doi.org/10.1016/j.tvjl.2006.09.006] [PMID: 17095270]

[4] Djungu DF, Retnani EB, Ridwan Y. *Thelazia rhodesii* infection on cattle in Kupang district. Trop Biomed 2014; 31(4): 844-52.
[PMID: 25776611]

[5] Mastropaolo M, Nava S, Guglielmone AA, Mangold AJ. Developmental changes in salivary glands of nymphs and adults of the spinose ear tick *Otobius megnini*. J Parasitol 2011; 97(3): 535-7.
[http://dx.doi.org/10.1645/GE-2616.1] [PMID: 21506856]

[6] Panadero-Fontán R, Otranto D. Arthropods affecting the human eye. Vet Parasitol 2015; 208(1-2): 84-93.
[http://dx.doi.org/10.1016/j.vetpar.2014.12.022] [PMID: 25620292]

[7] Otranto D, Traversa D. eyeworm: an original endo- and ecto-parasitic nematode. Trends Parasitol 2005; 21(1): 1-4.
[http://dx.doi.org/10.1016/j.pt.2004.10.008] [PMID: 15639731]

[8] Shen J, Gasser RB, Chu D, *et al.* Human thelaziosis--a neglected parasitic disease of the eye. J Parasitol 2006; 92(4): 872-6.

[http://dx.doi.org/10.1645/GE-823R.1] [PMID: 16995411]

[9]   Kasaija PD, Estrada-Peña A, Contreras M, Kirunda H, de la Fuente J. Cattle ticks and tick-borne diseases: a review of Uganda's situation. Ticks Tick Borne Dis 2021; Sep;12(5): 101756.

[10]   Nava S, Mangold AJ, Guglielmone AA. Field and laboratory studies in a Neotropical population of the spinose ear tick, *Otobius megnini*. Med Vet Entomol 2009; 23(1): 1-5.
        [http://dx.doi.org/10.1111/j.1365-2915.2008.00761.x] [PMID: 19067794]

[11]   Strydom T, Lavan RP, Torres S, Heaney K. The Economic Impact of Parasitism from Nematodes, Trematodes and Ticks on Beef Cattle Production. Animals (Basel) 2023; 13(10): 1599.
        [http://dx.doi.org/10.3390/ani13101599] [PMID: 37238028]

[12]   Takeuchi-Storm N, Moakes S, Thüer S, *et al.* Parasite control in organic cattle farming: Management and farmers' perspectives from six European countries. Vet Parasitol Reg Stud Rep 2019; 18: 100329.
        [http://dx.doi.org/10.1016/j.vprsr.2019.100329] [PMID: 31796188]

[13]   Krametter-Froetscher R, Leschnik M, Hoegler S, Loewenstein M, Baumgartner W. Occurrence of the ear-mite *Raillietia auris* in cattle in Austria. Vet J 2006; 171(1): 186-8.
        [http://dx.doi.org/10.1016/j.tvjl.2004.09.014] [PMID: 16427597]

[14]   Veloso FP, Rodrigues FS, Madureira RC, Piranda EM, Tavares LER, Paiva F. *Raillietia auris* (Mesostigmata: Raillietiidae) in cattle in the state of Mato Grosso do Sul, Brazil. Rev Bras Parasitol Vet 2022; 31(2): e003122.
        [http://dx.doi.org/10.1590/s1984-29612022032] [PMID: 35674533]

[15]   Duarte ER, Hamdan JS. Otitis in cattle, an aetiological review. J Vet Med B Infect Dis Vet Public Health 2004; 51(1): 1-7.
        [http://dx.doi.org/10.1046/j.1439-0450.2003.00719.x] [PMID: 14995970]

[16]   Navarro R, Wahlen K, Streiff D, Ketzis JK. Pilot Study: Occurrence of Ear Mites and the Otic Flora in Domestic Ruminants on St. Kitts. Vet Parasitol Reg Stud Rep 2017; 10: 18-9.
        [http://dx.doi.org/10.1016/j.vprsr.2017.06.010] [PMID: 31014591]

[17]   Costa AL, Leite RC, Faccini JLH. Preliminary investigations on transmission and life cycle of the ear mites of the genus *Raillietia trouessart* (Acari: Gamasida) parasites of cattle. Mem Inst Oswaldo Cruz 1992; 87 (Suppl. 1): 97-100.
        [http://dx.doi.org/10.1590/S0074-02761992000500019] [PMID: 1343805]

[18]   Asmare K, Abebe R, Sheferaw D, Krontveit RI, Barbara W. Mange mite infestation in small ruminants in Ethiopia: Systematic review and meta-analysis. Vet Parasitol 2016; 218: 73-81.
        [http://dx.doi.org/10.1016/j.vetpar.2016.01.017] [PMID: 26872931]

[19]   Jimena ON, Laura JM, Elena MMR, Alonso NHJ, Teresa QMM. Association of *Raillietia caprae* with the presence of Mycoplasmas in the external ear canal of goats. Prev Vet Med 2009; 92(1-2): 150-3.
        [http://dx.doi.org/10.1016/j.prevetmed.2009.08.002] [PMID: 19733407]

[20]   Pérez de León AA, Mitchell RD III, Watson DW. Ectoparasites of Cattle. Vet Clin North Am Food Anim Pract 2020; 36(1): 173-85.
        [http://dx.doi.org/10.1016/j.cvfa.2019.12.004] [PMID: 32029183]

[21]   Christensen CM. External parasites of dairy cattle. J Dairy Sci 1982; 65(11): 2189-93.
        [http://dx.doi.org/10.3168/jds.S0022-0302(82)82481-8] [PMID: 6130107]

[22]   Duarte ER, Melo MM, Hamdan JS. Epidemiological aspects of bovine parasitic otitis caused by *Rhabditis* spp. and/or *Raillietia* spp. in the state of Minas Gerais, Brazil. Vet Parasitol 2001; 101(1): 45-52.
        [http://dx.doi.org/10.1016/S0304-4017(01)00492-7] [PMID: 11587832]

[23]   Verocai GG, Fernandes JI, Correia TR, Melo RM, Alves PA, Scott FB. Otite parasitária bovina por nematóides rhabditiformes em vacas Gir no estado do Rio de Janeiro, Brasil [Bovine parasitic otitis due to rhabditiform nematodes in Gyr cows from the State of Rio de Janeiro, Brazil]. Rev Bras Parasitol Vet 2007; 16(2): 105-7. Portuguese.

[PMID: 17706013]

[24]   Sobral SA, Ferreira BS, Senna CC, *et al. Rhabditis* spp., in the Espírito Santo, State of Brazil and evaluation of biological control. Rev Bras Parasitol Vet 2019; 28(2): 333-7.
        [http://dx.doi.org/10.1590/s1984-29612019020] [PMID: 31188945]

[25]   Sobral SA, Ferraz CM, Souza RIL, *et al.* Association between *Duddingtonia flagrans*, dimethylsulfoxide and ivermectin for the control of *Rhabditis* spp. in cattle. Trop Anim Health Prod 2022; 54(4): 198.
        [http://dx.doi.org/10.1007/s11250-022-03197-5] [PMID: 35666291]

[26]   Sivajothi, S., Swetha, K. & Reddy, B.S. Rare case of *Thelazia* infection in a Jersey cow—a report from Andhra Pradesh, India. Comp Clin Pathol 2023; 32: 515-7.

[27]   do Vale B, Lopes AP, da Conceição Fontes M, Silvestre M, Cardoso L, Coelho AC. Thelaziosis due to *Thelazia callipaeda* in Europe in the 21st century—A review. Vet Parasitol 2019; 275: 108957.
        [http://dx.doi.org/10.1016/j.vetpar.2019.108957] [PMID: 31630050]

[28]   Cotuțiu VD, Ionică AM, Dan T, Cazan CD, Borșan SD, Culda CA, Mihaiu M, Gherman CM, Mihalca AD. Diversity of *Thelazia* spp. in domestic cattle from Romania: epidemiology and molecular diagnosis by a novel multiplex PCR. Parasit Vectors 2023; Nov 3;16(1): 400.

[29]   Vohradsky F. Clinical course of *Thelazia rhodesii* infection of cattle in the Accra plains of Ghana. Bull Epizoot Dis Afr 1970; 18(2): 159-70.
        [PMID: 5526752]

[30]   Prange H, Kokles R, Zimmermann G. Klinische Beobachtungen und Untersuchungen zur Ätiologie bei enzootisch auftretenden Keratokonjunktivitiden des Rindes unter Berücksichtigung von Thelazien [Clinical observations and studies regarding the etiology of enzootically occurring bovine keratoconjunctivitis, with particular consideration of *Thelazia*]. Monatsh Veterinarmed 1968; 23(18): 692-8. German.
        [PMID: 5693312]

[31]   Otranto D, Tarsitano E, Traversa D, De Luca F, Giangaspero A. Molecular epidemiological survey on the vectors of *Thelazia gulosa*, *Thelazia rhodesi* and *Thelazia skrjabini* (Spirurida: Thelaziidae). Parasitology 2003; 127(4): 365-73.
        [http://dx.doi.org/10.1017/S0031182003003913] [PMID: 14636023]

[32]   Giangaspero A, Traversa D, Otranto D. Ecologia di *Thelazia* spp. e dei vettori in Italia [Ecology of *Thelazia* spp. in cattle and their vectors in Italy]. Parassitologia 2004; 46(1-2): 257-9. Italian.
        [PMID: 15305729]

[33]   Demiaszkiewicz AW, Moskwa B, Gralak A, *et al.* The Nematodes *Thelazia gulosa* Railiet and Henry, 1910 and *Thelazia skrjabini* Erschov, 1928 as a Cause of Blindness in European Bison (Bison bonasus) in Poland. Acta Parasitol 2020; 65(4): 963-8.
        [http://dx.doi.org/10.1007/s11686-020-00243-w] [PMID: 32613456]

[34]   Otranto D, Cantacessi C, Testini G, Lia RP. *Phortica variegata* as an intermediate host of *Thelazia callipaeda* under natural conditions: Evidence for pathogen transmission by a male arthropod vector. Int J Parasitol 2006; 36(10-11): 1167-73.
        [http://dx.doi.org/10.1016/j.ijpara.2006.06.006] [PMID: 16842795]

[35]   Bani Hassan E, Moshaverinia A, Sheedfar F, *et al.* A report of the unusual lesions caused by *Thelazia gulosa* in cattle. Vet Parasitol Reg Stud Rep 2017; 7: 62-5.
        [http://dx.doi.org/10.1016/j.vprsr.2016.12.006] [PMID: 31014660]

[36]   Otranto D, Tarsitano E, Traversa D, Giangaspero A, De Luca F, Puccini V. Differentiation among three species of bovine Thelaziosis (Nematoda: Thelaziidae) by polymerase chain reaction–restriction fragment length polymorphism of the first internal transcribed spacer ITS-1 (rDNA). Int J Parasitol 2001; 31(14): 1693-8.
        [http://dx.doi.org/10.1016/S0020-7519(01)00279-X] [PMID: 11730798]

[37] Bradbury RS, Gustafson DT, Sapp SGH, *et al.* A Second Case of Human Conjunctival Infestation With Thelazia gulosa and a Review of *T. gulosa* in North America. Clin Infect Dis 2019; 70(3): ciz469.
[http://dx.doi.org/10.1093/cid/ciz469] [PMID: 31638142]

[38] Yadav S.N., Ahmed N., Bordoloi G., Sarma M., Thakuria P., Nath A.J. (2020). Therapeutic Efficacy of Ivermectin against Thelaziasis in Cattle. Agricultural Science Digest. 2021; 41: pp. 260-1.
[http://dx.doi.org/10.18805/ag.D-5198]

[39] Giangaspero A, Otranto D, Vovlas N, Puccini V. *Thelazia gulosa* Railliet & Henry, 1910 and *T. skrjabini* Erschow, 1928 infection in southern Europe (Italy). Parasite 2000; 7(4): 327-9.
[http://dx.doi.org/10.1051/parasite/2000074327] [PMID: 11147042]

[40] Kennedy MJ, MacKinnon JD. Site segregation of *Thelazia skrjabini* and *Thelazia gulosa* (Nematoda: Thelazioidea) in the eyes of cattle. J Parasitol 1994; 80(4): 501-4.
[http://dx.doi.org/10.2307/3283182] [PMID: 8064515]

[41] Kennedy MJ. Prevalence of eyeworms (Nematoda: Thelazioidea) in beef cattle grazing different range pasture zones in Alberta, Canada. J Parasitol 1993; 79(6): 866-9.
[http://dx.doi.org/10.2307/3283723] [PMID: 8277378]

[42] Khedri J, Radfar MH, Borji H, Azizzadeh M. Epidemiological Survey of Bovine Thelaziosis in Southeastern of Iran. Iran J Parasitol 2016; 11(2): 221-5.
[PMID: 28096856]

[43] Anderson RC. Nematode parasites of vertebrates: their development and transmission. 2000.
[http://dx.doi.org/10.1079/9780851994215.0000]

[44] Telmadarraiy Z, Kooshki H, Edalat H, Vatandoost H, Bakhshi H, Faghihi F, Hosseini-Chegeni A, Oshaghi MA. Study on Hard and Soft Ticks of Domestic and Wild Animals in Western Iran. J Arthropod Borne Dis 2022; Sep 30;16(3): 225-32.

[45] Diyes GCP, Rajakaruna RS. Seasonal dynamics of spinose ear tick *Otobius megnini* associated with horse otoacariasis in Sri Lanka. Acta Trop 2016; 159: 170-5.
[http://dx.doi.org/10.1016/j.actatropica.2016.03.025] [PMID: 27012721]

[46] Diyes GCP, Rajakaruna RS. Life cycle of Spinose ear tick, *Otobius megnini* (Acari: Argasidae) infesting the race horses in Nuwara Eliya, Sri Lanka. Acta Trop 2017; 166: 164-76.
[http://dx.doi.org/10.1016/j.actatropica.2016.11.026] [PMID: 27871776]

[47] Shepherd JG. Mating, Sperm Transfer and Oviposition in Soft Ticks (Acari: Argasidae), a Review. Pathogens 2023; 12(4): 582.
[http://dx.doi.org/10.3390/pathogens12040582] [PMID: 37111468]

[48] Ariyarathne S, Apanaskevich DA, Amarasinghe PH, Rajakaruna RS. Diversity and distribution of tick species (Acari: Ixodidae) associated with human otoacariasis and socio-ecological risk factors of tick infestations in Sri Lanka. Exp Appl Acarol 2016; 70(1): 99-123.
[http://dx.doi.org/10.1007/s10493-016-0056-z] [PMID: 27382981]

[49] Deepthi B and Yalavarthi Y. Eye Worm infection in a Cattle - A Case Report, Vet. World 2012; 5(4): 236-7.

[50] Hiepe T. Advances in control of ectoparasites in large animals. Angew Parasitol 1988; 29(4): 201-10.
[PMID: 3072885]

[51] Byford RL, Craig ME, Crosby BL. A review of ectoparasites and their effect on cattle production. J Anim Sci 1992; 70(2): 597-602.
[http://dx.doi.org/10.2527/1992.702597x] [PMID: 1347767]

[52] Campero LM, Basso W, Moré G, *et al.* Neosporosis in Argentina: Past, present and future perspectives. Vet Parasitol Reg Stud Rep 2023; 41: 100882.
[http://dx.doi.org/10.1016/j.vprsr.2023.100882] [PMID: 37208088]

[53]   Ahmed H, Afzal MS, Mobeen M, Simsek S. An overview on different aspects of hypodermosis: Current status and future prospects. Acta Trop 2016; 162: 35-45.
[http://dx.doi.org/10.1016/j.actatropica.2016.05.016] [PMID: 27260666]

[54]   Otranto D, Strube C, Xiao L. Zoonotic parasites: the One Health challenge. Parasitol Res 2021; 120(12): 4073-4.
[http://dx.doi.org/10.1007/s00436-021-07221-9] [PMID: 34142224]

[55]   Ai L, Chen SH, Chen JX. [Progress on functional genomics of some important zoonotic parasites]. Zhongguo Ji Sheng Chong Xue Yu Ji Sheng Chong Bing Za Zhi 2011; 29(1): 58-63.
[PMID: 21823328]

CHAPTER 8

Parasites of the Respiratory System

Fathy Ahmad Osman[1,*]

[1] *Animal Health Research Institute, Department of Parasitology, Agricultural Research Center, Egypt*

Abstract: The breeding of livestock, particularly cattle, is one of the oldest agricultural activities that have been used to raise farmers' living standards all over the world, particularly in developing nations, however, this activity faces a number of challenges, one of which is the risk of disease transmission to the cattle. Numerous diseases can reduce an animal's productivity; harm its overall health, or even cause their death. Parasites are one of the greatest challenges to the development of cattle husbandry. One of these diseases is caused by parasitic agents, especially respiratory tract disease. There are numerous ways that these parasites can spread from one animal to another and affect cattle both internally and outwardly. In this section of the book, parasites that affect the respiratory system are discussed from the aspect of clinical, treatment, and control measures. These parasites can be classified as primary parasites that directly infect the respiratory system, secondary parasites that infect other parts of the body but also cause respiratory problems, or tertiary parasites that cause respiratory problems while they are passing through or developing. Parasites are considered the most challenging infections because the clinical symptoms are typically subclinical.

Keywords: Livestock rearing, Parasitic agents, Respiratory disease, Parasite, Cattle.

INTRODUCTION

Cattle livestock rearing is one of the world's most traditional forms of agriculture. Most rural households in developing countries, particularly in Africa, keep cattle, and it has proven to be quite resilient to prior economic crises [1, 2], where cattle production provides food and income to both urban and rural inhabitants, cattle livestock production is a crucial aspect of agriculture and has a significant impact on a country's natural economy, Therefore, the management's key responsibility in the cattle sector is to maintain breeds that are free of disease, especially the parasitic disease. Cattle are still susceptible to disease and have a range of diseases with different etiological reasons. One of the main obstacles to the

* **Corresponding author Fathy Ahmad Osman:** Animal Health Research Institute, Department of Parasitology, Agricultural Research Center, Egypt; E-mail: fathyosman69@yahoo.com

expansion of cattle husbandry is parasites. These parasites have an impact on cattle both internally and externally, and there are several ways in which they might transfer from one animal to another. Parasites that represent a risk to the respiratory system are one of the many etiological variables that lead to respiratory diseases in cattle. The way that respiratory parasites affect cattle varies [3, 4]. Some like *Dictyocaulus viviparus*, live in the respiratory tract as adults, while others, like *Ascaris* species, *Ancylostoma* species, and *Strongyloides* species, do not, but do pass through the tract while migrating. While others, like *Fasciola species*, may enter the system accidentally. The respiratory tract involving both the upper and lower respiratory tracts is affected by a parasite agent; according to clinical standards, a parasite respiratory infection can cause either mild coughing, while the main clinical signs of concurrent bronchopneumonia include dyspnea, nasal discharge, weight loss, fever, and death. The severity of the clinical symptoms depends on the number of parasites present and the region of the tract that they commonly infect [5, 6]. It is also influenced by individual differences among hosts in the morphological and physiological characteristics of the respiratory tract or in the way, an infection is responded to. The history of grazing and clinical symptoms may be utilized to make the diagnosis, and several methods of fecal analysis and postmortem examination can be used to confirm the presence of a respiratory parasite, although clinical signs, the time of year, and grazing history are often enough to make the primary diagnosis. The parasite affecting the respiratory system of cattle can be classified into three groups as follows: (1), Primary parasites of the respiratory system, (2), parasites that affect the lungs through normal migration or proliferation and (3), Parasites of another organ system that produce respiratory symptoms. Cattle become infected when they consume grass that has been contaminated by infectious larvae that have been excreted in the feces of other diseased animals. In mild, moist conditions, these larvae are more likely to survive on the grass. The current warm and rainy weather conditions are favorable for this situation, thus caution is suggested. After being exposed to lungworms, animals typically develop resistance to re-infection. However, if young calves are not exposed, elderly cattle may develop a clinical condition [7, 8]. Further lungworm exposure is necessary to maintain immunity. Both elderly cattle who have never been exposed to the disease before and those whose immune systems have weakened because they have not been exposed again are being diagnosed with it more frequently. Both deworming all cattle right before the rain starts at the end of the dry season and deworming all cattle at the end of the rainy season to prevent a significant parasite burden while grazing, are effective approaches to managing and preventing parasitic respiratory diseases. These actions are essential to reducing pasture pollution, providing a balanced diet to keep animals healthy, and helping them develop the necessary resistance to external infections, but a vaccination that offers cattle significant parasite protection is the more effective course of action [9, 10].

Primary Parasite of the Respiratory System

Husk Disease

(Verminous bronchitis, Verminous pneumonia 'hoose').

Definition

Parasitic disease of the lower respiratory tract is characterized by a persistent cough, particularly at night during larval migration, dyspnea, and a normal body temperature but concurrent bacterial or viral infections can complicate the condition and cause the body temperature to rise [11].

Etiological Agent

Nematode parasites (*Dictyocaulus Viviparus*), which is a member of the subfamily Trichostrongyloidea.

Life Cycle

The adult worm in the lung lays eggs containing larvae, which cough and swallow. Eggs hatched into L1 larvae, which passed with feces and developed into second-stage larvae and third-stage larvae. The third stage larvae (infective stage) can attach to (*Pilobolus fungal*) sporangium growing on feces to become aerosolized and widely spread in the environment. The sensitivity of infective larvae to dehydration is high. Therefore, most of them die after 2-3 weeks in the summer if conditions are dry, although survival in autumn can be much longer [12]. During grazing, cattle ingest infective third-stage larvae with the herbage, and the third-stage larvae travel to the lung through the lymphatic system, where they mature into adults and show respiratory symptoms.Cattle that have been exposed to lungworms often become resistant to re-infection. However, if young calves are not exposed, old cattle could become clinically sick. Further lungworm exposure is necessary to maintain immunity [13] (Fig. **1**).

Epidemiology

Cattle infection with lungworms occurs in temperate regions with considerable intense irrigation. Despite the fact that ideal conditions can accelerate a rapid increase in pasture larval numbers, changes in temperature and rainfall can significantly modify the amount of infectious larvae present in pasture. Infected animals can support a small number of adult worms and hypobiotic larvae that can survive overwinter into the next year, while at really cold temperatures, the majority becomes nonviable. The most significant source of lungworm larval contamination of pasture, as opposed to larvae surviving at pasture over time, is silent carriers of lungworm, which are the most significant source of larval contamination of pasture [14].

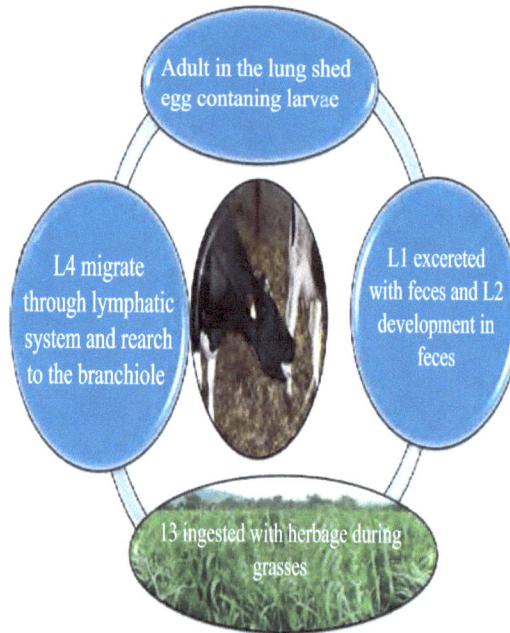

Fig. (1). Life cycle of lungworm in cattle.

Transmission

Once the larvae are contagious, the primary method of transmission is mechanical spreading away from the feces, where rain or the release of fungal sporangia from the Philobolus genus are two methods of dispersal processes. If an animal has not been exposed to infective larvae within the preceding six months, swallowed infective larvae move to the lungs and cause a robust immune response that is temporary [15]. Non-immune animals placed on contaminated pastures might potentially get serious illnesses.

Pathogenesis

Calves typically become infected during their first pasture season, although older cattle can also become infected (Fig. **2**). Depending on their location in the respiratory tract, how many infected larvae are eaten, and the animal's immune response, lungworms may be harmful, where the primary lesion during the prepatent stage of infection is bronchiole obstruction caused by an eosinophil infiltration in response to the developing larvae; this results in constriction of the airways and collapse of alveoli distal to the obstruction and the pathogenic effect varies depending on the infection stage (Table **1**).

Table 1. Clinical signs in different stages of verminous bronchitis.

Phase	Period After Infection	Life Cycle	Pathogenesis	Clinical Signs
Penetration phase	1-7 days	Larva penetrate intestine and migrate to lung	No clinical signs	Nil
Pre-patent phase	8-25 days	L4 enter alveoli	Larvae in lower airway (inflammation), around 15 day begin migrate to bronchi.	Cough being with exercise and decrease milk production.
Patent phase	26-60 days	Adult worm in lung and trachea and laying egg.	Bronchitis; Frothy mucus in upper airways Pneumonia; Collapsed area around the infected bronchi.	Productive cough, labored fast breathing and decrease milk production.
Post patent phase	61-90 days or after	Recovery phase after adult worm expelled.	Lung tissue inflammation, dissolution and aspiration of dead worm materials.	Cough, decrease milk production.

Pre-patent Phase

The animal can die during the pre-patent phase from severe pulmonary edema and interstitial emphysema [16].

Patent Phase

With the exacerbation of bronchitis, plasma cells, eosinophils, and lymphocytes will develop in the wall of the bronchus, and a frothy mucus, cellular exudate, and adult stage of nematodes will develop in the lumen. The bronchial inflammation and the ensuing response make the airways more resistant to pulmonary edema, and interstitial emphysema.

Post-patent Stage

Most animals recover, barring the development of a secondary infection in the wounded lungs [17].

Clinical Signs

The animal suffers from mild coughing, respiratory distress, with inclined respiratory rates (Table **1**). Initial breathing is quick and shallow with a cough that is made worse by physical activity [18] (Fig. **3**).

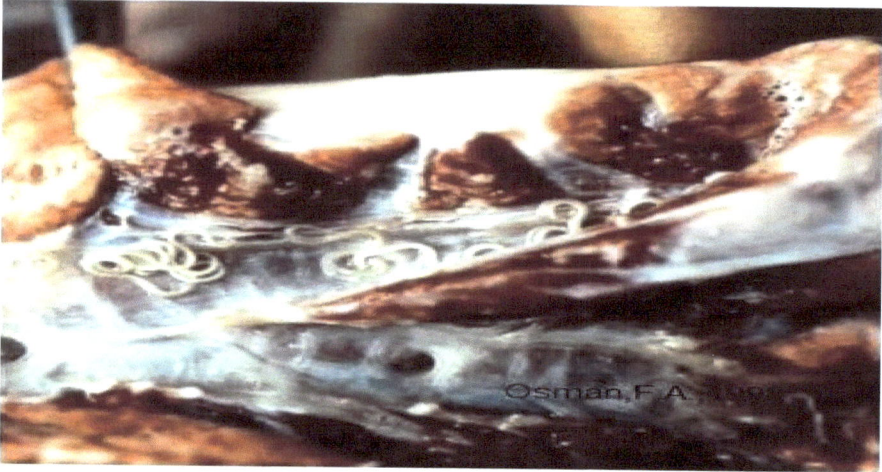

Fig. (2). Adult lungworms in bronchi.

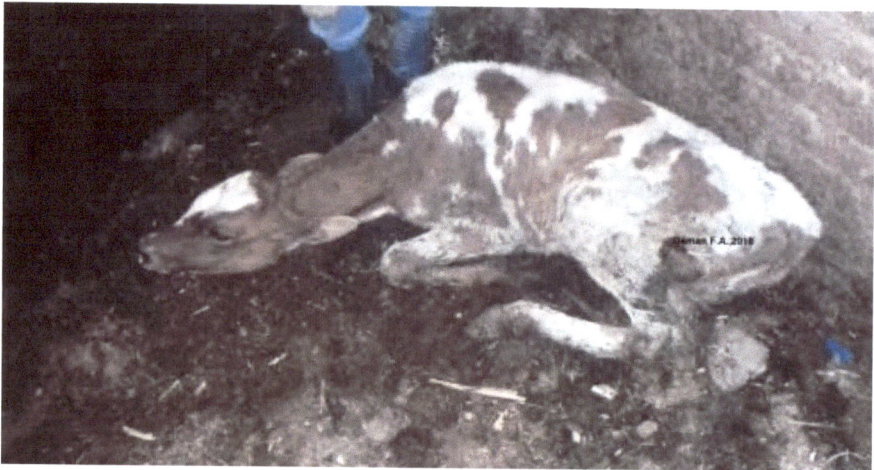

Fig. (3). Calve infected with lungworm. Showing respiratory clinical signs.

Diagnosis

The diagnosis of lungworms represents a significant problem for veterinarians in confirming the disease. The initial diagnosis is based on both clinical signs and epidemiology features of the disease. Differential diagnoses are for cattle respiratory disease. While laboratory testing is necessary for confirming diagnosis (the identification of larvae in fecal samples and/or antibodies in blood serum).

A. Fecal examination; (The preferred technique for locating and identifying parasite larvae is the Barman technique). These techniques are prone to false negative results because larvae of *D.viviparous* are not typically seen in the animal feces of animals in the pre-patent or post-patent phase [19].

B. Serological analysis; Antigen antibodies detection. By using more sophisticated technology like ELISA, antibodies against *Dictyocaulous Viviparus* in serum or milk samples can be found. Although antibodies have limited diagnostic utility since (1) they can still be detectable for a few months after the host has recovered from original infections, and (2) minimal, ELISA was prone to producing false negative results. Furthermore, despite efforts to address these deficiencies, the bulk milk ELISA's sensitivity is too low for accurate herd diagnosis [20].

C. Radiography and bronchoscopy; May also be beneficial in diagnosis.

D. Postmortem examination; This should involve scanning the trachea for lesions and adult worms, especially near the bifurcation, worm adults are seen in bronchi in the early stages -infection.

E. Histological examination; In various phases of lungworm infection, histologic sections from lesions or study of bronchial mucus smears may be needed to make the diagnosis.

Treatment

Lungworms can be managed with a variety of anthelmintics as macrocyclic lactones (ivermectin, doramectin, eprinomectin, and moxidectin) and benzimidazoles (fenbendazole, oxfendazole, and albendazole), which are applied in cattle and are most effective against all infections. In addition to anti-inflammatory, supportive saline solution and antibiotic therapy for any bacterial infections were also required [21].

Control

The two main ways for controlling lungworm infection are vaccination and/or anthelmintic prophylaxis.

Vaccination

For lungworm infections, oral vaccinations are accessible in Europe. Two doses of irradiation infectious larvae are given, the second dosage being given for two weeks before the start of grazing [22]. The two doses are given four weeks apart.

Anthelmintic Prophylaxis

Anthelmintic prophylaxis is the cornerstone of eliminating bovine lungworms with the added benefit of eradicating GI nematodes [23]. Treatments (Two or three) during the grazing season are effective when using persistent anthelmintic (ivermectin, doramectin, moxidectin, and eprinomectin). These medications may even induce immunity to the parasite by halting the progression of infections.

Nasal Schistosomiasis in Cattle

Snoring disease

Definition

Parasitic disease affecting cattle, clinically characterized by their long-term impact on production and growth.

Etiological Agent

Trematode parasite (Blood fluke), known as *Schistosomes spp.*, is a member of the family Schistosomatidae, and are dioeciously host [24]. Parasites are unavoidable parasites of animals' circulatory systems. The mature female is borne in a ventral groove and is more slender than the male. About 19 species reported to naturally infect animals, 8 parasites of ruminants have received particular attention, mainly because of their recognized veterinary significance, where they coexist, some of these species are known to interact, and interbreeding between species has been documented.

Intermediated Host

The freshwater snail (*Indoplanorbis exustus*) acts as an intermediate host.

Life Cycle

Eggs excreted with feces of infected animals when finding fresh water hatch into miracidium, which in snails change into cercaria. They exit the snail during the pre-patent stage (45-70 days), depending on the species, and swim around freely in the water for many hours before dying. Infections occur by oral ingestion and/or skin penetration when cattle are drinking or grazing and cercaria transport through the blood and lymph to their sites of predilection as cercariae change into adult worms [25]. Evidence suggests that *S. haematobium*, a human parasite, is naturally hybridized with *S. mattheei, S. bovis*, and *S. curassoni*. It is important to note that hybridizing human schistosomes and ruminants requires a host exchange between *S haematobium* in domestic animals and *S. mattheei*, *S. bovis*, or *S. curassoni* in humans (Fig. **4**).

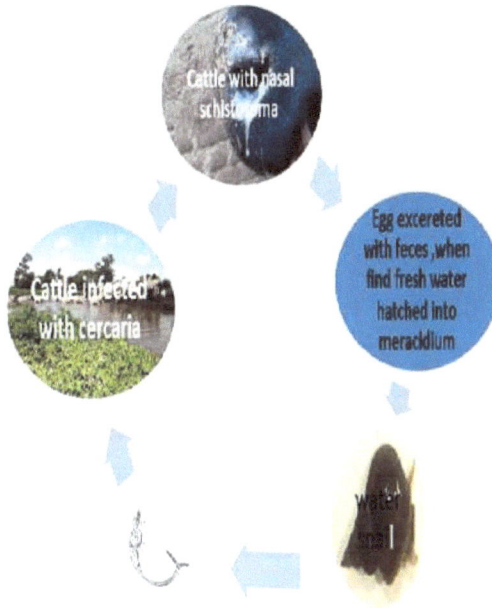

Fig. (4). Life cycle of nasal *Schistosoma* in cattle.

Epidemiology

Cattle schistosomes can arise intermittently throughout their range. The rates of infections in cattle can range from 40% to 70% in places with good conditions and the spread of these schistosomes may be directly impacted by the expanded host range and variations in the distribution of host observed in Africa [26].

Immunity

There is compelling evidence that cattle have developed an acquired immunity to the infection of *Schistosoma spp.* Studies on naturally infected animals that partially protect against reinfection demonstrate the importance of acquired resistance to schistosomes [22].

Clinical Signs

Snoring sickness is often a chronic disease, most animals do not show adequate symptoms to distinguish it from other respiratory illnesses. The main pathogens are eggs and adult flukes are seen in nasal mucosal blood vessels [27]. Rupture of abscesses, the release of eggs, pus, and hemorrhagic and/or mucopurulent nasal discharge is a common symptom, as nasal granulomas and fibrosis, which resemble cauliflower-like growths on the nasal mucosa, which lead to partial nasal obstruction and snoring develop [28]. Anorexia, progressive emaciation, dyspnea, and snoring are common symptoms of affected cattle. Other symptoms include nasal congestion, thick mucus nasal discharge on both sides and rhinitis, which results in excessive mucus-purulent nasal discharge.

Diagnosis

Case history and clinical symptoms can be used to make a preliminary diagnosis, but a confirmatory diagnosis should be based on laboratory tests and the presence of oocytes [29]. The fecal swab, filtration, sedimentation, rectal and liver biopsy, and miracle hatching tests are the most commonly used methods for detecting oocyte excretion in field settings. Several sero-diagnostic techniques have been allowed to diagnose schistosomiasis. Serology may not always be able to identify acute *S. bovis*. infection. However, it is helpful to identify chronic diseases in a sero-epidemiological examination by identifying species and their close evolutionary relatives, and molecular analysis can be used to diagnose diseases.

Treatment

Treatment with Anthiomaline (Lithium antimony thiomalate), begins with injection (15ml, I/M), after receiving the first dose of anthiomaline, the affected cattle respond, and the size of the nasal granular tumor will decrease. If necessary, anthiomaline injection can be given again at weekly intervals to reduce the size of the nasal granular tumor and stop the snoring or noise. Usually, it takes two or three shots to achieve complete recovery with Praziquantel (30 mg/kg, Po, in cattle) two doses for 3-5 weeks . Praziquantel is only used in China, where infected cattle are an important source of human diseases. While in India, all the infected cattle that were brought to veterinary care were administered Praziquantel or Anthiomaline, at a dose of 20 mg/kg of body weight [30].

Control

Avoiding grazing animals near water channels where infected snails are present, as well as routine deworming and treatment of animals at the early stage of infection, will help control schistosomiasis in cattle. Other controlling measures include the mechanical removal of snail traps. The use of ecological strategies to combat the snails, including drainage and the elimination of water weeds has also been effective.

Mammomonogamiasis

Syngamoniasis

Definition

Parasitic disease affects the respiratory systems of these animals (Cattle, sheep, goats, deer, cats, orangutans, and elephants), and is characterized clinically by chronic cough and symptoms like asthma.

Etiological Agent

Parasite belongs to the family Syngamidae (Nematodes), which typically live in the trachea, bronchus, or larynx of the upper respiratory tract and identified by the typical slender shape and are crimson in color (bloodsucking), their body is covered in a flexible but very tough cuticle, just like other roundworms, the genus Mammomonogamus contains a number of species, but *M. larynges* are the one that is most frequently encountered. The parasites can also infect people; approximately 100 human cases have been reported globally.

Definitive Host

The primary hosts are birds; however, ruminants (such as cattle, sheep, goats, and deer), cats, orangutans, and elephants are also regarded as the most important hosts.

Intermediate Host

It is unknown but the intermediate hosts may be arthropods, snails, or earthworms.

Infective Stage

It can be larvae, adult worms, or embryonated eggs.

Life Cycle

Mammomonogamus spp. the life cycle is not entirely understood for ruminants like cattle, definitive hosts are thought to exist. *M. laryngeus* is the most prevalent species; however, it rarely causes infections in people. Two current theories that explain the potential life cycle of parasites, particularly in endemic locations, may benefit medical diagnostics [31] (Fig. **5**).

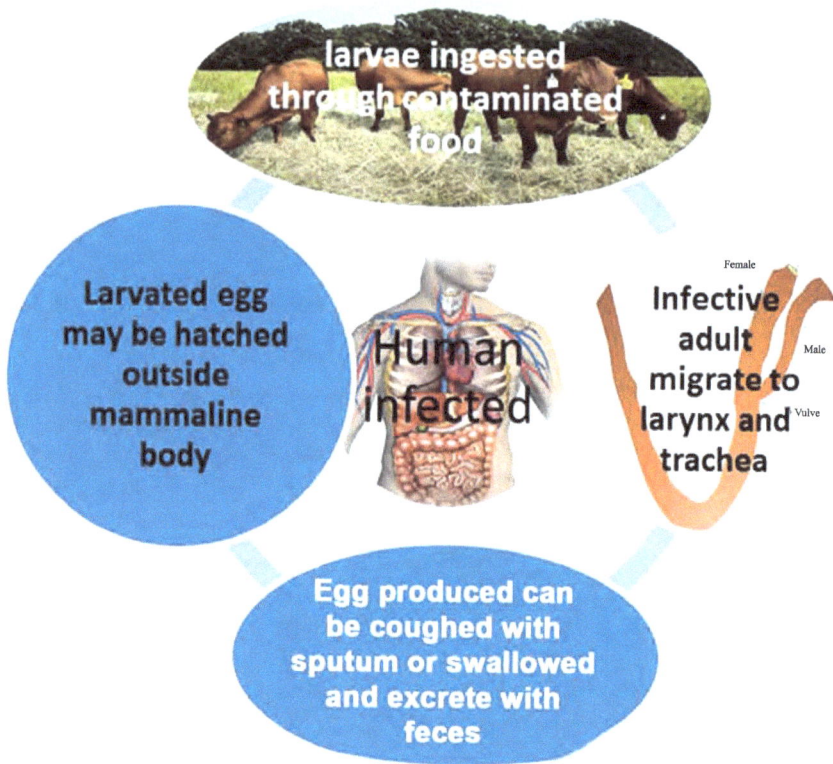

Fig. (5). Life Cycle of *Mammomonogamus spp.*

Hypothesis 1

An infection of the mammomonogamus can occur if the mature worm is consumed through contaminated food or water, infectious pathogens enter the trachea through the larynx and then proceed to the mucosal walls of the respiratory system. Following sexual reproduction, the worms start to lay their eggs in the host's respiratory system. The eggs either excrete from the diseased host's body or are swallowed. Therefore, the development of eggs into larvae does not occur within the host body [12].

Hypothesis 2

The infectious agents (infectious larvae or embryonated eggs) move to the intestinal area, migrate along the intestinal walls, and then move through the mesenteric veins to the alveolar area, where the eggs or larvae grow into an adult worm in seven days. The larynx is where the adult worms rise and begin to reproduce. The female worm's eggs leave the host's body through feces or sputum. The eggs change into larvae after three weeks [12].

Transmission

The female worm's eggs leave the host's body through feces or sputum, three weeks later, the eggs molt and change into larvae. (Fig. **5**) Life Cycle of *Mammomonogamus spp.*

Pathogenesis

The condition caused by *M. laryngeus*, appears as respiratory asthma-like symptoms and coughing only after the worms have grown to adult and obstructed the bronchial airways, where bronchial inflammation may result from the worms' potential for attaching the mucosal walls and devouring red blood cells. The incubation phase follows infection and normally lasts 6 to 11 days. This supports the second explanation, which proposes a probable pulmonary cycle as the cause of the symptoms one- to two-week delay.

Clinical Signs

Chronic coughing and symptoms like asthma are the main signs, where parasites typically live in the upper respiratory tract in the trachea, bronchus, or larynx. In severe cases of infection, worms may go further into the trachea, and bronchi and partially obstruct the airways. The majority of cases evolve into a chronic cough and, occasionally, hemoptysis, if left untreated, these symptoms include a low-grade fever that lasts for several months, weight loss, and pneumonitis but not anemia.

Diagnosis

Case history and clinical signs are used to make the initial diagnosis, but adult worms must be recovered and removed using forceps, a bronchoscope, or endoscopic tools to make the final diagnosis. However, if worms are firmly affixed to the bronchial walls, removal may be challenging. Another reliable evidence of infection is the identification of *M. laryngeus* eggs in feces (which are ovoid to ellipsoid, non-operculated, and 40 x 80 m in size, with thicker shells than those of hookworm eggs, and they have spicules spanning 23 to 30 m in length). Eosinophilia varies from case to case, making it impossible to use it as a reliable indicator of the severity of an infection, where some instances with numerous pairs of worms had low amounts of eosinophils; others with only one pair had quite high levels [14].

Treatment and Control

Since the life cycle is not clear, no preventive and control measures can be suggested but parasitic infections can be treated with several anthelmintic active components (albendazole, mebendazole, thiabendazole, and ivermectin). Also a unique treatment plan must be developed by the veterinary practitioner because the majority of commercial anthelmintics are not authorized for use against this worm and theses worms cannot currently be controlled biologically, *i.e.*, by using their natural enemies.

Parasites of another Organ System that Produces Respiratory Symptoms Toxocariasis

Neoascaris vitulorum

Definition

Parasitic disease can harm lung tissues by migration of parasite larvae. Young calves frequently suffer from high death rates as a result, along with financial losses. Although it can be found all over the world, it is more prevalent in parts of Africa, America, and Asia that have humid tropical or subtropical temperatures (Fig. **6**).

Etiological Agent

Toxocariosis is mostly caused by nematode parasite (*Toxocara vitulorum*), which lives as adults inside the lumen of the small intestine, but migratory larvae can also be detected in the lungs, trachea, bronchi, liver, kidneys, mammary glands, and other organs. It is white in color, with males reaching lengths of up to 25 cm and females reaching lengths of up to 30 cm.

Life Cycle and Transmission

The life cycle of parasites is linear, where the host can become infected by consuming live larvae eggs from contaminated sources during grassing (Horizontal transmission), and/or they can contract the infection by (vertical transmission), first suckling of colostrum from the infected mother. Larvae secreted in milk for up to 3–4 weeks following parturition, migrate through the hepato-trachea in calves under 6 months old. Also calves older than 6 months of age can become infected by horizontal transmission [4], but this infection rarely leads to patency. The somatic migration of the larvae occurs in these older calves and is halted in certain tissues, mostly the liver, lungs, muscles, brain, kidney, and peripheral lymph nodes. In female calves, these larvae are latent until late in the pregnancy, when they begin to develop again and migrate to the mammary gland around the time of delivery, allowing transmission through the milk. In endemic areas with inadequate control measures, the infection rate can reach up to 100% of the calves (Fig. **3**).

Clinical Signs

Clinical symptoms of the larvae's migration, which can seriously damage various organs in adult cattle, particularly the lungs, are rare because most calves spontaneously recover by the time they are 3 to 5 months, but the infected calf may have a normal body temperature or a slight rise, feces were muddy in color, had an offensive odor, semi-solid in consistency, and streaked with blood [8].

Diagnosis

The case history and clinical signs come first, as the breath of affected animals occasionally has a scent resembling acetone smell, in addition to cough and semi-solid feces or diarrhea. When newborn calves' feces are examined, *T. vitulorum* eggs can be found and used to make an accurate diagnosis (eggs measure 69-95 mm by 60-77 mm, are nearly spherical, colorless, sub-globular, and have thick, coarsely pitted shells, containing a solitary cell and have a thick, pitted membrane). However, pregnant cows may carry dormant larvae in their tissues to their offspring even if there are no visible eggs in their feces [11].

Treatment

It is advised to treat 10- to 16-day-old calves with an anthelmintic therapy that works well against immature parasites. By using this approach, the environment is far less contaminated, and a huge number of immature or mature parasites are prevented from having a detrimental effect.

> **N.B** -Pyrantel pamoate (25 mg/Kg BW.PO), along with supportive therapy (Normal saline and multivitamin), and the same dose was repeated after 7 days. Compounds like Levamisole, Febantel, and Oxfendazole can be tried but they may not expel all the worms.

Strongyloidiasis

Definition

Parasitic disease typically parasitizes the small intestine of cattle and is characterized clinically by diarrhea, and malnutrition, especially in young calves, respiratory disorders are caused by a parasite's larva migrating through the parenchyma tissue of the lung (Fig. **7**).

Etiological Agent

A nematode parasite named, *Strongyloides papillosus*, is a widely distributed intestinal nematode of cattle and small ruminants.

Epidemiology

The prevalence of *S. papillosus* has been reported to vary according to age groups, management systems, areas, and climates. It was discovered that 4-20% of 4-month-old dairy calves in Costa Rica were infected [12]. In southern Japan, during the damp and muggy summer months, calves have experienced high levels of illnesses [15]. *S. papillosus* was found in 10-53% of 1-month-old beef calves during housing in central Germany; however, during the grazing season, the prevalence decreased to 6% [18]. Groups living on wood shavings, high temperatures, and humidity are thought to be contributing factors to the parasite's environmental amplification and host hyperinfection.

Life Cycle

1-*Strongyliodes papillosus* has both a free-living and intra-host life cycle and the prepatent period is around nine days long.

A-Free-living life cycle

In the environment, L3 larvae can develop into adult male and female worms that reproduce sexually to create eggs.

B- Intra-host life cycle

Cattle can be infected through penetration of third-stage larvae into the animal's epidermis as well as through ingestion of infective larvae when eating, or drinking. The duodenum is where these larvae mature into adult females that can produce parthenogenetic eggs. High temperatures and humidity accelerate the maturation of soil eggs to infective L3 in less than 28 hours, making it easier for the ruminant host to become infective (highly infective).

Transmission

The host can get infected by oral ingestion or penetration of skin by infective larvae (L3) of S. *papillosus* that are contaminated by the pasture. The activation of encysted L3 in mother tissues can also infect calves through milk sucking.

Clinical Signs

Clinically, strongyloidiasis is characterized by diarrhea, elongated fecal pellets at the end, dehydration, anorexia, anemia, and respiratory disorders. Severely infected calves initially exhibited increased respiration before dying, but their body temperatures remained close to normal, and abnormal lung sounds and general spasms were noted [13]. All of the animals die within 3-4 minutes of showing the first respiratory symptoms [11], and different tachy- and brady-arrhythmia patterns were seen 1-2 days prior to death [16]. Rapid mortality may occur during the patent phase (8-14 days), while the pre-patent period in cattle infections is characterized by cough. Dead calves that were 3-4 months old and seemed to be in good health are frequently discovered; the causes of cardiac sudden death are still unknown. Heifer sudden death is typically a few days to a few weeks preceded by severe premature udder growth caused by congested mammary glands and mild ductal hyperplasia. Some of the parasitized living animals showed a comparable expansion of the mammary glands.

Pathogenesis

The larvae travel through the blood to the heart, after which they go on to the lungs, where they cough and swallow, disrupting breathing [10]. Where harmful effects of infected animals were caused by gastrointestinal motor abnormalities. Little is known about the mechanisms that cause gastrointestinal motor disruption but paralytic ileus is recorded, hypothesized that sudden death would be caused by a lethal arrhythmia caused by a parasite-associated cardiac toxin, and paralytic ileus.

Diagnosis

1. A preliminary diagnosis is based on the case history and clinical symptoms, however, a precise diagnosis requires a fecal examination to find larval eggs(40–50 um in diameter with thin shell), and/ or larvae when passed in the feces. The floating technique may not be completely sensitive and turn out to be negative, that is used to evaluate the contents of the colon, and a few feet of the proximal duodenum from a calf is submitted to a parasitology lab for detection and identification of adult female *S. papillosus* (do not freeze). Fecal samples from dead groups should also be taken in acute death cases when there is a strong suspicion of *S. papillosus* infection to improve the likelihood of making a diagnosis. More sophisticated methods, such as ELISA and PCR, are used for confirmatory diagnosis.
2. Post-mortem examination: Post-mortem investigations frequently reveal no evident abnormalities but affected heifers revealed prematurely bilaterally symmetric mammary gland hypertrophy.

3. Histological findings in affected calves frequently included generalized mammary gland vascular congestion, interstitial edema, bleeding with ductal hyperplasia and mild multifocal cardiomyocyte degeneration was present.

Treatment

Macrocyclic lactones, the most widely used treatments for *S. papillosus,* including ivermectin, doramectin, and moxidectin, are powerful anthelmintic drugs that can effectively treat and/or totally prevent early harm caused by *S. papillosus.* Deaths ceased within 24 hours, and by 7 days after deworming, breast growth had drastically decreased and seemed nearly normal. Albendazole is also effective [8].

Prevention and Control

Treatment applications should be supported by research. To keep bedding dry, use a ceiling fan, stay away from sawdust, or regularly replace the litter. The first general preventive action is to avoid mass rearing of native calves in a pen or mass deworming before grouping. To prevent illness and the spread of diseases among the group, calves with high counts of eggs (EPG > 10,000) should get efficient anthelmintic treatment.

Bunostomosis

(Hookworm infection)

Definition

Parasite disease is characterized clinically by anemia, black, tarry feces in calves, dehydration, weakness, loss of appetite, stunted growth, weight loss, bottle jaw, and respiratory disorders due to damage of lung tissues by larvae migration. Furthermore skin-penetrating larvae can result in dermatitis, which includes itchiness, swelling, redness, and thickness, as well as hair loss, a rough coat, and harmed hooves.

Etiological Cause

A blood-feeding nematode parasite known as the bovine hookworm (*Bunostomum phlebotomum*), which parasitizes the small intestines of cattle, buffalo, and yaks and is the primary cause of significant disease in cattle breeding (Huang and Shen, 2006; pp. 323–324). The hookworm is a white, long (3 cm), and sturdy worm. The small intestine is the preferred location for adult parasites, while skin, blood, lungs, and trachea may all contain larvae momentarily.

Life Cycle and Transmission

Depending on the parasite species and the host, the prepatent phase lasts 7 to 9 weeks. Calves develop an immune to infection quickly. No intermediary hosts are involved in the direct life cycle of any *Bunostomum* species. In the host's intestine, adult females lay eggs that are expelled out with the feces, in the environment, the eggs can release the L1-larvae, which, in favorable conditions (hot and humid conditions), mature into infective L3-larvae in a period of 5 days; in cold weather, this process takes substantially longer. These infectious larvae can persist on pastures for up to two months in warm conditions. In areas with a moderate climate (like Europe, Canada, *etc.*), they do not persist during the winter. The two most common ways for cattle infection are through their skin penetrations and through swallowing infected larvae from contaminated pasture and/or water. When a larva enters the skin, it enters the bloodstream, travels to the lungs, crosses the lung tissue, enters the trachea and mouth (*via* coughing, expectorations, *etc.*), and eventually enters the intestine after being ingested and settling in the duodenum as adults, where the females also begin to lay eggs [7].

Clinical Signs

The infective third-stage larvae of *B. phlebotomum* can enter the host's body through the mouth or skin and travel through the bloodstream and lungs before settling in the duodenum as adults.

General Signs

Adult worms' powerful mouth capsules leave behind heavy intestinal wall sores that frequently result in intestinal blood vessel rupture and subsequent bleeding, hence, infected cattle have anemia, weight loss, growth retardation, and even death in severe infection (Gao *et al.* 2014, pp. 92–100), where 50 to 200 worms infected calves can induce anemia, while over 2000 worms can be killed to calves, include diarrhea (sometimes mucous or hemorrhagic), dehydration, loss of appetite, weakness, weight loss or slowed growth, and bottle jaw.

Dermatitis Symptoms

Skin allergy at the site of penetration (including swelling, itching, redness, and thickness), rough coats, hair loss, and damaged hooves.

Respiratory Signs

Symptoms of respiratory problems (persistent cough, sneezing, and rhinitis) are caused by larvae migrating through the lung tissue.

Diagnosis

Perspective diagnosis can be made through case history and clinical signs, while accurate diagnosis depends on fecal and molecular diagnosis. Unfortunately, to date, the diagnosis of hookworm infection remains largely based on microscopic examination of feces and is often mistaken even by professional microscopists for possible environmental cross-contamination of eggs of *Bunostomum spp* [6]. For diagnosis and epidemiological research, it is now essential to develop a more effective and reliable method to detect and distinguish *B. phlebotomum* eggs or larvae, and accomplishing this goal is only possible by using molecular approaches. The eggs feature tough egg shells that commonly have detritus stuck to them, are ovoid but unevenly shaped, measure 55 x 95 micrometers, have a sticky surface on the shell, and contain 4 to 8 cells when shed.

Treatment and Control

Bunostomum spp. can be controlled with anthelmintics, although it is more feasible to employ dry bed grounds for long-term environmental cleanup. In areas where anthelmintics are frequently used, the parasite has nearly disappeared, but in other areas, it should be considered as a potential cause of anemia.

Parasite affecting the respiratory system through larvae migration and/or proliferation

Hydatid disease (Echinococcosis) Definition

A nearly universal zoonotic parasitic disease, known as hydatid cyst (Echinococcosis), typically affects any organ in the body, especially the liver and lungs of domestic animals and people, and produces cysts, and has economic significance due to condemnation of edible offal, primarily liver, lung and other organs or even whole carcasses.

Etiological Agent

The larval stages of cestodes belonging to the genus Echinococcus (family Taeniidae), where the adult worms live in the intestine of dogs and other carnivores. There are two species of medical and public health relevance namely, *Echinococcus granulosus* and *Echinococcus multilocularis*, which cause cystic echinococcosis and alveolar echinococcosis, respectively. Both illnesses are serious and dangerous, but the latter is more so because it has a high fatality rate and a poor prognosis. When inadequately treated, these illnesses, which are new or re-emerging diseases, are a significant public health concern (Fig. **8**).

Life Cycle

The parasite's larval stage "hydatid cyst" develops in cattle as an intermediate host, in addition to dogs and other carnivores, which are the only definitive hosts for the tapeworm, where the adult worms living in their small intestine, eggs, and/or proglottids segment are expelled with feces. The egg hatches generally in the small intestine after being ingested by an intermediate host (such as cattle, goats, sheep, swine, horses, camels, or humans) and releases an oncosphere that penetrates the intestinal wall and thereby travels through the blood to numerous organs, particularly the lung, and liver. The oncosphere transforms into a cyst in these organs, which grows over time. Within the cyst, protoscolices and daughter cysts emerge. By consuming the organs of the infected cattle that contain cysts, the final host contracts the infection. Protoscolices evaginate after consumption and adhere to the intestinal mucosa and they need 32 to 80 days to reach adult stages.

Clinical Symptoms

The disease often remains asymptomatic for years before the cysts grow large enough to cause symptoms in the affected organs, where when the lung is impacted, respiratory disorders are the most frequent clinical symptoms, while cyst rupture can result in a host reaction that includes fever, urticarial, eosinophilia, perhaps anaphylactic and cyst dissemination.

Diagnosis

Diagnosis in cattle must be carried in abattoirs, in addition to a reliable recording system that remains the most practical option. However, misdiagnosis can occur when a macroscopic diagnosis is employed without histological confirmation. which includes false positives for various diseases that resemble cysts and false negatives for microscopic cysts that are still forming. Such error positives have been linked to caseous lymphadenitis as a common culprit. Attempts to create immunodiagnostic testing for cattle have likewise failed. Diagnostic ultrasound examination has also been used; however, its sensitivity is limited. This is partly owing to the high levels of ultrasonic attenuation in the lung tissue, which prevents pulmonary cysts from being detected unless they are close to the organ's perimeter

Treatment

Treatment of hydatid cyst may applied to humans but in cattle, it is frequently difficult. In humans, it occasionally necessitates significant surgery and/or protracted medication therapy, which is summarized in 4 different ways: surgery;

anti-infective drug therapy; and "watch and wait" percutaneous treatment and management of hydatid cysts. The decision must be mostly based on the cyst's ultrasound imaging, using a stage-specific methodology, as well as the available medical infrastructure and human resources. Early diagnosis, and drastic (tumor-like) surgery, followed by anti-infective prophylaxis with albendazole, remain the cornerstones of treatment for alveolar echinococcosis. Radical surgery can be curative if the lesion is contained [12].

Control and Prevention

Dogs should not be fed offal of infected herbivores by keeping them away from abattoirs. Regularly administer praziquantel-containing wormers to dogs (at least once every six weeks). After handling dogs, always wash your hands with soap and water.

Sarcocystosis

Definition

Sarcocystosis is a cyst-forming coccidian parasite disease that affects domestic animals and occasionally humans, clinically characterized by producing moderate respiratory disorders when lung tissue is affected.

Etiological Agent

Sarcocystosis is caused by a coccidian parasite called *Sarcocystis spp*. There are more than 250 different Sarcocystis species known, but some of them have veterinary importance, where these species use cattle and water buffalo as intermediate hosts [18]. Cattle are infected by *Sarcocystis cruzi, Sarcocystis hominis,* and *Sarcocystis hirsuta* [5].

Sarcocysts containing bradyzoites are infectious for the carnivore host. The bradyzoites are not infectious for the intermediate host and sporocysts are not infectious for the definitive host. Thus, the parasite has a strict 2-host life cycle. With few known exceptions, Sarcocystis species are host-specific. "Immunization" using small doses of sporocysts appears to prevent the development or reduce the severity of clinical disease in cattle when challenged with large doses later (premunitive immunity).

Life Cycle

Sarcocystis has an indirect life cycle that often involves two hosts: the intermediate host (the prey), which supports asexual reproduction and the generation of muscle cysts, and the final host (the predator or scavenger), which supports intestinal sexual reproduction and produces adult parasites. The parasite produces oocytes during sexual reproduction (gametogony) in the enterocytes of the small intestine of the definitive host. Both individual sporocysts and sporulated oocysts, which have two sporocysts, can transit in feces. Four sporozoites and a refractile residual body are present in sporocysts. Sporocysts that the intermediate host (for *S. hominis*, cattle) has consumed burst, releasing sporozoites. First-generation schizonts are produced when sporozoites reach the endothelial cells of blood arteries and undergo schizogony. First-generation merozoites enter blood vessels and tiny capillaries. Invading muscle cells, the second-generation merozoites grow into Sarcocystis which contain bradyzoites, the infective stage for the final host. Cattle acquire infection by ingesting feed and water contaminated with sporocysts, sporozoites are liberated from sporocysts and initiate a complex asexual cycle. The sporozoite migrates from the intestine to extra-intestinal tissues. The sporozoite nucleus divides into many lobes, eventually forming merozoites. The multilobed dividing stage is called schizont. The schizonts are formed in a variety of cells, including vascular endothelial cells, somatic cells, and neuronal cells, depending on the species of Sarcocystis. After a few cycles of schizonts, the parasite encysts, usually in a myocyte, first forming metrocytes that give rise to bradyzoites. The encysted stage is called a sarcocyst [4]. A sarcocyst may take a month or more to mature and become infectious for the carnivore host. Mature sarcocysts can contain numerous bradyzoites, and the sarcocysts may grow in size for years to become macroscopic.

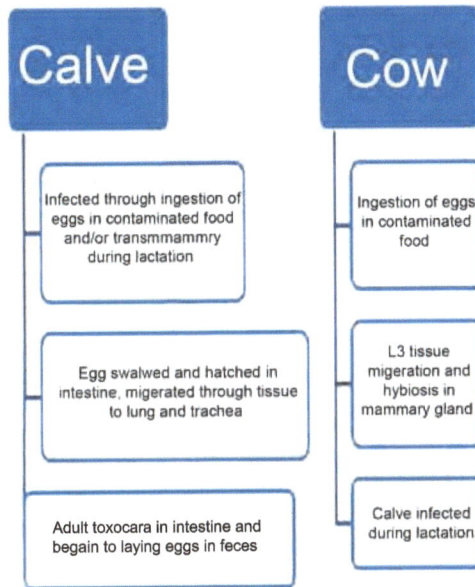

Fig. (6). The life cycle of *Toxocara vitulorum*.

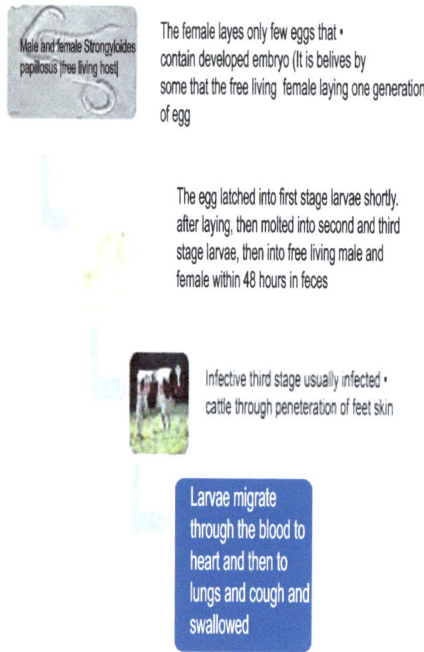

The female layes only few eggs that •
contain developed embryo (It is belives by
some that the free living female laying one generation
of egg

The egg latched into first stage larvae shortly.
after laying, then molted into second and third
stage larvae, then into free living male and
female within 48 hours in feces

Infective third stage usually infected •
cattle through peneteration of feet skin

Larvae migrate
through the blood to
heart and then to
lungs and cough and
swallowed

Fig. (7). Life cycle of *strongyliode. papillouses* in cattle.

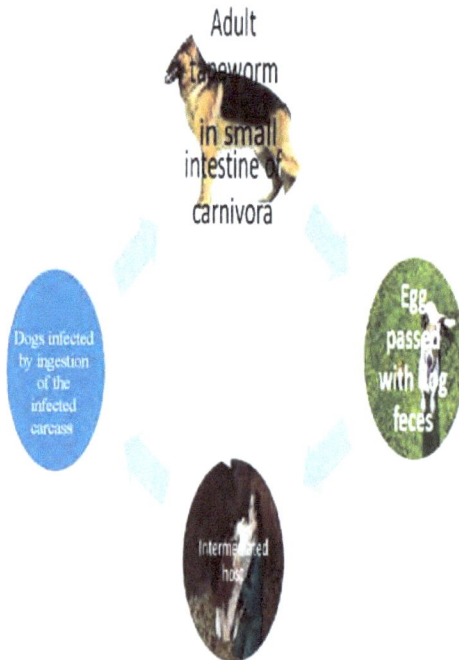

Fig. (8). Life Cycle Echinococcus.

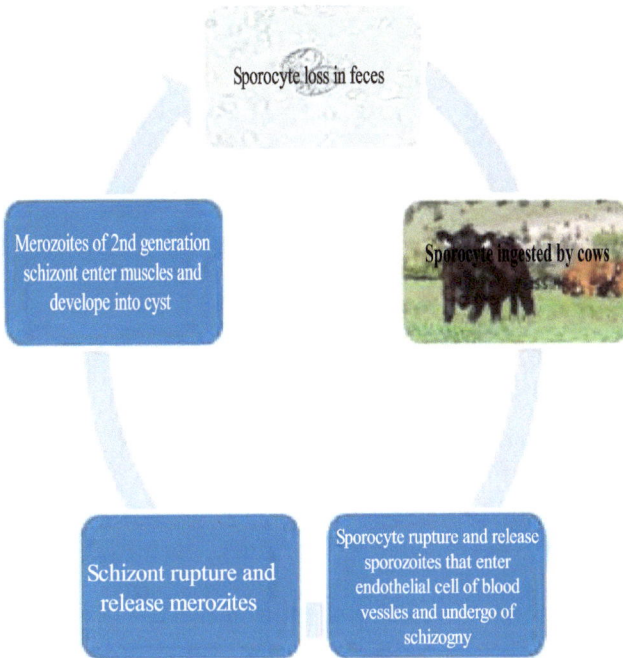

Fig. (9). Life cycle of sarcocyste in cattle.

Clinical Signs

In general, the majority of animals do not show any clinical symptoms, but when lung tissue is impacted, cattle may display loss of appetite, fatigue, diarrhea, weight loss, weakness, muscle twitching, and/or respiratory signs. Sporocyst consumption by pregnant cattle can result in stillbirth or abortion, and those consuming a lot of sporocysts risk dying. The dose of sporocysts and the host's immunological state may be the two most crucial variables in the emergence of clinical illness. Some animals that die of sarcocystosis have indications of internal bleeding. Pathologic changes in the myocardium and skeletal muscles were more pronounced in cows with lymphatic leukemia (Fig. **9**).

Diagnosis

Case history and clinical symptoms were used to make a preliminary diagnosis, but a postmortem investigation allowed for an accurate diagnosis by locating cysts inside the lung tissue, cysts in cattle can have a wide range of shapes and sizes, ranging from microscopic to grossly apparent. Grossly apparent cysts that resemble white rice grains, are long and threadlike, or are even rounded according to the *Sarcocystis* species.

Treatment and Prevention

There is no therapy for sarcocystosis in cattle, and there are no current initiatives to stop sarcocystosis in wild animals that roam freely. To manage this disease in cattle, proper sanitation is crucial. In order to eliminate the germs, meat cannot be frozen before cooking; neither people nor carnivore animals consume raw meat, offal that has suffered severe damage is deemed unfit for ingestion and condemned organs should not be left out for scavengers to eat; instead, they should be buried or burned [7].

CONCLUSION

The cattle pulmonary system can be affected by a variety of parasites. Parasites of the respiratory system of cattle are directly related to asymptomatic to severe infections associated with metastrongyloidea nematodes. Parasites inflicting respiratory infections are emerging in nature. Besides, helminths, mites, and pentastomida are also seen in the respiratory tract. The site of predilection varies from genera and species ranging from nasal cavities, and sinuses to the pulmonary artery, or lung parenchyma. Prevention and proper controlling strategies are needed to combat parasitic infection in the respiratory tract.

REFERENCES

[1]   Agrawal MC, Alwar VS. Nasal schistosomiasis: A review. Helminthological Abstract 1992; 61: 373-84.

[2]   Banerjee PS, Agrawal MC. Epizootiological studies in bovines on fluke infections with special reference to schistosomiasis. Indian Vet J 1992; 69: 215-20.

[3]   Beaver PC, Jung RC, Wayne E. Clinical parasitology. Philadelphia: Lea and Febiger 1984.

[4]   Dimitrijević B, Borozan S, Katić-Radivojević S, Stojanović S. Effects of infection intensity with Strongyloides papillosus and albendazole treatment on development of oxidative/nitrosative stress in sheep. Vet Parasitol 2012; 186(3-4): 364-75.
        [http://dx.doi.org/10.1016/j.vetpar.2011.11.017] [PMID: 22130332]

[5]   Dubey JP, Speer CA, Fayer R. Sarcocystosis of Animals and Man. Boca Raton, Florida: CRC Press Inc. 1989; pp. 113-20.

[6]   Dubey JP, Lindsay DS. Neosporosis, toxoplasmosis, and sarcocystosis in ruminants. Vet Clin North Am Food Anim Pract 2006; 22(3): 645-71.
        [http://dx.doi.org/10.1016/j.cvfa.2006.08.001] [PMID: 17071358]

[7]   Gao JF, Zhao Q, Liu GH, *et al.* Comparative analyses of the complete mitochondrial genomes of the two ruminant hookworms *Bunostomum trigonocephalum* and *Bunostomum phlebotomum*. Gene 2014; 541(2): 92-100.
        [http://dx.doi.org/10.1016/j.gene.2014.03.017] [PMID: 24625354]

[8]   Huang B, Shen J. Classify atlas of parasites for livestock and poultry in China. Beijing: Chinese Press of Agri SciTechnol 2006; pp. 323-4.

[9]   Holzhauer M, Holland WG, Ploeger HW. Preventive vaccination of lactating and pregnant heifers against lungworm: safety and protection in three dairy herds. Tijdschr Diergeneeskd 2005; 130(3): 74-7.

[PMID: 15717444]

[10]   Holzhauer M, van Schaik G, Saatkamp HW, Ploeger HW. Lungworm outbreaks in adult dairy cows: estimating economic losses and lessons to be learned. Vet Rec 2011; 169(19): 494.
[http://dx.doi.org/10.1136/vr.d4736] [PMID: 21856653]

[11]   Jäger M, Gauly M, Bauer C, Failing K, Erhardt G, Zahner H. Endoparasites in calves of beef cattle herds: Management systems dependent and genetic influences. Vet Parasitol 2005; 131(3-4): 173-91.
[http://dx.doi.org/10.1016/j.vetpar.2005.05.014]

[12]   Jiménez AE, Fernández A, Alfaro R, *et al.* A cross-sectional survey of gastrointestinal parasites with dispersal stages in feces from Costa Rican dairy calves. Vet Parasitol 2010; 173(3-4): 236-46.
[http://dx.doi.org/10.1016/j.vetpar.2010.07.013] [PMID: 20810217]

[13]   Kobayashi I, Horii Y. Gastrointestinal motor disturbance in rabbits experimentally infected with *Strongyloides papillosus*. Vet Parasitol 2008; 158(1-2): 67-72.
[http://dx.doi.org/10.1016/j.vetpar.2008.08.017] [PMID: 18845397]

[14]   Kim HY, Lee SM, Joo JE, Na MJ, Ahn MH, Min DY. Human syngamosis: the first case in Korea. Thorax 1998; 53(8): 717-8.
[http://dx.doi.org/10.1136/thx.53.8.717] [PMID: 9828862]

[15]   Laabs EM, Schnieder T, Strube C. *In vitro* studies on the sexual maturation of the bovine lungworm *Dictyocaulus viviparus* during the development of preadult larvae to adult worms. Parasitol Res 2012; 110(3): 1249-59.
[http://dx.doi.org/10.1007/s00436-011-2622-y] [PMID: 21858477]

[16]   Mahieu M, Naves M. Incidence of *Toxocara vitulorum* in Creole calves of Guadeloupe. Trop Anim Health Prod 2008; 40(4): 243-8.
[http://dx.doi.org/10.1007/s11250-007-9094-1] [PMID: 18557186]

[17]   McLeonard C, van Dijk J. Controlling lungworm disease (husk) in dairy cattle. In Pract 2017; 39(9): 408-19.
[http://dx.doi.org/10.1136/inp.j4038]

[18]   Mmbengwa V, Nyhodo B, Myeki L, van Ngethu X, Schalkwyk XH. Communal livestock farming in South Africa: does this farming system create jobs for poverty stricken rural areas. Sylwan 2015; 159: 176-92.

[19]   Nakanishi N, Nakamura Y, Ura S, *et al.* Sudden death of calves by experimental infection with *Strongyloides papillosus*. III. Hematological, biochemical and histological examinations. Vet Parasitol 1993; 47(1-2): 67-76.
[http://dx.doi.org/10.1016/0304-4017(93)90176-N] [PMID: 8493768]

[20]   Qadri K, Ganguly S. Occurrence of Schistosoma nasal infection in crossbred cattle: a case study. IIAOB Journal 2016; 7(7): 10-1.

[21]   Ranjan S, DeLay R. Therapeutic and persistent efficacy of moxidectin 1% non-aqueous injectable formulation against natural and experimentally induced lung and gastrointestinal nematodes in cattle. Vet Parasitol 2004; 120(4): 305-17.
[http://dx.doi.org/10.1016/j.vetpar.2004.01.017] [PMID: 15063941]

[22]   Ravindran R, Kumar A. Nasal schistosomiasis among large ruminants in Wayanad, India. Southeast Asian J Trop Med Public Health 2012; 43(3): 586-8.
[PMID: 23077837]

[23]   Roberts JA, Fernando ST, Sivanathan S. *Toxocara vitulorum* in the milk of buffalo (*Bubalus bubalis*) cows. Res Vet Sci 1990; 49(3): 289-91.
[http://dx.doi.org/10.1016/0034-5288(90)90061-8] [PMID: 2267418]

[24]   Sreeramulu P. Epizootiology of nasal schistosomiasis in bovines in Andhra Pradesh. Indian Vet J 1994; 71(10): 1043-4.

[25]   Sumanth S, D'Souza PE, Jagannath MS. A study of nasal and visceral schistosomiasis in cattle slaughtered at an abattoir in Bangalore, South India Rev Sci Tech off Int Epiz 2004; 23(3): 937-42.

[26]   Taira N, Ura S. Sudden death in calves associated with *Strongyloides papillosus* infection. Vet Parasitol 1991; 39(3-4): 313-9.
[http://dx.doi.org/10.1016/0304-4017(91)90048-Z] [PMID: 1957491]

[27]   Thienpont D, Rochette F, Vanparijs OFJ. diagnosing helminthiasis by carpological examination. Beerse, Belgium: Janssen Research Foundation 1986; 205.

[28]   Ura S, Nakamura Y, Tsuji N, Taira N. Sudden death of calves by experimental infection with *Strongyloides papillosus*. II. Clinical observations and analysis of critical moments of the disease recorded on videotape. Vet Parasitol 1992; 44(1-2): 107-10.
[http://dx.doi.org/10.1016/0304-4017(92)90148-3] [PMID: 1441181]

[29]   Ura S, Taira N, Nakamura Y, Tsuji N, Hirose H. Sudden death of calves by experimental infection with Strongyloides papillosus. IV. Electrocardiographic and pneumographic observations at critical moments of the disease. Vet Parasitol 1993; 47(3-4): 343-7.
[http://dx.doi.org/10.1016/0304-4017(93)90035-L] [PMID: 8333139]

[30]   Van Aken D, Lagapa JT, Dargantes AP, Vercruysse J. *Mammomonogamus laryngeus* (Railliet, 1899) infections in cattle in Mindanao, Philippines. Vet Parasitol 1996; 64(4): 329-32.
[http://dx.doi.org/10.1016/0304-4017(95)00933-7] [PMID: 8893487]

[31]   Wang CR, Gao JF, Zhu XQ, Zhao Q. Characterization of *Bunostomum trigonocephalum* and *Bunostomum phlebotomum* from sheep and cattle by internal transcribed spacers of nuclear ribosomal DNA. Res Vet Sci 2012; 92(1): 99-102.
[http://dx.doi.org/10.1016/j.rvsc.2010.10.024] [PMID: 21094506]

CHAPTER 9

Parasites of Liver and Pancreas

Bhupamani Das[1],*, Ayushi Nair[2], Mayank Prajapati[3] and Pallabi Pathak[4]

[1] *Department of Clinics (Veterinary Parasitology), College of Veterinary Science & Animal Husbandry, Kamdhenu University, Sardarkrushinagar, Gujarat, India*

[2] *College of Veterinary Science & Animal Husbandry, Kamdhenu University, Sardarkrushinagar, Gujarat, India*

[3] *Department of Medicine, College of Veterinary Science & A.H., Kamdhenu University, Sardarkrushinagar, Gujarat, India-385506*

[4] *Lakhimpur College of Veterinary Science, Assam Agricultural University, Joyhing, Lakhimpur, Assam, India*

Abstract: Infestation with parasites is incredibly widespread on a worldwide scale. Nematodes, cestodes, and trematodes are three types of helminths (parasitic worms) that can infect the liver and hepatobiliary systems. The host immunological response to the larvae or adult worms is the main source of morbidity and mortality from these infections. Asymptomatic carriage to cirrhosis and decompensated liver disease are the two extremes of parasitic disease presentations. Improvements in medical therapy, widespread screening and chemoprophylaxis, and the creation of preventative vaccination techniques are the main topics of current basic science and clinical research. This chapter discusses the general morphology, pathology, clinical symptoms, diagnosis, and treatment aspects of liver and pancreas-associated parasites of cattle.

Keywords: Cattle, Control, Disease, Diagnosis, Liver, Parasite, Pancreas.

INTRODUCTION

Food animals have always been the main source of milk and meat. Notwithstanding these, the growth and development of healthy ruminants have not been completely utilised by poorer countries due to obstacles such as famine, bad management, and infections. The liver, the largest organ in the body, carries out several metabolic, excretory, synthetic, detoxifying, and catabolic functions. On the other hand, the pancreas creates and secretes digestive enzymes that support an animal's digestive system as a whole. Diseases, such as pancreatic and liver parasite infections, can have a detrimental impact on animal reproduction

---

** **Corresponding author Bhupamani Das:** Department of Clinics (Veterinary Parasitology), College of Veterinary Science & Animal Husbandry, Kamdhenu University, Sardarkrushinagar, Gujarat, India; E-mail: bhupa67@gmail.com*

Tanmoy Rana (Ed.)

and productivity. Rumination in large, intensive systems makes ruminants more susceptible to parasitic helminths. The usual clinical consequences observed in ruminants are decreased rates of development, reproduction, feed conversion, genetic potential rate, and milk or meat output. The economic consequences of ruminant husbandry include decreased genetic potential rate, feed conversion, development, reproduction, and lower milk or meat output; on the other hand, abnormal signs of the gastrointestinal and cardiovascular systems are frequently observed clinically. Owners of ruminants lose money in the majority of infections and fatalities. Understanding the interplay between nutrition, livestock management, and parasitism is key to limiting economic loss.

Parasites that Directly Affect the Liver and Pancreas

Fasciola gigantica

Introduction

Fasciola gigantica is a well-known parasite of domesticated ruminants that cause major economic losses in some nations' cattle and sheep industries [1]. Clinical symptoms of digestive inefficiency can be seen in both young calves suffering from acute liver disease and older cattle suffering from chronic liver disease [2]. *F.gigantica* metacercariae ingestion by the ultimate host causes excystation and the release of freshly excysted juveniles (NEJs), which burrow through the duodenum wall into the peritoneum (Fig. **1**). They then go to the liver, where they penetrate the liver capsule. After passing through the liver for 11 weeks, the juvenile flukes grow in the bile ducts 12-16 weeks after infection (WPI), when they start laying eggs [3]. The complicated life cycle of *F. gigantica* requires an intermediary host, the family of aquatic snails Lymnaeidae, which reproduces asexually, and an initial vertebrate host, in which the liver flukes reproduce sexually [4, 5].

Morphology

The morphological characteristics and sizes of adult *Fasciola* species differ. *F. gigantica*, which measures 7.5 cm in length and 1.5 cm in breadth (Fig. **2**) [6], is larger than the two enormous leaf-shaped worms. These multiply in the gall bladder and biliary ducts of the main host (Fig. **3**). Although *Fasciola* spp. are hermaphrodites, meaning they may reproduce by self-fertilization, the most frequent method of reproduction is cross-fertilization between two adult flukes, contributing to the gene polymorphism seen in these species [7].

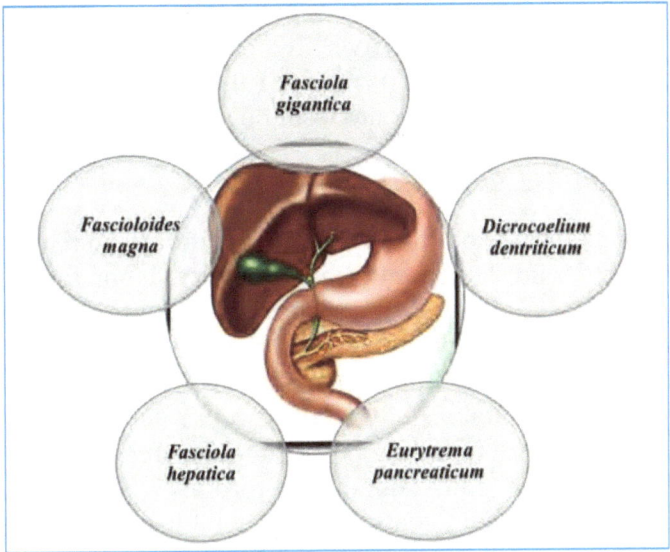

Fig. (1). Parasites that directly affect liver and pancreas of cattle.

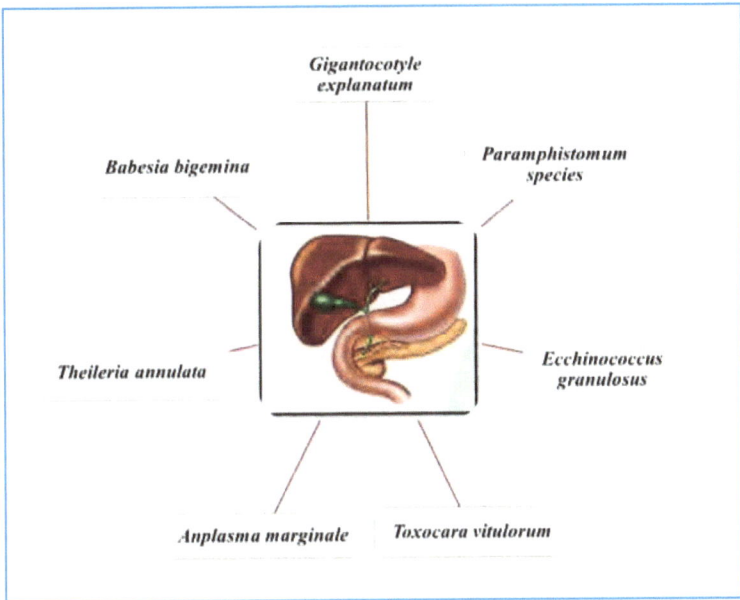

Fig. (2). Parasites that indirectly affect liver and pancreas of cattle.

Lifecycle

The flukes can lay up to 25,000 eggs a day and stay in their host for decades [8]. The intestine releases these eggs, which are then expelled into the surrounding area. After a week of consumption, the parasite passes through the peritoneum and the Glisson's capsule to reach the liver parenchyma. The juvenile fluke grows quickly as it passes through the liver by consuming host tissue cells and eventually blood [9, 10]. These activities are the primary cause of most of the clinical symptoms associated with acute fasciolosis.

Pathogenesis and clinical signs

In domestic ruminants, acute or chronic fasciolosis results in reduced weight gain, decreased milk yield, and decreased female fertility, labor force, and mortality. After a significant but brief intake of metacercariae, acute fasciolosis brought on by juvenile fluke migration appears as an epidemic. A combination of improper fluke management strategies and particular seasonal and meteorological variables sometimes lead to fluke intake. It typically occurs when overcrowding and/or drought drive cattle to graze in highly polluted moist areas [11]. Acute fasciolosis can cause gastrointestinal pain and discomfort as well as jaundice in some animals, especially in sheep and goats, but in other animals, the disease may cause no clinical symptoms before the animal dies. Sometimes the liver capsule bursts open, allowing fluid to enter the peritoneal cavity and potentially fatal peritonitis. The most common kind of illness in cattle is the chronic one, which arises from a few flukes that eventually infect the bile duct. The result is a chronic wasting disease because liver flukes are acquired gradually over several months or even years. The symptoms of chronic fasciolosis might vary based on when the parasite enters the hepatic bile duct, but they usually include diarrhea, constipation, bottle jaw, weight loss, and anemia. Fluke infection can diminish milk production and fertility and predispose to numerous disorders due to reduced liver function. Animals affected find it difficult to travel.

Diagnosis and treatment

Based on grazing history, clinical symptom observations, past knowledge of the disease's frequency in a particular habitat, and seasonal incidence, a tentative diagnosis of fasciolosis can be established. Conversely, the presence of immature and adult flukes in the liver, postmortem examination of sick animals, and the presence of Fasciola eggs in faeces are the basis for confirming the diagnosis. Animals treated with flukicides—compounds harmful to flukes such as triclabendazole and bithionol—are commonly employed.

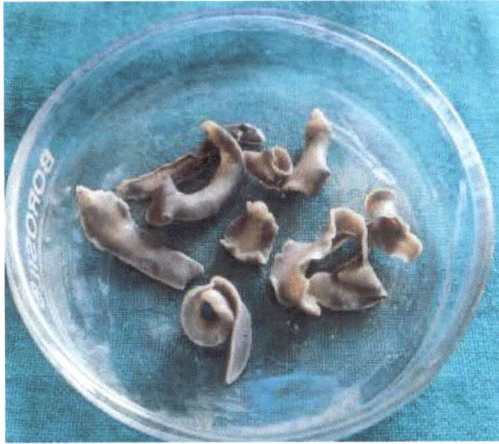

Fig. (3). *Fasciola gigantica* collected from the liver of cattle.

Fasciola hepatica

Introduction

One of the most significant flukes that affect domestic ruminants globally is *fasciola hepatica*, which causes liver fluke illness (liver rot, fascioliasis). Cattle are more susceptible to chronic liver fluke illness, which is rarely deadly. Sheep and camels are more susceptible to acute and subacute disease, which frequently results in death. *F. hepatica* is a leaf-shaped worm that grows in the liver of many animals, primarily cattle and sheep and is between 2 and 4 cm (0.8 and 1.6 inches) long. Cattle served as the definitive host for *Fasciola hepatica*, while the snail served as the intermediate host and the human served as an unintentional host [12, 13]. Rarely are these parasites identified at ectopic areas within the host body; instead, they typically reside in the hepatobiliary system of the affected animal [14].

Morphology

Fasciola hepatica is one of the world's largest flukes, measuring 30 mm in length and 13 mm in width. It is leaf-shaped, with a pointed rear (posteriorly) and a wide front (anteriorly). The oral sucker is a small but forceful projection at the anterior end of a cone-shaped projection. The acetabulum, which is placed anteriorly, is a larger sucker than the oral sucker.

Lifecycle

Miracidia develop in as short as 9-10 days after eggs are released in the faeces (at 22-26°C [71.6-78.8°F]; little development takes place below 10°C [50°F], even though eggs can last at least two years. Only in water do eggs hatch, and miracidia only last for around three hours. *Lymnaeid* snails are infected by miracidia, which cause asexual sporocysts, rediae, daughter rediae, and cercariae phases of development and multiplication. Cercariae arise from snails, encyst on aquatic plants, and develop into metacercariae after 6-7 weeks (or longer if temperatures are low). By hibernating in the winter, infected snails can prolong the developmental phase. Infection of the definitive host by *F. hepatica* occurs following the consumption of metacercariae, the infective stage, distributed on pasture. Once the metacercariae have made their way into the small intestine, NEJs (newly excysted juveniles) hatch and move through the peritoneum for 4-6 days (in the early stages of illness) until they recover and reach the liver capsule. Juvenile flukes begin in the liver migrating and eating throughout the liver parenchyma. In this phase, haemorrhagic tracts and the early phases of tissue healing are visible. The flukes appear eight to ten weeks later and reach the bile ducts, where they develop and begin egg-laying.

Pathogenesis and clinical signs

Fascioliasis is caused by an infection of the liver fluke *Fasciola hepatica*, which is spread through eating contaminated watercress or other water plants. Abdominal pain and hepatomegaly are two clinical symptoms.

Diagnosis and treatment

Triclabendazole has been the drug of choice for the treatment of *F. hepatica* infection for several decades because, unlike other flukicides, it may target early immature, immature, and mature flukes. Nonetheless, the use of this medicine in dairy cattle is limited in some nations. Furthermore, there is an increase in triclabendazole-resistant liver fluke populations [15], which complicates the control of fasciolosis in farmed ruminants.

Fascioloides magna

Introduction

The trematode *Fascioloides magna*, often known as the huge liver fluke of ungulates, is found around the world, including some regions of Canada. It predominantly parasitizes free-ranging ungulates, notably elk, caribou, and white-tailed and mule deer in Canada (definitive hosts), but it can also infect cattle (referred to as "dead-end" hosts) and sheep (referred to as "aberrant" hosts) on occasion. A snail serves as an intermediary host during the indirect life cycle, which is essentially the same as that of *Fasciola hepatica*. Metacercariae found on aquatic plants are consumed to infect the mammalian hosts. If cattle and sheep live in the same habitat as infected species, they can contract the parasite, however, the infection only very rarely manifests in these domestic hosts, associated with the broad and a typical migrations of sheep, morbidity and mortality in sheep. The vast and abnormal movements of the immature flukes have been linked to sheep morbidity and mortality. When pre-adult or adult parasites are trapped in fibrous-walled cysts in the liver parenchyma, cattle are frequently more tolerant of infection. *F. magna* in cattle is frequently a byproduct of slaughter in Canada, despite the fact that nothing is known about the consequences the flukes might have on live cattle during production. There is no evidence that *Fascioloides magna* is zoonotic [16].

Morphology

F. magna is an oval, up to 100 mm long, 2-4.5 mm thick, and 11-26 mm wide species that differ from other *Fasciola* spp. by its size and absence of an anterior projecting cone. White-tailed deer, elk, and caribou are the reservoir hosts in the US and Canada, whereas red deer and fallow deer are the reservoir hosts in Europe, where it has been imported. It is present in both domestic and wild ruminants.

Lifecycle

The life cycle is similar to that of *Fasciola* spp., with the prepatent period being 30 weeks long and a 7-month lifespan for the complete cycle. Although flukes can mature in cattle, this rarely happens because of the powerful encapsulation response that creates a closed cyst.

Pathogenesis and clinical signs

The appropriateness of the host species and the number of flukes have an impact on the pathology and any clinical symptoms linked to *F. magna*. The adult flukes dwell singly or in pairs in thin-walled cysts in the liver parenchyma of the "normal" definitive hosts. These cysts cause a localised inflammatory response, which is occasionally worsened by pressure atrophy of the surrounding tissues. The inflammation frequently prevents these cysts from draining properly, causing them to fill with a black fluid that contains flukes and eggs. Hepatic fibrosis can be brought on by persistent infections. The parasites are found as thick-walled cysts in the hepatic parenchyma of "dead-end" hosts, such as cattle, along with black, viscous fluid. Rarely do these cysts communicate with the biliary system, and rarely are eggs discovered in the faeces [16]. The risk of infection is modest, and the main losses are liver damage and, albeit rarely, death. Encapsulations do not take place in sheep and goats, and the parasites travel throughout the liver and other organs, wreaking havoc. A tiny number of parasites can kill because they migrate widely. Alpacas and llamas do not frequently develop *F. magna* infection, and when they do, their immune systems react similarly to those of cattle. When parasites infect cervids, there is little tissue reaction and the cysts are made of thin, fibrous tissue and connect to the bile ducts. Histological examination of diseased livers reveals dark, sinuous pathways created by the migration of immature flukes in all species.

Diagnosis and treatment

F. magna eggs resemble those of *Fasciola hepatica* eggs, but faecal sedimentation is of limited utility because eggs are typically not passed by cattle, sheep, alpacas, or llamas. For a certain diagnosis, the parasites must be recovered during necropsy. The possibility of *F. magna* illness should be considered when domestic ruminants and cervids graze in the same area. Cattle might get mixed infections of *F. hepatica*. Rafoxanide has been effective in treating naturally occurring infections in cattle. The best course of action is to avoid infections because no medication is 100% successful, and treatment should begin 8-10 weeks after the height of snail activity. Cervids are necessary for the completion of the life cycle; control may be achieved if they are kept out of places where cattle and sheep graze. The other techniques of control are the same as for *F. hepatica* [16].

Dicrocoelium dentriticum

Introduction

The trematode *Dicrocoelium dendriticum*, often known as the lancet fluke or lancet fluke, is a common ruminant parasite, however, humans can be unintentional final hosts. A zoonotic parasite called *Dicrocoelium dendriticum* infects ruminants and causes liver fluke disease. It is widespread throughout the world [17 - 19]. Dicrocoeliasis is a parasite illness that has been detected in America, Asia, North Africa, and Europe. Weight loss, growth delay, anaemia, digestive problems, edema, decreased milk production, and costs associated with anthelminthic treatment are typical symptoms of infection in ruminants and, rarely, humans [20 - 23]. The consumption of raw or undercooked diseased liver may cause fictitious infections [24].

Morphology

The lancet liver fluke is a flat, transparent, spindle-shaped parasite. The oral and ventral suckers are similar. The ventral sucker is found in the worm's first third. The gut does not stretch all the way to the fluke's tail. The testes are clearly seen in the fluke's front section. They are found caudal to the ventral sucker, between the caecal branches. The ovary is near to the midline and caudal to them. The genital pore is situated directly in front of the ventral sucker. The vitellar glands are clearly visible at the lateral borders, posterior to the testes.

Lifeycle

D. dendriticum inhabits the bile ducts, canaliculi, and gallbladder of its hosts (cows, sheep, goats, and pigs) in the adult stage [25 - 27]. The first intermediate host in the life cycle of this parasite, which resides in the liver of its definitive host, is a gastropod snail, and the second intermediate hosts are ants. The parasite lives in its larval stages as sporocysts and cercariae in the hepatopancreas of terrestrial snails and as metacercariae in the abdomen and brain of ants (the second intermediate host). The parasite has a slight host specialisation, with a preference for ruminants, which can be considered the real host of origin, primarily sheep and goats, and secondly large ruminants such as cattle [28]. The majority of infections, particularly in cows, are asymptomatic, but the effect on the liver is dependent on the number of flukes and the duration of infection. Because the fluke migrates up the biliary duct but does not enter the gut wall or liver tissue, lengthy infections can result in bile duct hypertrophy and liver lesions even in the absence of symptoms, While *D. dendriticum* infections are normally asymptomatic, certain animals may develop anaemia, edema, emaciation, and liver cirrhosis. The detection of *D. dendriticum* flukes is mostly based on the recovery of adults in the liver during necropsy or the detection of eggs in animal faeces [29]. *D. dendriticum*, which can be overlooked in organ aspects due to its morphologically small size, causes both yield loss in live animals and liver destruction due to the damage it causes in the liver, and infection with this parasite in animals can cause disturbances in the body's natural chemistry.

Pathogenesis and clinical signs

Pathological changes in the liver caused by heavy infections include thickened main hepatic ducts with the enlargement of their mucosa, glandular proliferation, increase in connective and muscle tissue, cellular infiltration, and proliferation of small bile ducts [30, 31]. The small liver fluke's buccal stilets may irritate the bile duct surfaces, producing proliferation and alterations in the septal bile ducts of the lobular hepatic margins. Fibrosis and cirrhosis of the parenchyma have been documented in patients with long-term infection [30].

Diagnosis and treatment

The eggs of *D. dendriticum* are very tiny (40 25 mcm), asymmetrical, and yellowish-brown and contain a miracidium. To find *D dendriticum*, faecal flotation with a solution of high specific gravity (1.30-1.45) is advised. Albendazole at 15-20 mg/kg in a single dose or two doses of 7.5 mg/kg on subsequent days, or netobimin at 20 mg/kg, are effective *D. dendriticum* anthelmintic therapies (>90% decrease) in both cattle and sheep.

Eurytrema pancreaticum

Introduction

Eurytrema spp. is a prominent trematode pancreatic fluke that causes significant economic losses in ruminants. Eurytrematosis is a disease caused by *Eurytrema spp.* infection. The parasite stages of *Eurytrema spp.* have a normal tropism (predilection site) in the biliary or pancreatic duct of ruminants.

Morphology

Pancreatic flukes are 8-16 mm in length and 6 mm wide, with a thick body. In Madagascar, Europe, Asia, and South America (Brazil), they are parasites of the pancreatic ducts and, on rare occasions, the bile ducts of sheep, pigs, goats, buffalo, and cattle. The most significant species, *Eurytrema pancreaticum*, is a frequent parasite of ruminants and other herbivores in Asia and South America. It has also been found in Madagascar and Russia. *E. pancreaticum* infection can be detrimental to animal health, cause clinical and subclinical disorders, result in significant financial losses, increase medical expenses, and reduce overall production [32], it might be connected with animal deaths and decreased performance because of chronic pancreatitis [33]. *Eurytrema* spp. causes young animal growth retardation, progressive weakness, lower weight increases, feed conversion, malnutrition, and decreased milk supply. *Eurytrema spp.* was thought to be the most common fluke in ruminants. *E. pancreaticum* is a well-known internal parasite helminth found in the pancreas of cattle [34].

Lifecycle

The earliest intermediate hosts are terrestrial snails (*Bradybaena* spp.), then the cercariae are released onto herbage and consumed by grasshoppers (*Conocephalus* spp.) or tree crickets (*Oecanthus* spp.) After the animal consumes a metacercariae-infected grasshopper, the young flukes excyst in the duodenum and move to the pancreatic duct, where they mature. Domestic ruminants are typically infected by grazing on the second intermediate host carrying metacercariae. Domestic ruminants are typically infected by grazing on the second intermediate host carrying metacercariae. The ruminants could only consume the infected intermediate hosts since the fluke-infected grasshoppers were paralysed, feeble, and unable to jump away. When a cow consumes grasshoppers, metacercariae is established in the small intestine and pierce the wall. The fluke travels from the sheep's small intestine to the pancreas *via* the peritoneum. The immature fluke will travel through the pancreatic tissue before entering the biliary or pancreatic duct and maturing into a reproducing adult [32, 35].

Pathogenesis and clinical signs

According to a study [32], *Eurytrema spp.* fluke was detected in 92% of dead cattle. A study examined the eggs and miracidia of *E. coelomaticum* recovered from the pancreas of naturally infected calves [36]. Eurytrematosis not only reduces ruminant output, but it also requires public health care as a zoonosis. *E. pancreaticum* unintentionally infects cats as well as humans under these circumstances. Another study described a fluke found in stray cats, *Felis catus*, in Korea [37]. Some authors described a previous research of *E. pancreaticum* infection in which 15 mature flukes were detected in the pancreatic ducts of a 70-year-old Japanese woman in Fukuoka Prefecture, Japan [38].

Diagnosis and treatment

The distinctive eggs are found in the faeces and used to make the diagnosis. Treatment with albendazole (7.5 mg/kg for sheep and 10 mg/kg for cattle) or praziquantel (20 mg/kg, for 2 days) has allegedly been successful.

Parasites that Indirectly affect the Liver and Pancreas

Schistosoma spindale

Introduction

A species of digenetic trematode belonging to the Schistosomatidae family is called *Schistosoma spindale*. Visceral schistosomiasis is caused by *Schistosoma spindale*, which is present in the mesenteric veins of ruminants [39]. Bovine schistosomiasis is a trematode infection caused by the genus *Schistosoma* in cattle. *Schistosoma bovis* is found only in Ethiopia's northern, southwestern, eastern, and central regions. *Schistosoma bovis* causes a disease characterised by liver damage, rough coat, pale mucosa, severe emaciation, and decreased reproductive capacity, resulting in a significant economic downturn and public health crisis [40].

Morphology

There is bilateral symmetry in the adult worms. To adhere to objects and stabilise themselves, they have oral and ventral suckers. Male worms are fairly thick and range in length from 6 to 2.2 centimetres. The 1.2-2.6 centimeter-long female spends the majority of the life cycle in a structure known as a gynecophoral canal that runs the length of the animal's body. In order to go to the venules lining the colon or bladder to lay her eggs, the thinner female splits off from her mate.

Pathogenesis and Clinical Signs

In animals, it is characterised by regular diarrhoea with blood and mucous, colic, weight loss, and weakness [41, 42]. Ruminant liver and intestines were shown to have egg granulomas [43]. This disease is often chronic in character, and the majority of animals' symptoms are insufficient to distinguish it from other debilitating illnesses [44]. *Schistosoma spindale* lives in the mesenteric veins, and can cause diarrhoea (occasionally with blood traces and mucoserous discharge), anaemia, edema, excessive thirst, anorexia, and emaciation [45, 46]. The routine diagnosis of visceral schistosomiasis is primarily based on clinical symptoms and faecal investigation for parasite eggs. A freshwater snail called *Indoplanorbis exustus* serves as the first intermediate host for *Schistosoma spindale* and the other two *Schistosoma* species on the Indian subcontinent, where it may be the only naturally occurring host, Ruminants are *Schistosoma spindale's* (mostly) definitive hosts, and *Schistosoma spindale* infects them with intestinal schistosomiasis [47].

Lifecycle

Adult schistosomes are obligatory parasites of the vertebrate blood vascular system. Schistosomes are dioecious (unisexual) worms that have an indirect lifecycle, with water snails belonging to the genera *Bullinus* and *Planorbis* acting as intermediary hosts [48]. The disease's infective stage is matured cercaria, which after leaving the snail infects the final host by skin or mucus membrane penetration [49]. Visceral Schistosomes mature in the portal veins of the liver, mate, and migrate to the mesenteric veins, where egg production begins [50]. In the mesenteric vein, the female inserts her tail into the venule. The eggs are assisted in their penetration of the venule endothelium by their spines and proteolytic enzymes released by the unhatched miracidia [51]. The eggs laid by the female worm enter the vein wall and move to the intestinal lumen or the nasal cavity. (*S. nasale*) of the host are retained inside the body, and it is the retained eggs and larvae that cause the disease. Their products are responsible for the majority of Schistosomosis morbidity [52].

Diagnosis and treatment

The presence and identification of eggs in the affected animal's faeces should be used to confirm the diagnosis. Microscopic inspection of scrapings of the intestinal mucosa or of crushed liver tissue (both looking for eggs) may be easier at necropsy than macroscopic examination of the mesenteric veins for the presence of adult worms. In order to effectively treat schistosomiasis in cattle, praziquantel (25 mg/kg, PO, in water buffalo; 30 mg/kg, PO, in cattle) may need to be administered twice, spaced 3-5 weeks apart.

Gigantocotyle explanatum

Introduction

Gigantocotyle explanatum is a widespread digenetic trematode parasite that lives in the liver, bile duct, and gallbladder of domesticated animals. Although the adult parasite is non-pathogenic, its immature forms cause severe pathological illnesses [53]. *G. explanatum* is a prevalent parasite that is only found in Asian countries [54]. Pathologies caused by *G. expalanatum* include connective tissue proliferation, haemorrhage, hypertrophy, and hyperplasia in the bile duct, compromising the health and productivity of livestock animals [55]. Freshwater snails, primarily *Gyraulus convexiusculus*, act as intermediate hosts for *G. explanatum* [56]. Buffalo bile duct parasites develop plugs on the luminal surface *via* their acetabulum. The bile duct has histopathological alterations near the site of fluke attachment [53]. Secondary parasitic infections lower milk production, impair product quality and quantity and raise mortality rates [39, 57].

Morphology

A fleshy body with a massive ventral sucker in the back. The lobed testes are arranged diagonally (Fig. **4**). The ovary is located above the ventral sucker, behind the testes. Unbranched caeca in the intestines.

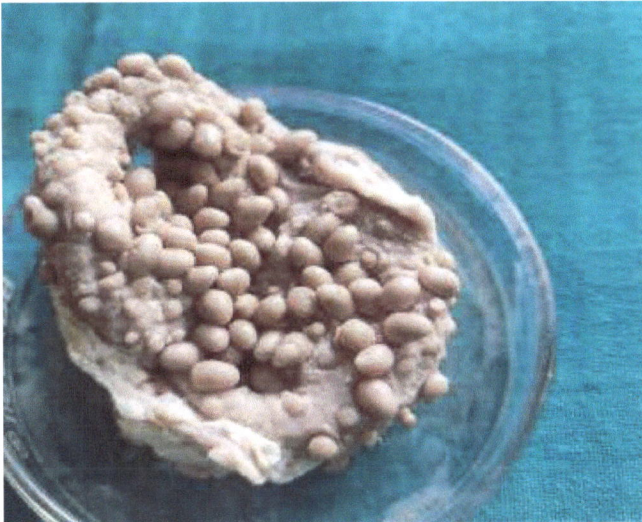

Fig. (**4**). *Gigantocotyle explanatum* from hepatobiliary system of cattle.

Lifecycle

The free-swimming larva called miracidium hatches out of the egg and penetrates the snails of the particular genus, where it undergoes a series of larval development, changing to sporocyst, redia, daughter redia, and ultimately cercaria. The parasite requires a snail as an intermediate host belonging to the genus *Lymnea*. The cercariae exit the snail and swim freely before becoming encrusted on plants and developing into metacercaria, where they remain until being consumed by the final host. The cyst wall breaks down in the buffalo intestine, allowing the juvenile trematodes to escape. The trematode enters the peritoneum through the intestinal wall, travels to the surface of the liver, and then enters and passes through the bile ducts.

Pathogenesis and clinical signs

Pathologies brought on by *G. expalanatum* include connective tissue proliferation, haemorrhage, hypertrophy, and hyperplasia in the bile duct, which have an impact on livestock animals' health and productivity. Amphistomes form "granulomatous nodules" at attachment sites that are heavily populated with inflammatory cells. Serum biochemical assays, including serum enzymes, can be used to assess the severity of the hepatic injury, the degree of cholestasis, and the liver's ability to synthesize substances.

Diagnosis and treatment

Normal methods for diagnosing *G. explanatum* include identifying worms in the liver during a post-mortem examination or performing a routine microscopic inspection of eggs discharged in faeces [58].

Paramphistomum spp.

Introduction

Paramphistomum is a genus of parasitic flatworms of the trematode family. It includes flukes, which mostly parasitize livestock ruminants, and some wild animals. They are the cause of the deadly disease paramphistomiasis, also known as amphistomosis, which primarily affects cattle and sheep [59]. These parasites' intermediate hosts are freshwater snails from the genera *Lymnae, Planorbis, Bulinus, and Fussaria* [39]. Paramphistomosis is found throughout the world's subtropical and tropical regions. The disease is a huge danger to the livestock sector, causing significant economic losses due to stunted growth, low food conversion rates, poor milk, meat, and wool production, and poor hide and skin quality [60 - 63]. Adult paramphistomes, the major parasites of the rumen and reticulum of ruminants, cause localised loss of rumen papillae, whereas juvenile flukes penetrate the mucosa of the duodenum and upper ileum to plug feed, causing necrosis and haemorrhagic ulcerations, known as duodenitis, which leads to severe pathological changes [39, 64]. Death from immature paramphistomes is extremely common, with estimates ranging from 80-90% in domesticated ruminants [65 - 67].

Lifecycle

Miracidia hatch in the water and infect planorbid or bulinid snails, with the snail shedding cercariae that encyst on the herbage, with the snail shedding cercariae that encyst on the herbage. The immature flukes excyst and reside in the small intestine for 3-6 weeks before migrating forward through the reticulum to the rumen in the ruminant host. 7-14 weeks after infection, eggs are produced. Sheep and calves that are infected can readily be identified by their symptoms, which include extreme anorexia, ineffective digestion, and frugal behavior. Fetid diarrhea is a clear sign that fluid faeces need to be checked for young flukes [68].

Pathogenesis and Clinical Signs

In livestock mammals, parasitic enteritis and anaemia generate significant output and economic losses. Immature flukes cause pathological signs. When the immature flukes begin to congregate in the intestine, it causes watery and fetid diarrhoea that is frequently associated with substantial mortality (up to 80-90%) in ruminants. At any given time, up to 30,000 flukes may aggregate and attack the duodenal mucosa, causing acute enteritis. Adult flukes are relatively harmless. Swelling, haemorrhage, discoloration, necrosis, bile duct hyperplasia, and fibrosis are all signs of significant liver tissue injury [69].

Diagnosis and Treatment

The huge, transparent, operculated eggs are easily identified; however, there may be no eggs in the faeces in acute paramphistomiasis. Fluid faeces examination may reveal juvenile flukes, many of which are passed in these circumstances. A necropsy is routinely used to make a diagnosis. In paramphistomiasis, oxyclozanide (20 mg/kg, repeated after 72 hours) appears to be helpful.

Echinococcus granulosus

Introduction

The tape worm parasite *Echinococcus granulosus* causes illnesses known by various names, including cystic hydatidosis, cystic echinococcosis (CE), and cystic hydatid sickness. There is evidence of the zoonosis known as CE occurring on each of the seven continents. The regions with the highest prevalence of cystic hydatid disease were those in South America, Eastern Europe, the Middle East, North Africa, and the Far East [70].

Morphology

The little tapeworm *E. granulosus* can grow to be between 3 and 6 mm long. It is made up of a neck, scolex, and three or four segments. On its rostellum, the scolex has four suckers and two rows of thirty to thirty-six hooks. The neck is described as broad and short. The segment in front is first immature then developed, and finally, if it is there, the third or fourth segment is a gravid segment. A gravid proglottid carries 823 eggs on average. In terms of length and width, the terminal segment is the longest.

Lifecycle

E. granulosus, sometimes known as the tapeworm, is a common cestode. The small intestine of canids, which are the ultimate host, is where adult worms are discovered. Humans are among the animals (intermediate hosts) whose tissues contain hydatid larvae. "Cystic echinococcosis" or "hydatidosis," an infection with the parasite's larval stage in the intermediate host, results in substantial financial losses in cattle production and a high burden of disease in people. Although the parasite is widespread throughout the world, it is more prevalent in areas where cattle breeding is done [71]. It spreads naturally between cattle, which are intermediate hosts infected by parasite eggs, and canids, definitive hosts with adult cestodes in the intestine and feces shedding parasite eggs, where the larval stage (metacestode) develops in the form of fluid-filled cysts in the liver, lungs, and other organs. Through the consumption of parasite cysts found in infected tissues of deceased animals, the infection is transferred to the definitive hosts.

Pathogenesis and clinical signs

Cattle with hydatid cysts often have fluid-filled structures, especially in the liver. These parasite-caused cysts began as fibrous capsules in the liver. Fibrogenesis is the host immune response of the liver to these parasites. One important kind of fibrogenic cell is the hepatic stellate cell (HSC), also called vitamin A-storing cells and found in the perisinusoidal area. The majority of hydatid disease losses are monetary in nature; these can be attributed to the harm done to domestic animals as well as potential prohibitions on the import and export of animals and their byproducts, especially from endemic areas [72, 73].

Diagnosis and treatment

The diagnosis of cystic echinococcosis (CE) in livestock is still mostly dependent on post-mortem inspection due to the lack of a sufficiently sensitive and specific pre-mortem practical alternative offered by current serodiagnostics, despite the disease's relatively low diagnostic sensitivity, especially in early infections. Grazing animals with hydatid cysts are not treated. The hearts, livers, and lungs are condemned if cysts are found during the killing.

Toxocara vitulorum

Introduction

Toxocara vitulorum is a nematode (roundworm) found predominantly in tropical and subtropical areas around the world [74]. The parasite undergoes arrested development in the somatic tissues of adult cattle before being transmitted through the intra-mammary route to nursing calves. Adult cattle are typically not pathogenic for the disease. However, if left untreated, it can be seriously detrimental to calves in tropical and subtropical areas with high death rates.

Morphology

Its adults are 15-30 cm long and leave leftovers in the host's small intestines [75, 76]. It is usually transferred transplacentally and *via* colostrum to calves, with water or feed infection being extremely rare [77 - 79]. *T. vitulorum* causes illness and mortality in calves, which become infected early after birth by consuming larvae secreted in colostrum and milk [80].

Lifecycle

Calves started to discharge eggs in their faeces between the ages of 16 and 23 days. The eggs released in faeces contain L1 larvae, which mature into L3 larvae in 2-4 weeks. L3-containing eggs do not hatch in the environment until they are consumed [75]. Larvae consumed by calves mature into adults in 3-4 weeks and begin shedding eggs in their faeces [81]. The mature worms of *T. vitulorum* are mostly found in suckling calves, which is a remarkable finding. Despite being the source of infection for the calves, the dam does not shed *T. vitulorum* eggs. This is because the larvae in the dam do not mature into adults and stay in the third stage. When a cow is pregnant, the larvae travel from the liver to the mammary gland and, just before parturition, to the milk, where they infect the calf [75].

Pathogenesis and clinical signs

T. vitulorum is one of the most dangerous parasites of young ruminants since it only lives in buffalo and bovine calves. Every day, an adult female *T. vitulorum* produces thousands of eggs. Egg fecundity ranges between 8000 and 100,000 eggs per gram of faeces every day [75, 82]. These eggs move through the faeces and, given favourable conditions such as enough moisture and a warm temperature, become infective in two to three weeks. Eggs' thick protective shell gives resistance to harsh environmental conditions such as chemical and physical assault, allowing eggs to remain infectious for many years [83]. As a consequence, infective eggs are abundant in pastures and other areas contaminated with calf faeces. When an infective stage egg is consumed by a host, the larvae hatch in the intestinal tract and move to the liver, lungs, and other tissues [84]. *T. vitulorum* larvae migrate, causing significant harm to several organs, particularly the liver and intestine. It is responsible for 11 to 50% of cow and buffalo calf mortality [85, 86]. Anorexia, stomach pain, diarrhoea or constipation, dehydration, weight loss or poor weight gain, and a butyric odour on the breath are common clinical findings in infected calves [82].

Diagnosis and treatment

Piperazine [87], pyrantel, febantel, and oxfendazole [75] are effective treatments for adult stage *T. vitulorum*. *T. vitulorum* third-stage larvae in the intestine can be treated with pyrantel and levamisole [75].

Toxoplasma gondii

Introduction

Almost all warm-blooded species, including livestock, are susceptible to infection by the zoonotic apicomplexan parasite *Toxoplasma gondii* [89, 90]. The definitive hosts of *T. gondii* are domestic cats and other felids. This suggests that the parasite can only complete its sexual life cycle in these species, as evidenced by the fact that only the faeces of infected felids can produce environmentally resistant oocysts [89]. The parasite infects these hosts *via* contaminated meat, milk, and water. Such contamination can occur with oocyst-contaminated consumables, which is a common pathway for farm animal contamination [88, 89].

Morphology

The trophozoites of *Toxoplasma gondii* measure 4-8 μm in length and 2-3 μm in width. They have a big nucleus, a blunt posterior end, and tapering anterior and posterior ends.

Lifecycle

Oocysts play an important role in the life cycle of *T. gondii*. They become infective to a wide range of warm-blooded intermediate hosts (livestock, synanthropic and wild dwelling animals such as rodents or birds, poultry, or people) after one to a few days of maturation (sporulation) in the environment [75 - 77]. In addition to oocysts, *T. gondii* has two other infective stages: tachyzoites and bradyzoites, the latter of which is seen in tissue cysts. Tachyzoites infiltrate and multiply in host cells after infection. This replication occurs solely within the parasite's parasitophorous vacuoles [90].

Pathogenesis and clinical signs

T. gondii was isolated from cattle for the first time in 1953, and cattle are now considered an intermediate host [91]. *T. gondii* infection in cattle can result in abortion, behavioural problems, and even death [92 - 94]. *T. gondii* infection in ruminants is a leading cause of miscarriages and stillbirths [95], causing enormous economic losses in the global sheep, goat, and cattle industries [96, 97]. It causes a wide range of symptoms, both non-specific (fever and dyspnea) and specific (fever, depression, lethargy, vomiting, diarrhoea, chorioretinitis, and lymphadenopathy) [98, 99].

Diagnosis and treatment

Toxoplasmosis is diagnosed by biologic, serologic, or histologic approaches or a combination of these methods. Toxoplasmosis clinical symptoms are nonspecific and insufficient to make a conclusive diagnosis. Indirect hemagglutination assay, indirect fluorescent antibody assay, latex agglutination test, or ELISA testing can be used to make an antemortem diagnosis. Toxoplasmosis treatment is rarely necessary. Sulfadiazine (15-25 mg/kg, PO, every 12 hours for 4 weeks) and pyrimethamine (0.44 mg/kg, PO, every 12 hours for 4 weeks) work synergistically to treat toxoplasmosis and are frequently used.

Babesia bigemina

Introduction

Babesiosis in cattle caused by intraerythrocytic hemoprotozoa *Babesia bigemina* is a tick-borne illness that affects cattle in tropical and subtropical Africa, Australia, North America, and Asia, including India. Major hosts and reservoirs for *B. bigemina* are cattle. It can grow to a size of up to two-thirds of the blood cell's diameter and is found in blood cells. It is spread by the common in the tropics *Boophilus* ticks.

Morphology

Babesia bigemina, a huge form measuring 4.5 μm × 2.0 μm. The parasites have the typical shape of a pear. Other shapes include oval, irregularly shaped, and round (2-3 μm in diameter).

Lifecycle

In the tick, the parasite goes through gamogony and sporogony in addition to merogony in the bovine. When an infected tick feeds on a bovine's blood, sporozoites are injected into the bloodstream. These sporozoites then invade erythrocytes and differentiate into trophozoites (T), which asexually divide into typically two merozoites. Eventually, merozoites leave erythrocytes and invade new ones to continue their replication cycle. Some merozoites stop dividing and change into gamonts or pre-gametocytes, which are then ingested by a tick. In the tick's gut, these pre-gametocytes then differentiate into gametes, also referred to as ray bodies which unite to produce a diploid zygote. Zygotes go through meiosis and produce motile haploid kinetes. These kinetes access the hemolymph, multiply through sporogony, and invade and replicate in a variety of tick organs, including the ovaries and eggs. In the salivary glands of the subsequent generation of larvae, kinetes change into sporozoites (transovarial transmission).

Pathogenesis and clinical signs

The erythrocyte stage of *B. bigemina* results in severe clinical symptoms in the infected cattle such as fever, anemia and haemoglobinuria [100]. Haemolytic anaemia, produced by the destruction and evacuation of parasitized and non-parasitized erythrocytes from the bloodstream, contributes to weakness and fatigue. In *Babesia*-infected cattle that survive the acute phase of the disease, there is a loss of condition [101]. Erythrocytes are destroyed in babesiosis by the physical effect of parasite multiplication [102], an increase in phagocytosis of erythrocytes by activated macrophages [103, 104], the production of an anti-erythrocyte antibody [105], and an increase in erythrocytic membrane. Babesiosis is distinguished by high fever and various degrees of hemolysis and anaemia. Anaemia can develop quickly. Clinical indicators can include pale mucous membranes, higher respiratory and heart rates, a decrease in appetite, a decrease in milk production, weakness, drowsiness, and other signs associated with anaemia or fever, such as miscarriages or temporarily impaired fertility in bulls. Jaundice can occur in animals infected with *B. bigemina*, especially when the clinical indications are less severe, and hemoglobinuria and hemoglobinemia are common.

Diagnosis and treatment

Babesiosis might be suspected based on clinical signs and history. Light microscopy of Giemsa-stained blood or organ smears is required to confirm the diagnosis. Molecular approaches, such as PCR tests, are more sensitive than optical microscopy and may be beneficial in detecting *Babesia* spp. as a carrier or during chronic infection. Diminazene is given to cattle at a dose of 3.5 mg/kg, IM, once. For therapy, 1.2 mg/kg SC imidocarb is given once.

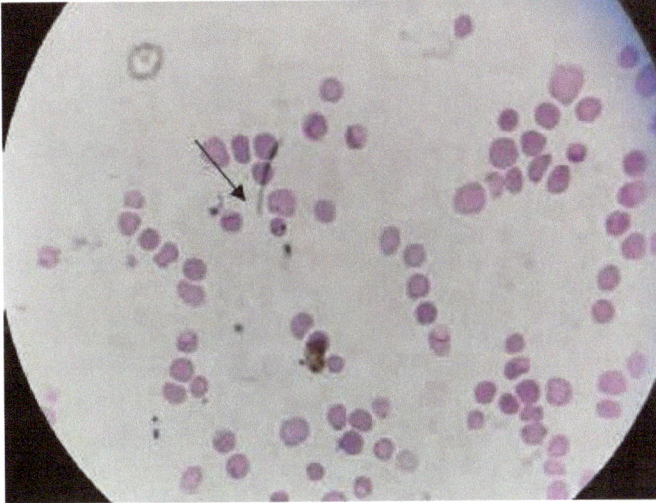

Fig. (5). *Theileria annulata* in the RBC in cattle.

Theileria annulata

Introduction

The tick-borne disease (TBD) known as "bovine tropical theileriosis," which results in large financial losses for the dairy and cattle industries, is caused by the hemoprotozoan parasite *Theileria annulata*. *T. annulata* is a parasite carried by ticks that causes tropical theileriosis. There are over 250 million cattle in southern Europe, North Africa, and Asia that could contract T. annulata. High death rates are the outcome [106, 107]. The world's regions with the highest rates of tropical theileriosis are Asia, the Middle East, southern Europe, and northern Africa [108, 109].

Morphology

T. annulata parasites in red blood were pear-seed, needle-shaped, rod-shaped, and cross-shaped. The cytoplasm was a bright blue colour, while the nucleus was a dark purple colour (Fig. **5**).

Lifecycle

The parasite goes through asexual developmental stages in mammal hosts and a sexual phase in tick vectors. The parasites reprogram multiple host signalling pathways and drive reproduction *via* poorly understood molecular processes after penetrating host leukocytes. *T. annulata* multiplication within red blood cells causes anaemia, which may increase the disease's pathophysiology. *Theileria* species are spread by the ixodid tick genera *Amblyomma, Haemaphysalis, Hyalomma,* and *Rhipicephalus*, and they infect a broad range of domestic and wild animals. The majority of these ticks are well-known for causing significant economic losses to the host disease outbreaks, fatalities, and crop loss in the agriculture business to skins and inadequate domestic animal production [110].

Pathogenesis and clinical signs

Tropical theileriosis is characterised by fever, mild nasal and ocular discharge, anorexia, salivation, enlargement of superficial lymph nodes, respiratory distress, acute anaemia, jaundice, and mortality due to hypoxia [111 - 113]. The most prevalent lesions were lymph node enlargement, spleen enlargement, pulmonary emphysema, and subcutaneous and intramuscular haemorrhages. There are excessive pericardial and pleural fluids, and the liver is larger than normal. The necropsy lesions, which included hepatomegaly, splenomegaly, and abomasal ulcers, are consistent with those reported by [114, 115], who suggested severe hepatobiliary system damage due to hypoxia caused by hemolytic anaemia and jaundice. The liver was friable, yellowish, and larger than normal, and the gall bladder was significantly distended with dark olive green or brownish-green bile. Tropical theileriosis was first diagnosed based on clinical symptoms and microscopic inspection of stained thin blood and lymph node smears [116].

Diagnosis and treatment

Buparvaquone is an effective medicine for treating tropical theileriosis in the early stages of illness; however, its relatively high cost limits its use globally.

Anaplasma marginale

Introduction

The pathogen rickettsial Bovine anaplasmosis, a hemolytic disease in calves transmitted by vectors, is caused by the parasite *Anaplasma marginale* (Rickettsiales: Anaplasmataceae) [117 - 120]. *A. marginale* is a global disease that attacks erythrocytes, resulting in fever, anemia, jaundice, abortion, and occasionally, fatality. Animals that contract the virus live their entire lives spreading it. Erythrocytes are the sole known location of *A. marginale* infection in cattle.

Morphology

Small, rounded specks of dark purple are seen around the edges of red blood cells. 1-2 microorganisms on average per red blood cell in up to 90% of red blood cells.

Lifecycle

It is possible for cattle to contract the parasite *Anaplasma marginale* from ticks. Once within the tick, the parasite can remain active for the duration of the tick's life cycle and spread several months later. *Anaplasma* grows in the circulation of vulnerable cattle after infection and binds to their red blood cells. While pregnant cows that survive almost invariably give birth throughout the course of their recovery from infection, infected bulls that do not die may remain sterile for up to a year. Rebuilding red blood cells and gaining lost weight requires at least two to three months of recovery.

Pathogenesis and clinical signs

Anaplasma species are the most prevalent tick-borne infections in cattle, with a high frequency in tropical and subtropical regions around the world [121]. When an acute infection occurs, 70% or more of the erythrocytes in these cells may become infected due to the presence of four to eight rickettsia in the membrane-bound inclusions (also known as initial bodies) [122, 123]. The proportion of erythrocytes that are parasitized grows geometrically when erythrocytic infection is identified. Following phagocytization of infected erythrocytes by bovine reticuloendothelial cells, mild to severe anemia and icterus without hemoglobinemia and hemoglobinuria emerge. Clinical signs in animals older than two years old may include fever, weight loss, abortion, lethargy, icterus, and frequent death [124]. Anaplasmosis causes progressive hemolytic anaemia and severe economic losses in tropical and subtropical areas [125]. Ticks are known carriers of *A. marginale*, and roughly 20 tick species have been identified as vectors of Anaplasmosis [126]. Bovine anaplasmosis is a devastating economic disease that causes losses in the dairy and beef industries due to decreased milk production, weight loss, abortion, jaundice, and, in some cases, death [127, 128]. The disease is mostly transmitted to cattle by ixodid ticks, although it can also be transmitted through fly bites and bloodstained objects such as needles, ear tags, and castration equipment. In some cases, placental transmission may play a role in the disease's epidemiology [129]. Fever, anaemia, weakness, swollen lymph nodes, abortion, decreased milk supply, and jaundice are all symptoms of anaplasmosis in cattle, which can be deadly in severe cases [130]. Cattle who recover from acute infection continue to be carriers for the remainder of their lives and can act as sources of infection for previously naive livestock groups, resulting in endemic infection or epizootics [131].The lesions are characteristic of those seen in animals with erythrophagocytosis-induced anemia. Cattle that die of anaplasmosis typically have severely anemic and jaundiced carcasses. Blood is fluid and thin. The spleen is typically big, mushy, and has noticeable follicles. The liver may have orange and yellow flecks. The gallbladder is frequently swollen and produces thick bile that is either dark or green. Lymph nodes in the mediastinum and liver are brown in color. In addition to petechial hemorrhages in the epi- and endocardium and serous effusions in body cavities, there is frequent evidence of acute GI stasis.

Diagnosis and treatment

Giemsa-stained blood smears and serologic tests such as ELISA are used to make the diagnosis. Antibiotics such as tetracycline and imidocarb are currently utilised in therapy. Treatment with these medications can totally clear infections, and the cattle are then immune to severe anaplasmosis for at least 8 months.

CONCLUSION

The liver is a unique organ immunologically since it has a lower immune activation level. For parasites that dwell in the liver, this creates the optimal conditions for them to develop into the next phases of their life stages. The parasites are able to avoid detection by the immune system when they migrate to the liver. It has been determined that the liver is a site of larval attrition in the cases of both *Schistosoma* species. In cattle, the pancreas is not a discrete organ; rather, it is dispersed widely and mesentery-adjusted to the duodenum. *Eurytrema* species in the pancreas cause loss of production in cattle. Thus, uncovering the molecular mechanisms underlying this attrition may help in the development of novel therapies.

REFERENCES

[1]   Mungube EO, Bauni SM, Tenhagen BA, Wamae LW, Nginyi JM, Mugambi JM. The prevalence and economic significance of *Fasciola gigantica* and *Stilesia hepatica* in slaughtered animals in the semi-arid coastal Kenya. Trop Anim Health Prod 2006; 38(6): 475-83.
[http://dx.doi.org/10.1007/s11250-006-4394-4] [PMID: 17243475]

[2]   Doyle E. Food borne parasites: a review of the scientific literature. Madison: Food Research Institute, University of Wisconsin 2003; p. 28.

[3]   Calvani NED, Šlapeta J. *Fasciola* species introgression: just a fluke or something more? Trends Parasitol 2021; 37(1): 25-34.
[http://dx.doi.org/10.1016/j.pt.2020.09.008] [PMID: 33097425]

[4]   Mas-Coma S, Valero MA, Bargues MD. Chapter 2. *Fasciola*, lymnaeidae and human fascioliasis, with a global overview on disease transmission, epidemiology, evolutionary genetics, molecular

epidemiology and control. Adv Parasitol 2009; 69: 41-146.
[http://dx.doi.org/10.1016/S0065-308X(09)69002-3] [PMID: 19622408]

[5]   Rondelaud D, Belfaiza M, Vignoles P, Moncef M, Dreyfuss G. Redial generations of *Fasciola hepatica* : a review. J Helminthol 2009; 83(3): 245-54.
[http://dx.doi.org/10.1017/S0022149X09222528] [PMID: 19203397]

[6]   Sumruayphol S, Siribat P, Dujardin JP, Dujardin S, Komalamisra C, Thaenkham U. *Fasciola gigantica, F. hepatica* and *Fasciola* intermediate forms: geometric morphometrics and an artificial neural network to help morphological identification. Peer J 2020; 8: e8597.
[http://dx.doi.org/10.7717/peerj.8597] [PMID: 32117632]

[7]   Cwiklinski K, Dalton JP, Dufresne PJ, *et al.* The *Fasciola hepatica* genome: gene duplication and polymorphism reveals adaptation to the host environment and the capacity for rapid evolution. Genome Biol 2015; 16(1): 71.
[http://dx.doi.org/10.1186/s13059-015-0632-2] [PMID: 25887684]

[8]   Boray JC. Experimental Fascioliasis in Australia. Adv Parasitol 1969; 7: 95-210.
[http://dx.doi.org/10.1016/S0065-308X(08)60435-2] [PMID: 4935272]

[9]   Bennett CE. Scanning electron microscopy of *Fasciola hepatica* L. during growth and maturation in the mouse. J Parasitol 1975; 61(5): 892-8.
[http://dx.doi.org/10.2307/3279230] [PMID: 1185431]

[10]   Han JK, Choi BI, Cho JM, Chung KB, Han MC, Kim CW. Radiological findings of human fascioliasis. Abdom Radiol (NY) 1993; 18(3): 261-4.
[http://dx.doi.org/10.1007/BF00198118] [PMID: 8508088]

[11]   Urquhart GM, Armour J, Duncan JL, Dunn AM, Jennings FW. Parasitology (2nd ed.), UK, Oxford Longman scientific and technical press. 1996; pp. 100-9.

[12]   Mas-Coma S, Bargues MD, Valero MA. Fascioliasis and other plant-borne trematode zoonoses. Int J Parasitol 2005; 35(11-12): 1255-78.
[http://dx.doi.org/10.1016/j.ijpara.2005.07.010] [PMID: 16150452]

[13]   Vaughan JL, Charles JA, Boray JC. Fasciola hepatica infection in farmed emus (*Dromaius novaehollandiae*). Aust Vet J 1997; 75(11): 811-3.
[http://dx.doi.org/10.1111/j.1751-0813.1997.tb15659.x] [PMID: 9404615]

[14]   Nguyen TGT, Van De N, Vercruysse J, Dorny P, Le TH. Genotypic characterization and species identification of *Fasciola* spp. with implications regarding the isolates infecting goats in Vietnam. Exp Parasitol 2009; 123(4): 354-61.
[http://dx.doi.org/10.1016/j.exppara.2009.09.001] [PMID: 19733565]

[15]   Kelley JM, Elliott TP, Beddoe T, Anderson G, Skuce P, Spithill TW. current threat of triclabendazole resistance in *Fasciola hepatica*. Trends Parasitol 2016; 32(6): 458-69.
[http://dx.doi.org/10.1016/j.pt.2016.03.002] [PMID: 27049013]

[16]   Pybus MJ. Liver flukes. In: Samuel WM, Ed. Parasitic Diseases of Wild Mammals. 2nd ed. Ames: Iowa State University Press 2001; pp. 121-49.
[http://dx.doi.org/10.1002/9780470377000.ch6]

[17]   Khanjari A, Bahonar A, Fallah S, *et al.* Prevalence of fasciolosis and dicrocoeliosis in slaughtered sheep and goats in Amol Abattoir, Mazandaran, northern Iran. Asian Pac J Trop Dis 2014; 4(2): 120-4.
[http://dx.doi.org/10.1016/S2222-1808(14)60327-3]

[18]   Kantzoura V, Kouam MK, Feidas H, Teofanova D, Theodoropoulos G. Geographic distribution modelling for ruminant liver flukes (*Fasciola hepatica*) in south-eastern Europe. Int J Parasitol 2011; 41(7): 747-53.
[http://dx.doi.org/10.1016/j.ijpara.2011.01.006] [PMID: 21329694]

[19]   Shinggu PA, Olufemi OT, Nwuku JA, Baba-Onoja EBT, Iyawa PD. Liver flukes egg infection and associated risk factors in white fulani cattle slaughtered in Wukari, Southern Taraba State, Nigeria.

Adv Prev Med 2019; 2019: 1-5.
[http://dx.doi.org/10.1155/2019/2671620] [PMID: 31016046]

[20] Karadag B, Bilici A, Doventas A, *et al.* An unusual case of biliary obstruction caused by *Dicrocoelium dendriticum*. Scand J Infect Dis 2005; 37(5): 385-8.
[http://dx.doi.org/10.1080/00365540510031430] [PMID: 16051581]

[21] Manga-González MY, González-Lanza C, Cabanas E, Campo R. Contributions to and review of dicrocoeliosis, with special reference to the intermediate hosts of *Dicrocoelium dendriticum*. Parasitology 2001; 123(7) (Suppl.): 91-114.
[http://dx.doi.org/10.1017/S0031182001008204] [PMID: 11769295]

[22] Otranto D, Traversa D. Dicrocoeliosis of ruminants: a little known fluke disease. Trends Parasitol 2003; 19(1): 12-5.
[http://dx.doi.org/10.1016/S1471-4922(02)00009-0] [PMID: 12488216]

[23] Ferreras-Estrada MC, Campo R, González-Lanza C, Pérez V, García-Marín JF, Manga-González MY. Immunohistochemical study of the local immune response in lambs experimentally infected with *Dicrocoelium dendriticum* (Digenea). Parasitol Res 2007; 101(3): 547-55.
[http://dx.doi.org/10.1007/s00436-007-0511-1] [PMID: 17393185]

[24] Di G. Liver fluke infections. In: Warrell DA, Cox TM, Firth JD, Eds. Oxford textbook of medicine. New York, USA: Oxford University Press 2010.

[25] Jeandron A, Rinaldi L, Abdyldaieva G, *et al.* Human infections with *Dicrocoelium dendriticum* in Kyrgyzstan: the tip of the iceberg? J Parasitol 2011; 97(6): 1170-2.
[http://dx.doi.org/10.1645/GE-2828.1] [PMID: 21736477]

[26] Beck MA, Goater CP, Colwell DD. Comparative recruitment, morphology and reproduction of a generalist trematode, *Dicrocoelium dendriticum*, in three species of host. Parasitology 2015; 142(10): 1297-305.
[http://dx.doi.org/10.1017/S0031182015000621] [PMID: 26059630]

[27] Ofori M, Bogoch II, Ephraim RKD. Prevalence of *Dicrocoelium dendriticum* ova in Ghanaian school children. J Trop Pediatr 2015; 61(3): 229-30.
[http://dx.doi.org/10.1093/tropej/fmv015] [PMID: 25828830]

[28] Mas-Coma S, Rodriguez A, Bargues MD, Valero MA, Coello JR, Angles R. Secondary reservoir role of domestic animals other than sheep and cattle in fascioliasis transmission in the Northern Bolivian altiplano. Res Rev Parasitol 1997; 57(1): 39-46.

[29] Otranto D, Traversa D. A review of dicrocoeliosis of ruminants including recent advances in the diagnosis and treatment. Vet Parasitol 2002; 107(4): 317-35.
[http://dx.doi.org/10.1016/S0304-4017(02)00121-8] [PMID: 12163243]

[30] Wolff K, Hauser B, Wild P. Dicrocoeliose des Schafes: Untersuchungen zur Pathogenese und zur Regeneration der Leber nach Therapie. Berl Munch Tierarztl Wochenschr 1984; 97(10): 378-87.
[PMID: 6517848]

[31] Camara L, Pfister K, Aeschlimann A. Analyse histopathologique de foie de bovin infesté par Dicrocoelium dendriticum. Vet Res 1996; 27(1): 87-92.
[PMID: 8620193]

[32] Schwertz CI, Lucca NJ, da Silva AS, *et al.* Eurytrematosis: An emerging and neglected disease in South Brazil. World J Exp Med 2015; 5(3): 160-3.
[http://dx.doi.org/10.5493/wjem.v5.i3.160] [PMID: 26309817]

[33] Su X, Zhang Y, Zheng X, *et al.* Characterization of the complete nuclear ribosomal DNA sequences of *Eurytrema pancreaticum*. J Helminthol 2018; 92(4): 484-90.
[http://dx.doi.org/10.1017/S0022149X17000554] [PMID: 28651672]

[34] Jiraungkoorskul W, Sahaphong S, Tansatit T, Kangwanrangsan N, Pipatshukiat S. Eurytrema pancreaticum: The *in vitro* effect of praziquantel and triclabendazole on the adult fluke. Exp Parasitol

2005; 111(3): 172-7.
[http://dx.doi.org/10.1016/j.exppara.2005.07.004] [PMID: 16125702]

[35]   Jang DH. Study on the Eurytrema pancreaticum: II. Life cycle. Kisaengchunghak Chapchi Dec 1969;
       7(3): 178-200.

[36]   Pinheiro J, Franco-Acuña DO, Oliveira-Menezes A, *et al.* Additional study of the morphology of eggs
       and miracidia of *Eurytrema coelomaticum* (Trematoda). Helminthologia 2015; 52(3): 244-51.
       [http://dx.doi.org/10.1515/helmin-2015-0039]

[37]   Chai JY, Bahk YY, Sohn WM. Trematodes recovered in the small intestine of stray cats in the
       Republic of Korea. Korean J Parasitol 2013; 51(1): 99-106.
       [http://dx.doi.org/10.3347/kjp.2013.51.1.99] [PMID: 23467726]

[38]   Ishii Y, Koga M, Fujino T, *et al.* Human infection with the pancreas fluke, Eurytrema pancreaticum.
       Am J Trop Med Hyg 1983; 32(5): 1019-22.
       [http://dx.doi.org/10.4269/ajtmh.1983.32.1019] [PMID: 6625056]

[39]   Soulsby EJ. Protozoa, Helminth and Arthropods of Man and domestic Animals. London: Bailliere
       Tindall Graay Coat Publisher 1982; pp. 236-51.

[40]   Hambali I, Adamu N, Ahmed M, *et al.* Sero-prevalence of *Schistosoma* species in cattle in Maiduguri
       metropolis and Jere local government areas of Borno State, Nigeria. J Adv Vet Anim Res 2016; 3(1):
       56-61.
       [http://dx.doi.org/10.5455/javar.2016.c132]

[41]   Vaidyanathan SN. *Schistosoma spindale* in a cow. Treatment with Anthiomaline. Indian Vet J 1949;
       26: 225-8.

[42]   Mohanty DN, Mohanty RK, Ray SK, Mohanty KM. A note on *Schistosoma spindale* infection in cattle
       and its successful treatment. Livestock Advisor 1984; 9: 37-9.

[43]   Fransen J, De Bont J, Vercruysse J, Van Aken D, Southgate VR, Rollinson D. Pathology of natural
       infections of Schistosoma spindale Montgomery, 1906, in cattle. J Comp Pathol 1990; 103(4): 447-55.
       [http://dx.doi.org/10.1016/S0021-9975(08)80032-1] [PMID: 2079559]

[44]   De Bont J, Vercruysse J. Schistosomiasis in Cattle. Adv Parasitol 1998; 41: 285-364.
       [http://dx.doi.org/10.1016/S0065-308X(08)60426-1] [PMID: 9734296]

[45]   Biswas H, Dey AR, Begum N, Das PM. Epidemiological aspects of gastro-intestinal parasites in
       buffalo in Bhola, Bangladesh. Indian J Anim Sci 2014; 84(3): 245-50.
       [http://dx.doi.org/10.56093/ijans.v84i3.38696]

[46]   Nithiuthai S, Anantaphruti MT, Waikagul J, Gajadhar A. Waterborne zoonotic helminthiases. Vet
       Parasitol 2004; 126(1-2): 167-93.
       [http://dx.doi.org/10.1016/j.vetpar.2004.09.018] [PMID: 15567584]

[47]   Liu L, Mondal MMH, Idris MA, *et al.* The phylogeography of *Indoplanorbis exustus* (Gastropoda:
       Planorbidae) in Asia. Parasit Vectors 2010; 3(1): 57.
       [http://dx.doi.org/10.1186/1756-3305-3-57] [PMID: 20602771]

[48]   Brown DS. Freshwater snails of Africa and their medical importance. London: Taylor & Francis;
       1994.
       [http://dx.doi.org/10.1201/9781482295184]

[49]   Aiello SE, Mays A. The Merck Veterinary Manual. 8 th ed. Merck and co., Inc., U.S.A: Whitehouse
       Station, N.J. 1998; pp. 29-31.

[50]   Bont JD. Cattle schistosomosis: host-parasite interactions [PhD thesis]. Ghent, Belgium: University of
       Ghent 1995; p. 223.

[51]   Urquhart GM, Armour J, Duncan JL, Jennings FW. Veterinary helminthology: Veterinary
       Parasitology. New York: Churchill Livingstone Inc. 1987; pp. 114-6.

[52]   Fekade D, Woldemichael T A, Tadele S. Pathogenesis and pathology of Schistosomosis. 5 th ed. Addis Ababa: Addis Ababa University printing Press. 1989; 34.

[53]   Malik SI. Histopathological studies on the digenetic trematodes in naturally infecting buffaloes [M.Phil thesis]. Rawalpindi, Pakistan: PMAS-Arid Agriculture University 2010; p. 3-5.

[54]   Smith MC, Sherman DC. Goat medicine, Lea & Febiger. Philadelphia: Waverly Company 1994; pp. 336-7.

[55]   Swarup D, Pachauri SP, Mukherjee SC. Prevalence and clinicopathology of naturally occurring fascioliasis and biliary amphistomiasis in buffaloes. Indian J Anim Sci 1987; 57: 252-7.

[56]   Patzelt R. Studies on epidemiology, pathogenesis, and therapy of gigantocotylosis in water buffalo in Punjab, Pakistan [PhD dissertation]. Berlin, Germany: Freie University 2002; p. 110-115.

[57]   Gupta PP, Singh B, Mandal PC, Gill BS, Grewal GS. A postmortem study of mortality pattern in adult buffaloes inPunjab. Indian J Anim Sci 1978; 48: 669.

[58]   Alim MA, Islam MK, Mondal MMH. A cross-sectional study on Fasciola gigantica and Gigantocotyle explanatum burdens in naturally infected buffaloes in Bangladesh. Bangladesh J Vet Med.; 2012, 3(1): 39-44.
        [http://dx.doi.org/10.3329/bjvm.v3i1.11343]

[59]   Horak IG. Paramphistomiasis of domestic ruminants. Adv Parasitol. 1971; 9: 33-72.
        [http://dx.doi.org/10.1016/S0065-308X(08)60159-1]

[60]   Bunza MD, Ahmed A, Afana S. Prevalence of paramphistomiasis in ruminants slaughtered at Sokoto Central Abattoir, Sokoto. Nigeria Journal of Basic and Applied Sciences 2008; 16: 287-92.

[61]   Kamaraj C, Rahuman AA, Bagavan A, *et al.* Evaluation of medicinal plant extracts against blood-sucking parasites. Parasitol Res 2010; 106(6): 1403-12.
        [http://dx.doi.org/10.1007/s00436-010-1816-z] [PMID: 20306205]

[62]   Sanchís J, Sánchez-Andrade R, Macchi MI, *et al.* Infection by Paramphistomidae trematodes in cattle from two agricultural regions in NW Uruguay and NW Spain. Vet Parasitol 2013; 191(1-2): 165-71.
        [http://dx.doi.org/10.1016/j.vetpar.2012.07.028] [PMID: 22902261]

[63]   Atcheson E, Lagan B, McCormick R, *et al.* The effect of naturally acquired rumen fluke infection on animal health and production in dairy and beef cattle in the UK. Front Vet Sci 2022; 9: 968753.
        [http://dx.doi.org/10.3389/fvets.2022.968753] [PMID: 36061117]

[64]   Biu AA, Abbagana A. Prevalence of paramphistomes in camels slaughtered at Maiduguri, Nigeria. Nigerian Journal of Parasitology 2007; 28(1): 44-6.
        [http://dx.doi.org/10.4314/njpar.v28i1.37858]

[65]   Juyal PD, Kasur K, Hassan S, Paramit K. Epidemiological status of paramphistomiasis in domestic ruminants in punjab. Journal of Parasite Distribution 2003; 231-5.

[66]   Ilha MR, Loretti P, Reis AC. Wasting and mortality in beef cattle parasitized by *Eurytrema coelamaticum* in the State of Parama. Southern Brazil Veterinary Parasitology 2005; 133: 49-60.
        [http://dx.doi.org/10.1016/j.vetpar.2005.02.013] [PMID: 16046069]

[67]   O'Shaughnessy J, Garcia-Campos A, McAloon CG, *et al.* Epidemiological investigation of a severe rumen fluke outbreak on an Irish dairy farm. Parasitology 2018; 145(7): 948-52.
        [http://dx.doi.org/10.1017/S0031182017002086] [PMID: 29143720]

[68]   Olsen OW. Animal Parasites: Their Life Cycles and Ecology (3 ed.). Dover Publications, Inc, New York/University Park Press, Baltimore, US. 1974; pp. 273-6.

[69]   Bilqees FM, Mirza S, Khatoon N. Paramphistomum Cervi Infection and Liver Tissue Damage in Buffaloes. VDM Verlag 2011; pp. 1-112.

[70]   Eckert J, Deplazes P, Craig PS, Gemmell M, Gottstein B. Echinococcosis in Animals: Clinical Aspects, Diagnosis and Treatment. In: Eckert J, Gemmell MA, Meslin FX, Pawlowski ZS, Eds.

WHO/OIE Manual on Echinococcosis in Humans and Animals: A Public Health Problem of Global Concern. Paris, France: W.O. Anim. Hlth 2001; pp. 72-99.

[71]   Deplazes P, Rinaldi L, Alvarez Rojas CA, *et al.* Global distribution of alveolar and cystic echinococcosis. Adv Parasitol 2017; 95: 315-493.
[http://dx.doi.org/10.1016/bs.apar.2016.11.001] [PMID: 28131365]

[72]   Battelli G. Echinococcosis: costs, losses and social consequences of a neglected zoonosis. Vet Res Commun 2009; 33(S1) (Suppl. 1): 47-52.
[http://dx.doi.org/10.1007/s11259-009-9247-y] [PMID: 19575305]

[73]   Sarıözkan S, Yalçın C. Estimating the production losses due to cystic echinococcosis in ruminants in Turkey. Vet Parasitol 2009; 163(4): 330-4.
[http://dx.doi.org/10.1016/j.vetpar.2009.04.032] [PMID: 19482428]

[74]   Starke WA, Machado RZ, Bechara GH, Zocoller MC. Skin hypersensitivity tests in buffaloes parasitized with *Toxocara vitulorum*. Vet Parasitol 1996; 63(3-4): 283-90.
[http://dx.doi.org/10.1016/0304-4017(95)00860-8] [PMID: 8966994]

[75]   Roberts JA. *Toxocara vitulorum*: treatment based on the duration of the infectivity of buffalo cows (*Bubalus bubalis*) for their calves. J Vet Pharmacol Ther 1989; 12(1): 5-13.
[http://dx.doi.org/10.1111/j.1365-2885.1989.tb00634.x] [PMID: 2704061]

[76]   Warren EG. Observations on the migration and development of *Toxocara vitulorum* in natural and experimental hosts. Int J Parasitol 1971; 1(1): 85-99.
[http://dx.doi.org/10.1016/0020-7519(71)90049-X] [PMID: 5170633]

[77]   Akyol CV. Epidemiology of *Toxocara vitulorum* in cattle around Bursa, Turkey. J Helminthol 1993; 67(1): 73-7.
[http://dx.doi.org/10.1017/S0022149X00012888] [PMID: 8509621]

[78]   Kassai T. Veterinary Helminthology. Boston, MS: Butterworth Heinemann 1999; pp. 102-3.

[79]   Roberts JA, Fernando ST, Sivanathan S. *Toxocara vitulorum* in the milk of buffalo (*Bubalus bubalis*) cows. Res Vet Sci 1990; 49(3): 289-91.
[http://dx.doi.org/10.1016/0034-5288(90)90061-8] [PMID: 2267418]

[80]   Ijaz M, Khan M S, Avais M, Ashraf K, Ali M M. Infection rate and chemotherapy of various helminths in goats in and around Lahore. Pak Vet J 2008; 28: 167-70.

[81]   Raza MA, Murtaza S, Bachaya HA, Dasatger G, Hussain A. Point prevalence of Haemonchosis in sheep and goats slaughtered at Multan abattoir. J Anim Plant Sci 2009; 19: 158-9.

[82]   Asif Raza M, Iqbal Z, Jabbar A, Yaseen M. Point prevalence of gastrointestinal helminthiasis in ruminants in southern Punjab, Pakistan. J Helminthol 2007; 81(3): 323-8.
[http://dx.doi.org/10.1017/S0022149X07818554] [PMID: 17711599]

[83]   Davila G, Irsik M, Greiner EC. *Toxocara vitulorum* in beef calves in North Central Florida. Vet Parasitol 2010; 168(3-4): 261-3.
[http://dx.doi.org/10.1016/j.vetpar.2009.11.026] [PMID: 20138706]

[84]   Jones JR, Mitchell ESE, Redman E, Gilleard JS. *Toxocara vitulorum* infection in a cattle herd in the UK. Vet Rec 2009; 164(6): 171-2.
[http://dx.doi.org/10.1136/vr.164.6.171] [PMID: 19202170]

[85]   Singh RP, Sahai BN, Jha GJ. Histopathology of the duodenum and rumen of goats during experimental infections with *Paramphistomum cervi*. Vet Parasitol 1984; 15(1): 39-46.
[http://dx.doi.org/10.1016/0304-4017(84)90108-0] [PMID: 6541393]

[86]   Alicata JE. Value of piperazine in the treatment of ascariasis in calves. J Parasitol 1959; 45: 48.

[87]   Tenter AM. *Toxoplasma gondii* in animals used for human consumption. Mem Inst Oswaldo Cruz 2009; 104(2): 364-9.
[http://dx.doi.org/10.1590/S0074-02762009000200033] [PMID: 19430665]

[88]   Dubey JP. Toxoplasmosis of Animals and Humans. 2nd ed., Boca Raton: CRC Press 2010.

[89]   Schlüter D, Däubener W, Schares G, Groß U, Pleyer U, Lüder C. Animals are key to human toxoplasmosis. Int J Med Microbiol 2014; 304(7): 917-29.
[http://dx.doi.org/10.1016/j.ijmm.2014.09.002] [PMID: 25240467]

[90]   Sanger VL, Chamberlain DM, Chamberlain KW, Cole CR, Farrell RL. Toxoplasmosis. V. isolation of toxoplasma from cattle. Javma-J. J Am Vet Med Assoc 1953; 123(917): 87-91.
[PMID: 13069361]

[91]   Liu WT, Lu YX, Lu LY, *et al.* Serological investigation of bovine Toxoplasmosis in some areas of Heilongjiang Province. Heilongjiang. Anim Sci Vet Med 2010; 53: 80-1. [In Chinese].

[92]   Ma YL, Wang WY, Cai XY, Liu BH, Xie AM. Preliminary investigation on the causes of abortion in cattle and sheep in Huzhu County. Chin. Qinghai. J Anim Vet Sci 2018; 48: 41-2. [In Chinese].

[93]   Chen Y, Huangfu HP, Shi DM, *et al.* Serological investigation of Toxoplasmosis in dairy cattle of part areas in Henan Province. Chin J Vet Med 2017; 53: 45-6. b [In Chinese].

[94]   Cenci-Goga BT, Rossitto PV, Sechi P, McCrindle CME, Cullor JS. Toxoplasma in animals, food, and humans: an old parasite of new concern. Foodborne Pathog Dis 2011; 8(7): 751-62.
[http://dx.doi.org/10.1089/fpd.2010.0795] [PMID: 21486145]

[95]   Kortbeek LM, De MELKER HE, Veldhuijzen IK, Conyn-Van Spaendonck MAE. Population-based Toxoplasma seroprevalence study in The Netherlands. Epidemiol Infect 2004; 132(5): 839-45.
[http://dx.doi.org/10.1017/S0950268804002535] [PMID: 15473146]

[96]   Radostits OM, Gay CC, Hinchcliff KW, Constable PD. Veterinary Medicine: A Textbook of the Diseases of Cattle, Horses, Sheep, Pigs and Goats. 10th ed. London, UK: Sounders 2006; pp. 1518-22.

[97]   Center for Disease Control and Prevention (CDC), United States. Available from: http://www.cdc.gov/ncidod/dpd/parasites/toxoplasmosis/default.htm

[98]   Rouatbi M, Amairia S, Amdouni Y, *et al. Toxoplasma gondii* infection and toxoplasmosis in North Africa: a review. Parasite 2019; 26: 6.
[http://dx.doi.org/10.1051/parasite/2019006] [PMID: 30767889]

[99]   Radostits OM, Gay CC, Blood DC, Hinchcliff KW. Veterinary Medicine. 9th ed. London, Philadelphia, New York: Baillier Tindall 2000; pp. 303-11.

[100]   Bock R, Jackson L, De Vos A, Jorgensen W. Babesiosis of cattle. Parasitology 2004; 129(S1) (Suppl.): S247-69.
[http://dx.doi.org/10.1017/S0031182004005190] [PMID: 15938514]

[101]   Ristic M, Kreier JP, editors. Babesiosis. In: Kreier JP, editor. Advances in parasitology. 1st ed. London: Academic Press 1980; p. 171-205.

[102]   Shoda LKM, Palmer GH, Florin-Christensen J, Florin-Christensen M, Godson DL, Brown WC. *Babesia bovis*-stimulated macrophages express interleukin-1beta, interleukin-12, tumor necrosis factor alpha, and nitric oxide and inhibit parasite replication *in vitro*. Infect Immun 2000; 68(9): 5139-45.
[http://dx.doi.org/10.1128/IAI.68.9.5139-5145.2000] [PMID: 10948137]

[103]   Court RA, Jackson LA, Lee RP. Elevated anti-parasitic activity in peripheral blood monocytes and neutrophils of cattle infected with *Babesia bovis*. Int J Parasitol 2001; 31(1): 29-37.
[http://dx.doi.org/10.1016/S0020-7519(00)00144-2] [PMID: 11165268]

[104]   Góes TS, Góes VS, Ribeiro MFB, Gontijo CM. Bovine babesiosis: Anti-erythrocyte antibodies purification from the sera of naturally infected cattle. Vet Immunol Immunopathol 2007; 116(3-4): 215-8.
[http://dx.doi.org/10.1016/j.vetimm.2006.12.011] [PMID: 17292487]

[105]   Lew-Tabor AE, Rodriguez Valle M. A review of reverse vaccinology approaches for the development of vaccines against ticks and tick borne diseases. Ticks Tick Borne Dis 2016; 7(4): 573-85.

[http://dx.doi.org/10.1016/j.ttbdis.2015.12.012] [PMID: 26723274]

[106] Zeb J, Shams S, Din IU, *et al.* Molecular epidemiology and associated risk factors of *Anaplasma marginale* and *Theileria annulata* in cattle from North-western Pakistan. Vet Parasitol 2020; 279: 109044.
[http://dx.doi.org/10.1016/j.vetpar.2020.109044] [PMID: 32032840]

[107] Bilgic HB, Karagenç T, Shiels B, Tait A, Eren H, Weir W. Evaluation of cytochrome b as a sensitive target for PCR based detection of *T. annulata* carrier animals. Vet Parasitol 2010; 174(3-4): 341-7.
[http://dx.doi.org/10.1016/j.vetpar.2010.08.025] [PMID: 20880635]

[108] Purnell RE. *Theileria annulata* as a hazard to cattle in countries on the northern Mediterranean littoral. Vet Res Commun 1978; 2(1): 3-10.
[http://dx.doi.org/10.1007/BF02291428]

[109] Bishop R, Musoke A, Morzaria S, Gardner M, Nene V. *Theileria* : intracellular protozoan parasites of wild and domestic ruminants transmitted by ixodid ticks. Parasitology 2004; 129(S1) (Suppl.): S271-83.
[http://dx.doi.org/10.1017/S0031182003004748] [PMID: 15938515]

[110] Omer OH, El-Malik KH, Magzoub M, *et al.* Biochemical profiles in Friesian cattle naturally infected with *Theileria annulata* in Saudi Arabia. Vet Res Commun 2003; 27(1): 15-25.
[http://dx.doi.org/10.1023/A:1022054522725] [PMID: 12625400]

[111] Osman SA, Al-Gaabary MH. Clinical, haematological and therapeutic studies on tropical theileriosis in water buffaloes (*Bubalus bubalis*) in Egypt. Vet Parasitol 2007; 146(3-4): 337-40.
[http://dx.doi.org/10.1016/j.vetpar.2007.03.012] [PMID: 17420101]

[112] Aulakh GS, Singla LD. Clinico-haematobiochemical observations on bovines naturally infected with *Theileria annulata.* J Vet Parasitol 2006; 20: 49-52.

[113] Sandhu GS. Histopathological, biochemical, and hematological studies in crossbred calves suffering from experimental tropical theileriosis [M.V.Sc thesis]. Ludhiana, India: Punjab Agricultural University 1996.

[114] Oryan A, Namazi F, Sharifiyazdi H, Razavi M, Shahriari R. Clinicopathological findings of a natural outbreak of *Theileria annulata* in cattle: an emerging disease in southern Iran. 2012; 112(1): 123-7.

[115] Tuli A, Singla LD, Sharma A, Bal MS, Filia G, Kaur P. Molecular epidemiology, risk factors and hematochemical alterations induced by *Theileria annulata* in bovines of Punjab (India). Acta Parasitol 2015; 60(3): 378-90.
[http://dx.doi.org/10.1515/ap-2015-0053] [PMID: 26204174]

[116] Bram RA. Tick-borne livestock diseases and their vectors. 1. *The global problem.* World Anim Rev 1975; 6: 1-5.

[117] Dumler JS, Barbet AF, Bekker CP, *et al.* Reorganization of genera in the families Rickettsiaceae and Anaplasmataceae in the order Rickettsiales: unification of some species of Ehrlichia with Anaplasma, Cowdria with Ehrlichia and Ehrlichia with Neorickettsia, descriptions of six new species combinations and designation of *Ehrlichia equi* and 'HGE agent' as subjective synonyms of *Ehrlichia phagocytophila.* Int J Syst Evol Microbiol 2001; 51(6): 2145-65.
[http://dx.doi.org/10.1099/00207713-51-6-2145] [PMID: 11760958]

[118] Kocan KM, Blouin EF, Barbet AF. Anaplasmosis control. Past, present, and future. Ann N Y Acad Sci 2000; 916(1): 501-9.
[http://dx.doi.org/10.1111/j.1749-6632.2000.tb05329.x] [PMID: 11193665]

[119] Schmidt HE. Anaplasmosis in cattle. J Am Vet Med Assoc 1937; 90: 723-36.

[120] Ruybal P, Moretta R, Perez A, *et al.* Genetic diversity of *Anaplasma marginale* in Argentina. Vet Parasitol 2009; 162(1-2): 176-80.
[http://dx.doi.org/10.1016/j.vetpar.2009.02.006] [PMID: 19285808]

[121] Richey EJ. Bovine anaplasmosis, In R. J. Howard (ed.),Current veterinary therapy food animal practice. The W B Saunders Co, Philadelphia,. 1981; pp. 767-72.

[122] Ristic M, Sibinovic S, Welter CJ. the United States: Livestock Sanitary Association 1968; pp. An attenuated *Anaplasma marginale* vaccine Proceedings of the 72nd Annual Meeting of. 56-69.

[123] Ristic M. Bovine anaplasmosis. In J Kreier (ed), Parasitic Protozoa. Academic Press, Inc., New York, N.Y. 1977; 4: pp. 235-49.

[124] Hairgrove T, Schroeder M E, Budke C M, Rodgers S, Chung C. Molecular and serological in-herd prevalence of *Anaplasma marginale* infection in Texas cattle. Prev Vet Med 2015; 119: 1-9.

[125] Ueti MW, Reagan JO Jr, Knowles DP Jr, Scoles GA, Shkap V, Palmer GH. Identification of midgut and salivary glands as specific and distinct barriers to efficient tick-borne transmission of *Anaplasma marginale*. Infect Immun 2007; 75(6): 2959-64.
[http://dx.doi.org/10.1128/IAI.00284-07] [PMID: 17420231]

[126] Hove P, Khumalo Z, Chaisi M, Oosthuizen M, Brayton K, Collins N. Detection and characterisation of *Anaplasma marginale* and *A. centrale* in South Africa. Vet Sci 2018; 5(1): 26.
[http://dx.doi.org/10.3390/vetsci5010026] [PMID: 29510496]

[127] Okafor C C, Collins S L, Daniel J A, Harvey B, Sun X. Factors associated with Seroprevalence of *Anaplasma marginale* in Kentucky cattle. Vet Parasitol Reg Stud Rep 2018; 13: 212-9.

[128] Aubry P, Geale DW. A review of bovine anaplasmosis. Transbound Emerg Dis 2011; 58(1): 1-30.
[http://dx.doi.org/10.1111/j.1865-1682.2010.01173.x] [PMID: 21040509]

[129] Kocan KM, de la Fuente J, Blouin EF, Coetzee JF, Ewing SA. The natural history of *Anaplasma marginale*. Vet Parasitol 2010; 167(2-4): 95-107.
[http://dx.doi.org/10.1016/j.vetpar.2009.09.012] [PMID: 19811876]

[130] Kocan KM, de la Fuente J, Coburn LA. Insights into the development of *Ixodes scapularis*: a resource for research on a medically important tick species. Parasit Vectors 2015; 8(1): 592.
[http://dx.doi.org/10.1186/s13071-015-1185-7] [PMID: 26576940]

[131] Tiele D, Sebro E, H/Meskel D, Mathewos M. Epidemiology of Gastrointestinal Parasites of Cattle in and Around Hosanna Town, Southern Ethiopia. Vet Med (Auckl). 2023 Jan 17;14:1-9

CHAPTER 10

Parasites of the Musculoskeletal System

Bhupamani Das[1,*] and **Ayushi Nair[2]**

[1] *Department of Clinics (Veterinary Parasitology), College of Veterinary Science & Animal Husbandry, Kamdhenu University, Sardarkrushinagar, Gujarat, India*

[2] *Department of Medicine, College of Veterinary Science & A.H., Kamdhenu University, Sardarkrushinagar, Gujarat, India-385506*

Abstract: Parasitic diseases are still a common occurrence in cow herds, both in conventional and organic systems, and understanding these diseases is a prerequisite for putting in place effective management measures and boosting farm profitability. The evolution of diagnostic techniques has allowed for a deeper understanding of the aetiology through the identification of parasite strains. Their epidemiology has altered over time in response to factors that are both human and environmental in origin. A reappraisal of the zoonotic danger of consuming beef has also been prompted by the recent rise of parasitic diseases including cysticercosis, sarcocystosis, toxoplasmosis, hydatidosis neosporosis, besnoitiosis, hypodermosis, toxocarosis, hookworm, and aberrant ascarid infection. The purpose of this book chapter is to focus on parasites that can directly or indirectly affect the musculoskeletal system, which can update our understanding of the state of parasite infections in cattle today.

Keywords: Cattle, Diagnostic techniques, Infection, Musculoskeletal system, Parasite.

INTRODUCTION

The musculoskeletal system is rarely involved in the presentation of parasite infections. The majority of these acute, subacute, and chronic illnesses are found in tropical and subtropical regions. They develop as a result of an immunological disorder or the invasion of a parasite into the musculoskeletal system's supporting structures. The daily activities of animals are negatively impacted by parasites that indirectly damage this system. These parasites enter the musculoskeletal system either through oral or cutaneous invasion. Few parasites have been found in the musculoskeletal system, according to reports. This chapter discusses major parasites that directly affect the musculoskeletal system of cattle as well as parasites that indirectly affect the musculoskeletal system.

---

* **Corresponding author Bhupamani Das:** Department of Clinics (Veterinary Parasitology), College of Veterinary Science & Animal Husbandry, Kamdhenu University, Sardarkrushinagar, Gujarat, India, E-mail: bhupa67@gmail.com

Transmission of Parasites through Musculoskeletal System

The process of transferring a parasite from one host to another is known as parasite transmission. It is understood that parasites can spread in two main ways: horizontally (from one person to another) and vertically (from one host generation to the next). Our ability to limit the spread of parasitic diseases depends on our ability to fully comprehend these transmission techniques, which are used by different parasites in various ways. Horizontal transmission necessitates time spent away from the host body and may be mediated by vector species, other hosts, or environmental factors. Therefore, a parasite must have developed the tools to exploit these in order to ensure transmission. On the other hand, parasites that use vertical transmission must adapt transmission methods from one generation to the next (Fig. **1**). In order to facilitate transmission, the parasite may then hijack or even take control of its host's physiology. It is feasible for some parasites to use both horizontal and vertical modes of transmission [1].

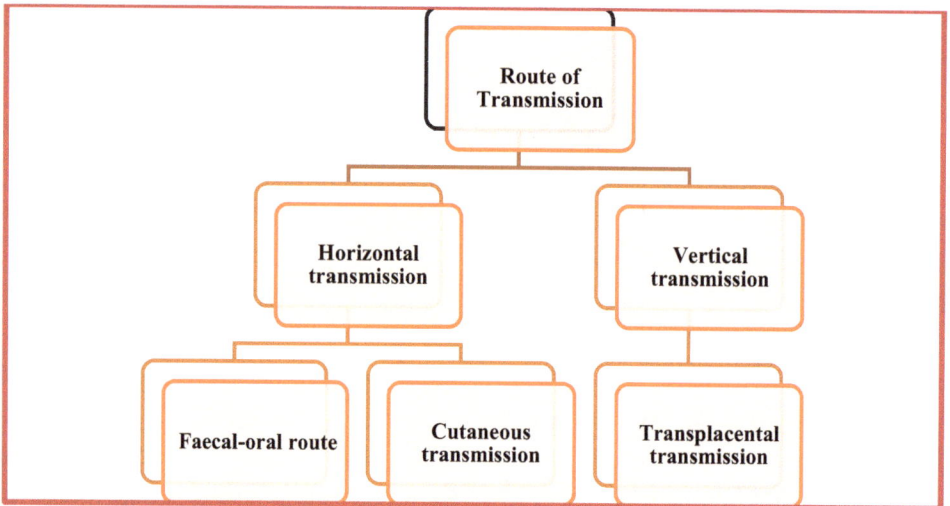

Fig. (1). Transmission pattern of parasites into the musculoskeletal system.

Horizontal Transmission

A. *Through oral route*: The most typical way that parasites are transmitted is orally, or *via* the faeco-oral route. By consuming food, water, or vegetables infected with parasite faeces, which contain the infective stages of the parasite, an infection is transferred orally.

B. *Cutaneous transmission*: The parasites can enter a person through unbroken skin (for example, hookworm can enter a person through the skin over feces-contaminated soil) or through the bite of bloodsucking insect vectors, which introduces the parasites into the body.

Vertical Transmission

Highly effective vertical transmission and transmission during pregnancy may be the most crucial distribution strategy in some parasites. This type of parasite is a major contributor to foetal infection during pregnancy, which results in abortion and musculoskeletal affection in cattle. Interesting issues are raised about the ways in which this parasite manipulates pregnancy to pass from generation to generation. It might happen through exogenous transplacental transmission from eating oocysts while pregnant or endogenous transplacental transmission from activating a quiescent stage during pregnancy. In order to control these economically significant parasites, an understanding of these pathways is crucial.

Impact on the Musculoskeletal System

In cattle, parasites migrate into different muscles and skeletal systems of the body, generally after entering through various transmission routes. In the migratory process, the main pathogenesis starts in the form of gelatinous tracts to the formation of cysts of varying sizes. The human and other carnivore gets the infection after consuming the infective stage in the form of meat.

Parasitic Diseases that Directly Affect the Musculoskeletal System

Taenia Saginata

In cattle with metacestodes of the human tapeworm *Taenia saginata*, cysticercosis most commonly affects the various muscles [2]. The cysticerci are usually discovered during meat examination at the regularly inspected localization sites, such as the heart, skeletal muscle, and diaphragm [3]. Meat containing living cysticerci, such as the meager beef in *T. saginata* that is consumed raw or improperly cooked can cause the disease. The larval or metacestode forms of *T. saginata* are called cysti, which are oval, transparent cysts with clear fluid that are about 5 X 10 mm in size and contain an opaque, invaginated protoscolex that is visible inside [4]. The only naturally vulnerable ultimate host for any species of Taenia is humans. Following ingestion by the host, the cysticercus evaginates in the small intestine of humans and develops over the course of two to four months to become a fully differentiated adult tapeworm. Infections with *T. saginata* are typically isolated. The tapeworm attaches to the intestinal mucosa of the jejunum by the scolex, and then spends the majority of its length lying along the mucosa and following the small intestine loops. In *T. saginata*, between 10 and 15 terminal segments are lost on average per day before being evacuated. Segments of *T. saginata* have a tendency to voluntarily crawl out of the anus or away from the faecal bolus (adapted to cattle's open-range grazing behaviour). 50,000–100,000 eggs are transported in each phase. *Taenia* species' eggs are identical to one another; they are spherical, 30 to 40 kilometres in diameter, and have a double-walled membrane with radiating striae. Usually, the oncosphere, a six-hooked embryo, may be seen inside the egg. As soon as the eggs are released from the intermediate host, they become infectious for the intermediate host, and when consumed by a *T. saginata*-susceptible intermediate host (cattle), they "hatch." The hexacanth embryos hatch from the eggs, use their six hooklets to break through the intestinal wall, travel *via* blood or lymphatic vessels, and then make their way to muscle, subcutaneous tissue, or other organs where they continue to grow and develop into cysticerci. These formations have a lifespan of several years before degenerating into fibrotic and calcified forms. One of the most important factors in preserving the life cycles of *Taenia* species is the environmental contamination of human faeces. By grazing on the ground or consuming water or roughage contaminated with eggs from human faeces, cattle can contract *T. suginuta*. It can also be significant to consider the indirect pollution of pasture by poorly treated human waste. Other domesticated bovines, such as the water buffalo and yak, may also contract *T. saginata* larval infection, but ungulates rarely do [5]. The edible sections of the carcass, such as the liver, heart, tongue, lung, and kidney, as well as the masseter muscles, cardiac muscles, triceps muscles, thigh muscles, shoulder muscles, diaphragm, and intercostal muscles (Fig. **2**), are typically where the *T. saginata*metacestodes can be located [6]. Cysts most commonly proliferate in the masseter, triceps, heart, tongue, and thigh muscles, according to [6]. While Kumar and Gebretsadik Berhe (2008) reported cysts in the tongue (0.61%), masseter muscles (0.59%), shoulder muscles (0.26%), heart (0.26%), and liver (7.45%) [7], a study reported cysts in the heart (29.2%), shoulder (25.3%), masseter muscle (26.7%), tongue (10.4%), diaphragm (5.4%), liver (1.4%), lung (0.9%), and kidney (0.5%).

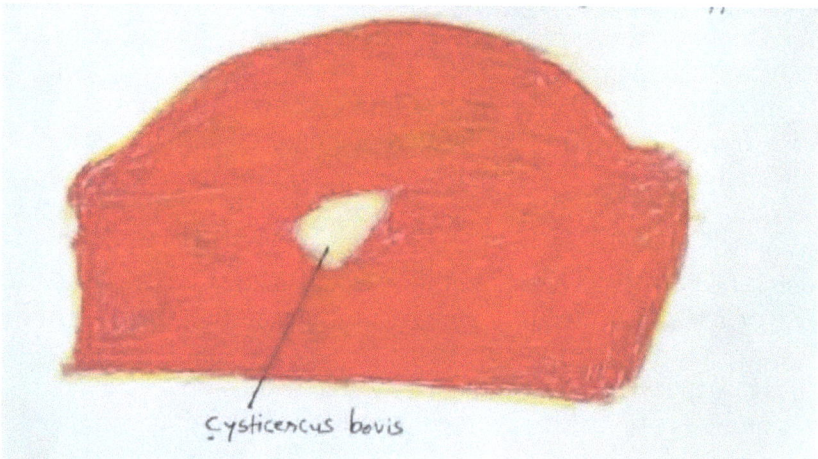

Fig. (2). *Cysticercus bovis* in muscle (Illustrated by Jayesh purohit).

The most common way to find bovine cysticercosis is postmortem investigation. When completely mature, *C. bovis* has a round or oval shape and is made up of a scolex that has invaginated a tiny fluid-filled vesicle [8]. About 10 weeks after infection, the cystic stage becomes infectious and can live for up to 9 months. It is crucial to distinguish between viable and dead cysts because only the former can infect humans. Viable cysticerci are pinkish-red in appearance, but dead, deteriorated, or calcified cysticerci plainly form recognisable areas of white and have fibrotic lesions. By preserving the cysts in cow bile for an extended period of time, the cysts' true vitality is determined [9]. The effectiveness of the meat inspection varies significantly from one abattoir to the next due to the fact that the identification of bovine cysticercosis by meat inspection greatly depends on the knowledge and motivation of the meat inspector [10]. Second, because national regulations or practical reasons prevent several incisions in the so-called regions of predilection, a sizable portion of infected carcasses remain undetected [9, 11]. The study determined that every part of a carcass has the same significance as a cysticerci predilection site and can be examined in the same way during routine meat inspections at slaughterhouses. It also suggested expanding the area and number of predilection sites to be observed, including the liver, forelimbs, lumbar, pelvis, tongue, lungs, neck and back, head, and diaphragm. The development of a viable sero-diagnostic test in the live animal would lead to changes in current meat inspection practices [8, 9].

Sarcocystis Species

Sarcocystosis is an intracellular infection caused by apicomplexan protozoans of the genus *Sarcocystis* (from the Greek sarkon for muscle and kystis for cysts). It is typically persistent and silent. The genus contains more than 120 recognised species, and the parasites often go through a lifetime of heteroxenous predator-prey and two hosts. The ultimate host is frequently a predator, whereas the intermediate host serves as its respective prey. Family Sarcocystidae members differ from their respective definitive and intermediate hosts' sexual and asexual generations in a variety of ways. Muscular and intestinal sarcocystosis are the two types of sarcocystosis that affect men. Asexual generations occur in the muscles (both skeletal and cardiac muscles) of intermediate hosts, which are typically herbivorous or prey animals, while sexual generations of gametogony and sporogony take place in the lamina propria of the intestine of definitive hosts, which are flesh-eating carnivores or omnivores. Because of this, *Sarcocystis* has an unavoidable two-host life cycle, with definitive hosts exhibiting intestine sarcocystosis and intermediate hosts exhibiting muscle sarcocystosis. Those who are certain hosts pass sporocysts in their faeces. When consumed by intermediate hosts, these become quickly infectious. Sporocysts in intermediate hosts' intestines burst, releasing sporozoites that proceed through an early stage of schizogony in the vascular endothelium of internal organs. Merozoites are released when schizonts burst, and these merozoites grow into cysts in the skeletal or cardiac muscles. These zoite-filled cysts, also known as sarcocysts, are often spindle-shaped. Intake of raw or undercooked meat containing sarcocysts causes the intestinal epithelium to begin gametogony and sporogony, which manifests as sporocysts in the stool [12]. The parasite reproduces sexually by gamogony in the intestine enterocytes of the final host. Eventually, the faeces shed into the environment include oocysts with two sporocysts (diagnostic stages for the final host), each of which is home to four sporozoites. Vascular endothelial cells undergo asexual schizogony after being ingested by the intermediate host of these infectious forms (oocysts/sporocysts). At that location, the first and second generations of merozoites emerge from schizonts and eventually enter muscle cells to produce the usual tissue sarcocysts. With the exception of humans, the final host frequently exhibits no symptoms of the non-invasive intestinal infection or relatively moderate illness. The intermediate host, which includes humans, on the other hand, typically exhibits prominent illness symptoms. Sarcocysts are most frequently seen in the gut, central nervous system, heart, tongue, oesophagus, diaphragm, and skeletal muscle (Fig. **3**) in the intermediate host [13].

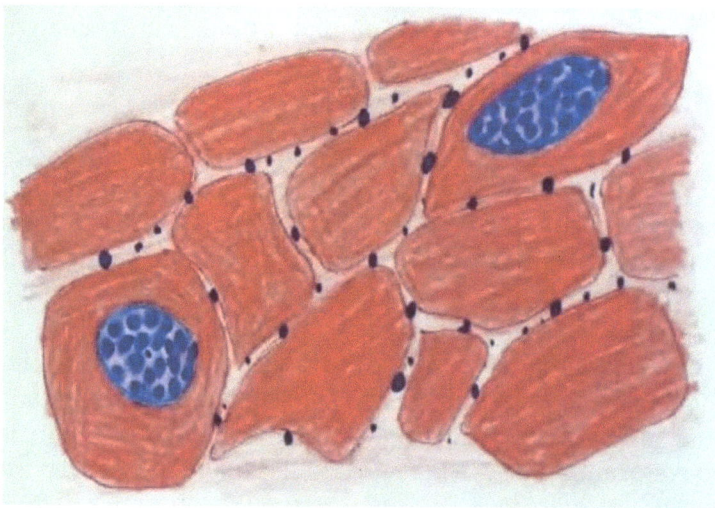

Fig. (3). Sarcocystis bradyzoite in muscle (Illustrated by Jayesh purohit).

The presence, structure, dimensions, and form of the parasite tissue cyst in the intermediate host are the primary diagnostic criteria. This is dependent on the host cell type, intermediate host species, and cyst maturation, though [13]. According to research using electron microscopy, the sarcocysts resemble those of the related apicomplexan parasite *Toxoplasma gondii* quite closely [14]. The cyst's shape is elongated to oval (typically 100–300 x 20–80 m, but can occasionally be considerably larger), and it has a wall thickness of 1-6 m. Internal villi and wall striations may or may not be present. Humans get intestinal, non-invasive sarcocystosis with watery diarrhoea, nausea, and other gastrointestinal symptoms when they consume raw or undercooked meat that is infected with the intracellular cystic stage of the parasite [13]. Humans can potentially unintentionally and seldom serve as intermediate hosts for an unidentified Sarcocystis species. The first human examples of this invasive sarcocystosis in Malaysia (1975–1992) were all discovered accidentally during autopsies or biopsies of members of various Malaysian ethnic groups [15].

Toxoplasma Gondii

Toxoplasma Gondii, which causes toxoplasmosis, is a common zoonotic parasite that can infect practically all warm-blooded species and has a high seroprevalence in the human population [16]. According to a study [17], cattle and sheep exhibit varied levels of susceptibility to *T. gondii* infection. Food is a key factor in toxoplasmosis transmission to humans from a variety of sources. Meat is of the biggest importance within the food category since it might contain bradyzoites inside tissue cysts, which might result in infection after consumption if the parasites are not killed by freezing or frying them first. A selection advantage over ancestral strains and closely similar parasites is provided by oral infectivity. The significance of meat as a risk factor for foodborne *T. gondii* infection, originally noted in a study [18], is explained by *T. gondii's* capacity to evade sexual propagation and infect hosts directly by ingestion of tissue cysts. After consuming sporulated oocyst (Fig. **4**) from soil, water, or plants, the intermediate host (Cattle) becomes infected [19]. Tachyzoites move to localise in the muscles and neurological system shortly after consumption. Finally, tissue cysts develop; some of which are bradyzoites. Clinical signs and abortion will not occur in cattle infected naturally with *T. gondii* [16]. However, beef has a unique place in toxoplasmosis epidemiology. Because beef is occasionally consumed raw or undercooked, it is crucial for the spread of *Toxoplasma* to humans. With significant regional variation, it is believed that this specific horizontal route of transmission accounts for up to 60% of *T. gondii* infections. Despite the possibility of abortion or the birth of frail lambs as a result of a first infection in pregnant sheep, these animals are thereafter shielded from other threats by the development of a potent immune system. However, abortion or perinatal mortality has not been documented in cattle, despite the fact that they can become infected easily. According to data [17], cattle respond to *T. gondii* infection more successfully than sheep do. Skeletal muscle cells, in addition to neurons, are thought to be the preferred cell type for parasite persistence during toxoplasmosis. Importantly, one of the main ways that *T. gondii* spreads to people may be due to the persistence of the parasite within this cell type *T. gondii* tissue cysts can be found in a variety of host organs during chronic toxoplasmosis. The quantity of tissue cysts, however, varies according to the host species and the kind of parasitized organ. It is unclear whether this results from a specific tissue tropism of *T. gondii*, a preference for the bradyzoite stage to form in particular organs and/or cell types, or a preference for the chronic stage to persist for a long time in some organs but not others [20]. According to a UK abattoir survey that used magnetic capture real-time PCR and amplicon sequencing to confirm the results, 1.79% of the diaphragm muscle samples tested positive for *T. gondii* [21]. Again, a different Iranian researcher discovered that imported cattle had a 26% prevalence of toxoplasma and native cattle had a 6% prevalence [22].

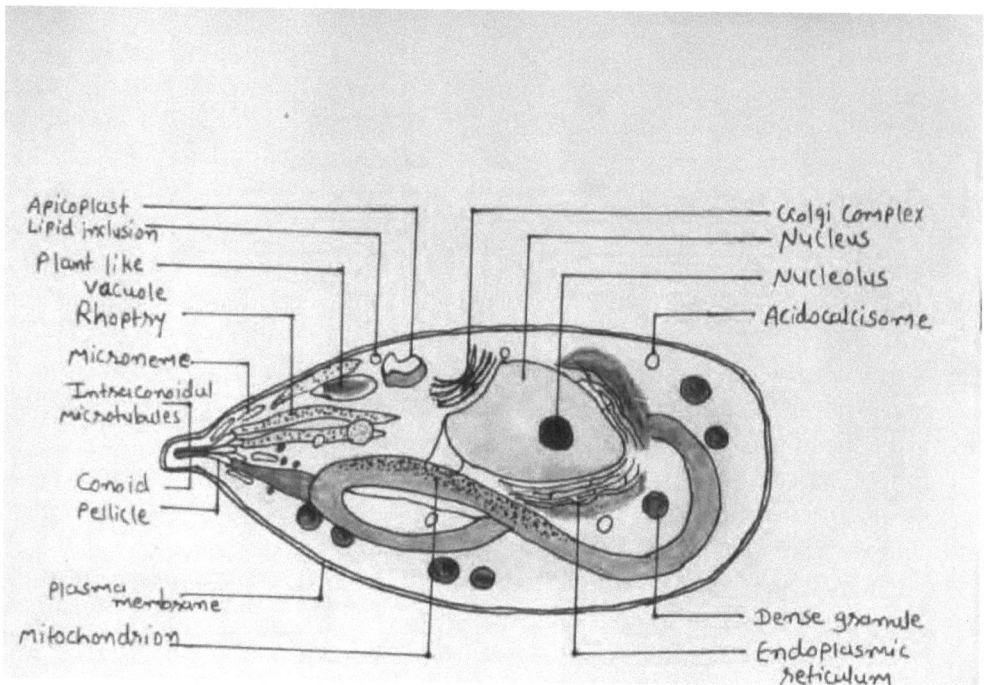

Fig. (4). Sporulated oocyst of *Toxoplasma gondii* (Illustrated by Jayesh purohit).

Most countries lack control programs along the meat production chain due to the small number of people at risk for disease, and prevention efforts instead rely primarily on educating those in at-risk groups and, in some cases, serological monitoring during pregnancy. For instance, pregnant women are frequently given advice on cat ownership and the intake of items that pose a health risk, such as raw or undercooked meat and unwashed fresh vegetables. The most crucial risk factors for *T. gondii* infection, however, are reportedly not known by all medical practitioners. Moreover, specialists disagree on the function of meat from various animal sources. While the significance of meat from bovines is not generally recognised, it has historically been recognised that sheep meat, along with goat meat and pork, is a highly contaminated source [18].

Ecchninococcus Granulosus

One of the most significant parasitic illnesses in cattle worldwide and one of the most common parasitic zoonoses is hydatidosis/cystic echinococcosis (CE), which is brought on by the larval stages of the tapeworm *Echinococcus granulosus* [23, 24]. The last stages of *E. granulosus* life cycle require two hosts. The primary intermediate hosts are livestock and humans, but carnivores are the definitive hosts because they house adult tapeworms in their intestines and excrete the parasite eggs with their faeces [25, 26]. Dogs have a significant impact on the disease's epidemiology. The dog consumes the leftovers and offal of domestic or wild herbivores raised for butchering or living in close quarters with humans and other domestic herbivores. The floors of homes, villages, and the surrounding environment are all contaminated by the dog's faeces. An intermediary host consumes the eggs, where the metacestode stages and protoscolices grow. Man is typically a dead-end intermediate host [26], and the cycle is complete when an intermediate host or its infected organ is consumed by an appropriate carnivore [27].

Hydatid cysts can form in the liver (Fig. **5**), lungs, or other organs as a result of infection in both people and animals [28]. Clinical symptoms in the intermediate hosts vary depending on the organs involved (where the cyst is located) and the severity of the infection, but typically no overt clinical symptoms are noticed. The majority of infections are only discovered at the abattoir, and the hydatid in the liver or lungs is typically tolerated without any clinical signs. When oncospheres have been transferred through the bloodstream to other organs, such as the kidney, pancreas, central nervous system, or marrow cavity of long bones, pressure from the growing cyst may cause a variety of clinical symptoms. Cysts in the lungs result in dyspnea, whereas those in the liver might result in hepatic insufficiency, gastrointestinal problems, and ascites. Cysts in the brain cause cerebral symptoms like blindness and paralysis. Depending on whether the liver or lungs are infected, the hydatid at its pulmonary or hepatic locations causes respiratory distress or belly enlargement in males who serve as intermediate hosts. There are at least 10 genetically distinct populations within the complex *E. granulosus*, and it is widely distributed due to the large variety of domestic and wild animal species that serve as intermediate hosts [27, 29]. A heavily infected dog may contain as many as 40000 tapeworms, shedding about 1000 eggs every two weeks, demonstrating the tremendous biotic potential of *E. granulosus* [30]. The eggs are assumed to be completely developed and infectious to an appropriate host when discharged, such as sheep, cattle, people, or other intermediary hosts. According to a study [31], echinococcus eggs are remarkably robust to a wide variety of temperatures. The gathering of baseline data is necessary before considering a justification for control programmes. In the Madhya Pradesh district of India [32], three cases of hydatid cysts were discovered in the liver and lung of cattle. Kebede *et al.* (2011) found 79/521 (15.2%) harboring hydatid cysts in cattle [33]. Hydatid disease of the musculoskeletal system has a radiological appearance that resembles tumours and other inflammatory disorders. Therefore, it might be challenging to make a clinical and radiological diagnosis of musculoskeletal hydatid disease prior to surgery. Different radiographic alterations could happen on a radiograph. It can mimic any type of nonspecific or specific osteomyelitis in circumstances of osteolytic and inflammatory alterations. When bone is eroded and destroyed, it can almost completely osteolyze, deform, and occasionally have radiologic characteristics that are mistaken for malignant bone tumours. The area of destruction can be more precisely identified using computed tomography (CT). CT and magnetic resonance imaging are mostly used to detect the extraosseous spread of hydatid disease in soft tissues [34].

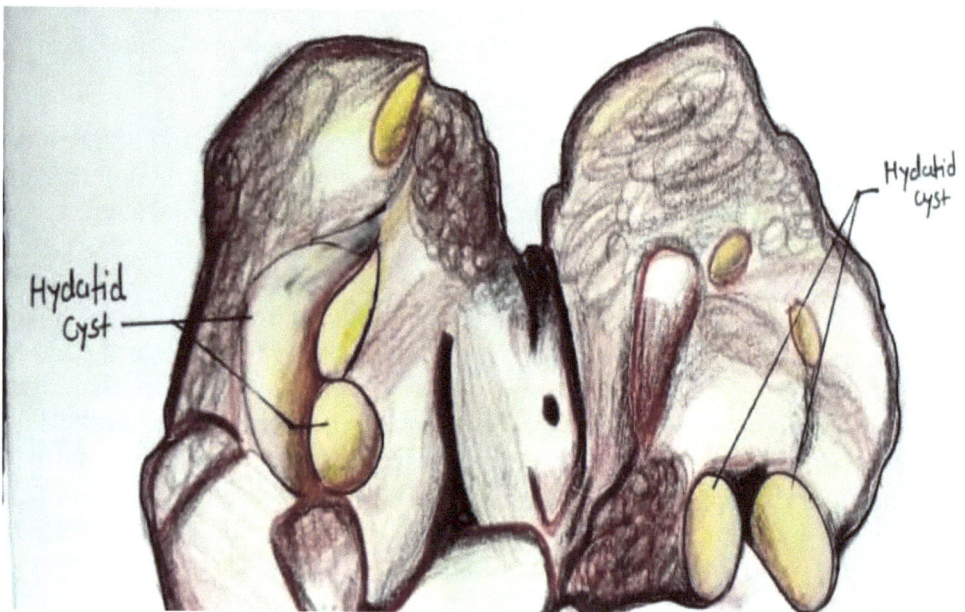

Fig. (5). Hydatid cyst in liver (Illustrated by Jayesh purohit).

Besnoitia Species

Bovine besnoitiosis is regarded as a reemerging illness. *Besnoitia besnoiti*, an obligate intracellular protozoan hastropism for skin and connective tissue, causes the infection that leads to bovine besnoitiosis, a developing illness. In cattle, it has been hypothesised that direct contact between infected and uninfected animals is the primary method of transmission. In the penile mucosa and vestibulum vaginae, tissue cysts can exist. These tissue cysts (Fig. **6**) can burst, and bradyzoites can pass across mucosal barriers. Therefore, natural breeding may promote the parasite's proliferation. Transmission might happen when different animals use the same needles or when insects (such *Stomoxys* or *Tabanus* species) bite them [35, 36]. The infectious form for intermediate hosts that can be transmitted orally is the oocyst, which sporulates in the environment. Intradermal bradyzoite inoculation resulted in a higher clinical score than subcutaneous or intravenous bradyzoite inoculation [37]. *Besnoitia besnoiti* reproduces asexually, primarily in endothelial cells of venous blood arteries [38]. *B. besnoiti* infection in cattle, the incubation period may last for two weeks to two months. Next, the progression of bovine besnoitiosis occurs in two phases that follow one another: febrile acute (anasarca) and chronic (scleroderma). Fever is the first symptom of the disease's acute stage, which may go unnoticed when tachyzoites invade blood vessel endothelia. The following edema causes an increase in vascular permeability. Vasculitis, thrombosis, and degenerative and fibrinoid necrotic vascular lesions also appear, primarily in the skin and testes. In this stage, symptoms like lameness, orchitis, hyperemia of the skin, and enlargement of the superficial lymph nodes may appear. The slow replication of bradyzoites inside tissue cysts with a preference for connective tissue, particularly the superficial layers of skin, mucous membranes of the upper respiratory tract, the vestibulum vaginae, and in males, the testes and epididymis, is what causes chronic infection. Pathognomonic tissue cysts can be seen in the scleral conjunctiva. Other common clinical indicators of the chronic stage include cutaneous abnormalities, such as thickening and folding of the skin in the scrotum and neck, loss of necrotic epidermis, and atrophy and induration of the bull testes. Vascular diseases in the scrotal skin and pampiniform plexus are likely to blame for male infertility. It can also proliferate in the skin, intermuscular connective tissue, ocular globe, superior respiratory tract, and testicles, as well as in arterial endothelium, macrophages, and fibroblasts [39, 40]. Both the acute and chronic stages of the illness might result in death. In severe cases, convalescence is sluggish despite low mortality. During acute and chronic infections, severely damaged bulls may become sterile. Affected animals carry the infection for life. The parasite DNA is found in mediastinal lymph nodes, liver, cardiac muscle, ovaries, uterus, masseter muscles, and tonsils. *Besnoitia besnoiti* cysts are still found in the lungs and vulva [41]. The cysts can be seen macroscopically and can have a diameter of up to 0.5 mm. Three different layers surround the tissue cysts, including a parasite-generated cyst wall on the luminal face of the parasitophorous vacuole membrane (PVM) containing the bradyzoites and connective tissue derived from the host encircling the infected host cell [42]. Immune cells such as macrophages and eosinophilic granulocytes appear to have invaded the superficial and, to a lesser extent, the deep dermis, expanding it and causing fibrosis [43, 44]. Agricultural productivity and animal health are impacted by tissue cyst development. Indirect fluorescent antibody test (IFAT), enzyme-linked immunosorbent assays (ELISA), Western blot, and skin biopsy—the gold standard—are the most popular and advised methods to detect bovine besnoitiosis [45 - 47]. The only vaccination for cattle management that is permitted everywhere is a live vaccine that Israel uses to immunise imported bulls. So, complete control depends only on precise diagnosis and herd management. Animals with clinical indications, such as tissue cysts in the vestibulum vaginae and poor body condition scores, should be targeted for slaughter. Unproductive cattle should also be culled, and sperm quality should be regularly checked before breeding season. Bovine besnoitiosis has a significant influence on the welfare and economic well-being of affected animals and farms. Mortality, decreased hide and meat value, male sterility, involuntary culling, and abortion are all related to losses [48].

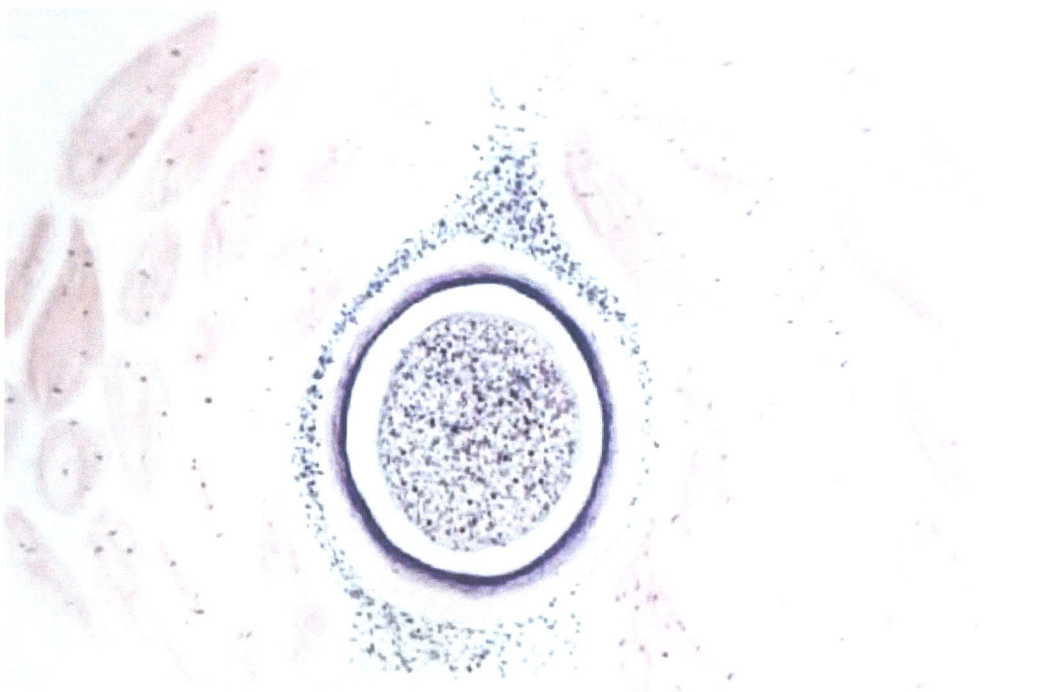

Fig. (6). *Besnoitia besnoiti* tissue cyst in affected cattle (Illustrated by Jayesh purohit).

Neospora Caninum

Neosporosis is a condition brought on by infection with protozoal parasites of the genus *Neospora*. Bovine abortion and slowly progressing myositis are the most frequently reported worldwide. *Neospora caninum* was described in puppies with encephalomyelitis and myositis for the first time in 1984 [49]. Calves younger than two months old have been recorded to exhibit symptoms. Ataxia, weight loss, and neurological problems are some of these symptoms. Reduced peripheral feeling and knee reflex are visible upon nervous system evaluation. Eyes in calves can be asymmetrical or projecting. On rare occasions, *N. caninum* can result in birth abnormalities such as scoliosis, hydrocephalus, and spinal canal narrowing [50]. The mode of transmission and tissue distribution of *N. caninum* in animals *via* the natural routes of transmission are poorly understood. The parasite can spread transplacentally to a variety of hosts, but in cattle, the vertical route is the primary route of transmission. According to several studies [51 - 55], carnivores can contract an infection by ingesting contaminated tissues. The dog, as a definitive host, sheds unsporulated oocysts in the environment [51, 52]. After 3 days in the environment, the oocysts (sexual stage) sporulate and divide into two sporocysts, each containing four sporozoites. Cattle, as intermediate hosts, consume oocysts found in contaminated food and water. Sporozoites are released into the intestine, where they penetrate cells and transform into tachyzoites (a rapidly dividing asexual phase). Tachyzoites have been discovered in brain cells, macrophages, fibroblasts, vascular endothelial cells, hepatocytes, and muscle cells (Fig. 7), including myocardium and the placenta [56, 57]. In cattle, *N. caninum* spreads quite effectively. Both horizontal and vertical transmission paths are crucial for infection and are necessary for the parasite's survival. When cattle consume *N. caninum* oocysts that have been sporulated, horizontal transmission occurs. During pregnancy, illness spreads from a persistently infected dam to her offspring *via* vertical transmission. Although vertical (endogenous transplacental) transmission can result in abortion, it usually results in the birth of a healthy calf with congenital infection [58 - 61]. Multifocal necrosis and extensive mononuclear infiltrations can be seen in numerous tissues in aborted fetuses with *N. caninum* infections. The heart, skeletal muscle, lung, and liver are only a few of the tissues that may experience the destruction of foetal cells and the ensuing lymphoid inflammation [62 - 64]. Both dairy and beef cattle experience abortions due to *Neospora caninum*. From the third month of pregnancy until term, cows of any age can abort. The majority of neosporosis-induced abortions take place between weeks 5 and 6. Foetuses can be born alive with clinical symptoms, stillborn, resorbed, mummified, autolyzed, or clinically normal but chronically infected. Abortions brought on by neosporosis happen all year round. Seropositive (antibody-carrying) cows are more likely to miscarry than seronegative (antibody-negative) cows, and this is true for both dairy and beef cattle. However, up to 95% of calves born to seropositive moms with congenitally infected remain clinically healthy. Congenital infection rates are often unaffected by the age of the dam, the number of lactations, or the history of abortion, but some findings suggest that vertical transmission is more effective in persistently infected cattle. Only cattle under 2 months old have been documented to exhibit clinical symptoms. Calves infected with *Neospora caninum* may exhibit neurologic symptoms, be underweight, be unable to stand or be born healthy. Both the forelimbs and the hindlimbs may be flexed or hyperextended. Ataxia weakened patellar reflexes, and a lack of conscious proprioception may all be discovered during a neurological examination. Calves' eyes may appear asymmetrical or have exophthalmia. *Neospora caninum* can occasionally lead to birth abnormalities such as hydrocephalus and spinal cord constriction. Both epidemic and endemic abortions are possible [65]. Up to 33% of dairy cow foetuses in contaminated areas have reportedly been found to miscarry within a few months. Neosporosis has been linked to repeated abortions in a modest percentage (5%) of cows [66] in most regions of the world [67 - 69]. A histologic examination of the foetus is required for a conclusive diagnosis of neosporosis, whereas testing the blood from an aborting cow simply indicates exposure to *N. caninum*. The finest specimens for diagnosis are the brain, heart, liver, placenta, and bodily fluids or blood serum. Diagnostic rates are higher when various tissues are tested. Neosporosis lesions can be detected in a variety of organs, however, the foetal brain is the organ that is most frequently afflicted. Focused encephalitis, which exhibits necrosis and non-suppurative inflammation, is the most typical neosporosis lesion [70]. Epizootics have a higher incidence of hepatitis than spontaneous abortions. The placenta contains lesions as well, but it can be challenging to locate protozoa. The laboratory, the stage of the fetus's autolysis, and the collection techniques all affect how effectively PCR diagnoses a condition. Although the greatest evidence for the cause of abortion at this time is the immunohistochemical detection of *N. caninum* in lesions, it is incredibly insensitive. In formalin-fixed, paraffin-embedded cow aborted brain tissue, *Neospora caninum* DNA can be found using PCR. Various ELISAs, the indirect fluorescent antibody test (IFAT), and the Neospora agglutination test (NAT) can all be used to identify *N. caninum* antibodies. Antibodies specific to N. caninum can be found using immunoblots. It is possible to diagnose *N. caninum* infection by looking for *N. caninum* antibodies in the foetus' serum, but a negative result is useless because the fetus's ability to produce antibodies depends on the stage of gestation, the amount of exposure, and the interval between infection and abortion. The diagnosis is improved by immunoblotting with an *N. caninum*-specific antigen. Peritoneal fluid is preferable to other body fluids for serologic diagnostics even if blood serum or any other foetus body fluid may be employed. Congenital infection can be diagnosed in calves using pre suckling serum. Due to the ambiguity of serologic diagnosis in chronically infected animals and the accessibility of sera from non-infected cattle, the definitive antibody level that should be regarded as diagnostic for neosporosis has not been established for bovines. Immunohistochemistry with *Neospora* antibodies is an efficient approach for identifying the parasites in both tissue cyst and tachyzoite stages in foetal tissues. *Neospora* immunohistochemistry works best on foetal brain slices, however, the parasites can also be found in the lung, kidney, and skeletal muscle. Mummified foetuses have been effectively treated using immunohistochemistry to detect *Neospora* infections, albeit the autolytic state of these foetuses reduces the diagnostic fidelity [71]. Reducing the number of infected cows in the herd and preventing the entrance of infected replacement cattle into the herd could be the main goals for infection control. The likelihood of a repeat abortion in cows with a confirmed *Neospora* abortion can be considered when making culling choices for these animals [72, 73].

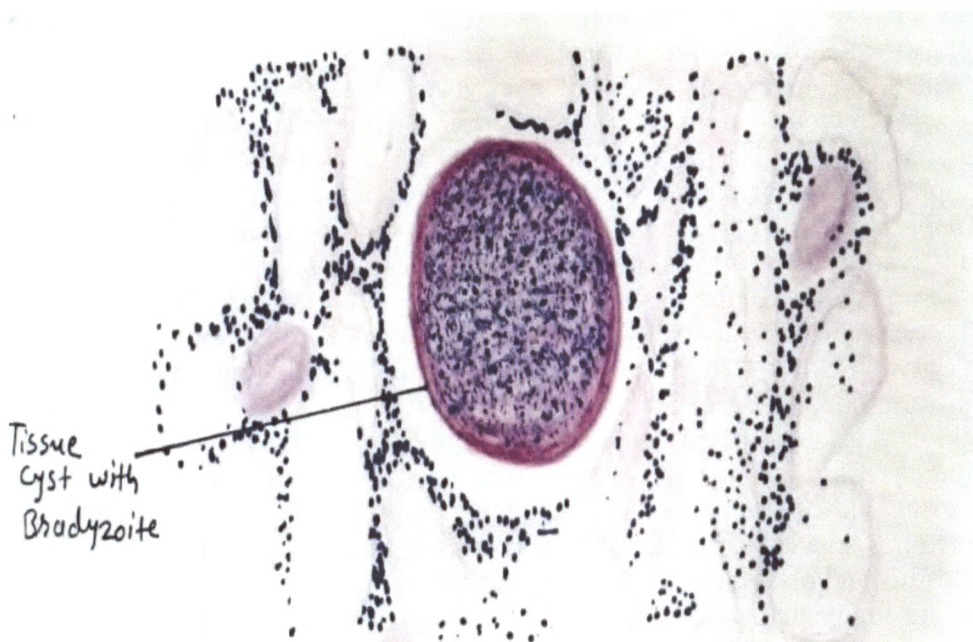

Fig. (7). Cyst of *Neospora caninum* in cattle tissue (Illustrated by Jayesh purohit).

Hypoderma Species

The term "warble fly" refers to big flies in the genus *Hypoderma* that parasitize cattle. Their larvae are frequently referred to as "cattle grubs" or "wolves," and they are also known by the names "heel flies," "bomb flies," and "gadflies." The ox warble fly, *Hypoderma bovis*, is one of the common species of warble fly. Bovine hypodermosis, often known as warble fly or bovine grub infestation, is a globally recognised veterinary disease. The Anglo-Saxon term for boil is warble [74]. Subcutaneous myiasis caused by *Hypoderma* species larvae in wild and farmed ruminants causes the conditions [75]. *H. bovis* eggs are placed singly on the animals' bodies and above their hocks [76] and the egg production ranges between 500 and 800 [77]. Adult *Hypoderma* live in the wild and do not consume animal products. After mating in the summer, females lay their eggs on the hairs of calves, typically on the lower portions of the body. The larva that has grown inside each egg hatches after a few days and enters the skin. *H. bovis* places a single egg on each hair. First-stage larvae (1 mm long), which hatch from the eggs in 3–7 days, crawl to the base of the hair shaft and pierce the skin. The first-stage larvae (L1) typically move along neural channels, connective tissue, or fascial planes between muscles. They exude proteolytic enzymes that help them migrate and activate the immune system. Following the nerves to the epidural fat, where the larvae spend the winter in *H. bovis*, successive larval migrations occur. To reach the diaphragm and the submucosa of the esophagus, where they overwinter, the larvae of *H. lineatum* follow connective tissue. Both species' larvae travel into the subcutaneous tissues along the back in the late winter and pierce the skin. They lay down and pupate on the earth after several weeks. The adult then takes flight. *H. lineatum* larvae move through the submucosal connective tissues of the oesophageal wall of the body and eventually reach the back of animals, whereas *H. bovis* larvae travel along nerve routes and reach the spinal canal. Young larvae of the warble fly (*H. bovis)* pierce the skin of cattle and move through the body for several months before resting beneath the skin of the animal's back. Each larva produces a distinct lump, or warble, from which a cattle grub emerges. The majority of them developed nodular eruptions on the back, thigh, and flank region and were found to have reduced their feed intake, as well as a severe fall in the milk yield of the affected milch cows. *H. bovis* larvae and their secretions in the epidural fat of the spinal canal are related to disintegrated connective tissue, fat necrosis, and inflammation in otherwise healthy cattle. The inflammation can sometimes spread to the periosteum and bone, resulting in a localised area of periostitis and osteomyelitis. The epineurium and perineurium may occasionally become implicated. Infestation of warble flies is regarded as one of the most economically significant ectoparasitic illnesses of cattle, goats, and sheep [78]. Warbles can be detected in the diseased animal's back from the tail head to the shoulders, as well as from the topline to about one-third of the way down the sides. Each warble has a breathing hole that ranges in size from a small slit to a circular (3-4 mm in diameter) aperture for more advanced larvae. Warbles can sometimes form huge, suppurating abscesses. The third-stage larvae's emergence, forced ejection, or death within the cysts usually results in the lesions healing without sequelae. Cattle carcasses and skins contaminated with cattle grubs display obvious signs of infestation and have a lower value. Damage to skin, gadding, decreased milk output, carcass depreciation resulting in butcher's jelly or licked meat, and other causes all contribute to economic losses caused by hypodermosis [79]. The most often used compounds to treat and control the condition are ivomec, moxidectin, doramectin, and eprinomectin [75]. Following frequent exposure to natural infestations, cattle develop resistance to Hypoderma spp [80, 81]. and artificial exposures [82, 83]. It has been discovered that older cattle have less *Hypoderma* spp. larvae than calves or yearlings, indicating the development of some form of immunity.

Parasitic Diseases that Indirectly Affect the Musculoskeletal System

Toxocara Vitulorum

Toxocara Vitulorum, a small-intestinal nematode, primarily affects cattle, buffalo, zebu, and infrequently sheep and goats in tropical and subtropical regions including Africa, India, and Asia. A direct life cycle is present in *Toxocara vitulorum*. Larvae can remain in milk for up to 3–4 weeks following parturition, and transmission is predominantly vertical through the milk. Larvae migrate through the liver and trachea in calves under 6 months old who have milk-borne infections. 3-4 weeks make up the pre-patent period. Through the consumption of larval eggs, calves older than 6 months old can get infected, however, this infection seldom leads to patency. The larvae in these older calves go through somatic migration, which is stopped in the tissues, primarily the liver and lungs, as well as the muscle, brain, kidney, and peripheral lymph nodes. Until late in pregnancy, when they begin to develop again and travel to the mammary gland around the time of delivery, these larvae are quiescent in female calves, allowing transmission through the milk.

Toxocara vitulorum has a similar life cycle to other *Toxocara* species, however, adult *T. vitulorum* are typically exclusively found in the duodenum of 3- to 10-week-old calves, which contract the infection while nursing. The larvae do not develop when embryonated eggs are consumed by a pregnant cow. Instead, they move *via* the liver, lung, various viscera, muscle, and mammary glands before entering the milk and colostrum (although the colostrum from water buffaloes appears to have very few larvae in it). Additionally, hypobiotic larvae revive and are able to access the mammary gland for up to three pregnancies. The first-week following calving is when milk contains the most larvae, while minor amounts can still be discovered up to 18 days later. *T. vitulorum* in calves often has a prepatent period of 21 to 28 days. The majority of calves stop shedding eggs between the ages of 2-4 months, while a small percentage may do so even up to 6 months. *T. vitulorum* transmission in utero is regarded as negligible or nonexistent. However, in a recent field research from Laos, 17% of calves that were too young to be infected in milk had eggs discovered in their faeces. This discovery has to be confirmed because it was impossible to rule out alternative scenarios (such as coprophagia or incorrect age estimations for the calves). T.

vitulorum eggs can reach the infective stage in the laboratory in 7–12 days at 28–30°C (82–86°F). *Toxocara* larvae are released in the intestines of most mammals, birds, and certain invertebrates from embryonated *Toxocara* eggs. The larvae do not finish their migration into the intestines of animals other than the final host. Instead, after breaking through the intestinal wall, they continue to move into the tissues. Most of all will likely eventually be encapsulated as hypobiotic larvae. Uncertainty surrounds how long these larvae can survive in different hosts. Small rodents can get infected for life, and dormant larvae have been discovered in experimentally infected macaques for at least 9 years. However, in experimentally infected pigs, hypobiotic larvae did not appear to endure for an extended period of time. Anorexia, symptoms of gastrointestinal pain, diarrhoea of various intensities, constipation, dehydration, steatorrhea, unfrugality, weight loss or poor weight gain, a poor hair coat, and a butyric odour on the breath are some of the clinical indicators that have been observed in spontaneously infected calves. Infected calves used in experiments have been reported to cough. Infrequent sequelae could result in intestinal blockage, volvulus or perforation, intussusception, or even death from some infections. There have also been reports of subclinical instances, which may be widespread in some herds, especially in otherwise healthy and well-fed calves. Moderate experimental infections in adult cattle and water buffalo are asymptomatic and likely comparable to natural infections. Large egg doses have been known to produce paralysis, conjunctivitis, and opisthotonos, while extremely large doses have caused fever, diarrhoea, and coughing. The presence of nematodes in the intestinal lumen is the most visible sign of enteric illness. Additionally, problems include mucoid enteritis, thickening of the intestinal walls, intussusception, obstruction of the pancreatic, bile, or gall bladder ducts, intestinal perforations, peritonitis, or blood loss into the peritoneal cavity may occur. Bruises are brought on by *Toxocara* larvae during their migration in the lungs, migrating larvae can cause petechial haemorrhages and multifocal, circumscribed white to grey foci (eosinophilic granulomas or accumulations of inflammatory cells). Some animals may have more significant hemorrhages, congestion, and/or signs of inflammation. Sometimes, larvae might be seen in the diaphragm and pleural cavity. On a histological examination, lesions such as interstitial pneumonitis, eosinophilic arteritis, and bronchiolitis, as well as enlargement and hyperplasia of the pulmonary arteries, may be visible. Additionally, secondary bacterial pneumonia is possible, particularly in young puppies. Other organs, especially the liver, may also exhibit white to grey foci, hemorrhagic (*e.g.*, petechial) lesions, as well as additional signs of tissue destruction (*e.g.*, edema, areas of necrosis or fibrosis, ascites). In the renal cortex of young dogs, granulomas containing larvae are infrequently discovered, frequently as an unanticipated result. There have been reports of ocular lesions such as orbital cellulitis and retinal damage. By identifying *T. vitulorum* eggs in faecal examination, a diagnosis can be made. The breath of diseased animals occasionally has a smell that is similar to acetone. *T. vitulorum* infections can be successfully treated with a variety of anthelmintics, including benzimidazoles and ivermectin. These medications can stop the larvae from developing into patency in calves when administered at 3 and 6 weeks of age [84].

Bunostomum Radiatum

Bunostomum is a huge (3 cm), robust, white worm that can infect calves and result in anaemia and black, and tarry faeces. Young calves kept in damp surroundings, especially in the tropics, may experience problems with infection because it can spread through ingestion or skin penetration. The eggs are huge, dark, and rectangular, similar to trichostrongyle-type eggs (that is, thin-shelled and segmented [100 x 50 μm], but they have rough eggshells that frequently have detritus adhering to them. *Bunostomum radiatum* adults live in the big intestine, specifically the caecum of cattle. The life cycle is similar to that of other intestinal nematodes, although transmission can occur through ingestion or skin penetration by infective L3 larvae. When larvae enter the gut, they penetrate the intestinal wall into the mucosa and moult to L4, emerging in 7 to 10 days in a susceptible host. They go through the pulmonary system, somatic tissue to the uterus, or mucosal tissue from either route of entrance. Colostrum may also contain larvae. The life cycle is completed by producing eggs in the intestine, which is the final stop. In hypersensitive hosts, however, nodules grow around the larvae. The larvae can live in the nodules for up to a year. Larvae can become arrested, encyst in mucosa or serosa, and finally result in the creation of unique, calcified nodules after reinfection and the development of partial immunity. Clinical indications of acute infection, such as watery, black, foetid diarrhoea, weight loss, and mortality, might result from an overly inflammatory reaction to the encystment of immature larvae. In chronic infection, calcified nodules may impair intestinal motility and result in intussusception [85].

Ascaris Suum

Ascarididae is a parasitic nematode family that is known as intestinal roundworms in humans and other animals. *Ascaris suum* has been observed migrating in the tissues of a variety of mammals [86 - 88]. After hatching in the large intestine, the larvae usually make their way through the liver to the lungs, where they can cause varied degrees of respiratory distress. It is now recognised that the lung of cattle serves as the animal's shock organ. and it has been recommended [89, 90] that infection with *A. suum* embryonated eggs caused fog-fever-like symptoms in calves. The migratory activity of *A. suum* in the liver causes a significant localised inflammatory response and, eventually, whitish fibrotic lesions known as milk spots or white spots, which are easily detected at slaughter. The lesions are classified as either superficial granulation tissue-type milk spots (small or large) with apparent grey-white interlobular septa or lymphonodular milk spots (elevated and spherical) [91]. Several incidences of clinical illness and even mortality in cattle have been reported due to A. suum, particularly in young stock. Acute respiratory distress, pneumonia, or death occurred 10 days after being exposed to pig dung in the feed or pig cages previously used for pigs [92 - 94]. On two dairy farms, heifers grazed pig slurry-fertilized pastures, resulting in an abrupt reduction in milk output, respiratory problems, and eosinophilia [95]. *A. suum* can cause significant clinical manifestations and reduce carcass quality in cattle and sheep; however, we expect the clinical impact of *A. suum* to be limited in areas of industrialized farming systems because most farms are specialised for a single type of livestock, and pig slurry is rarely applied on ruminant grazing areas.

CONCLUSION

A parasitic infection can result in a variety of illnesses because parasites or an immune system-mediated process can attack musculoskeletal systems. It is crucial to take parasite-induced symptoms into account when myositis, or vasculitis, formation of tissue cysts emerges in cattle or people living in endemic locations, as well as in certain populations in industrialised nations. Both internal and external parasites pose a threat to the cattle herd's health and ability to produce. Each one could have an effect on the operation by lowering performance or productivity or by making one more susceptible to illness and dying more frequently. Many of the productivity or performance losses frequently go unnoticed. Consequently, all beef operation herd health plans should include internal and exterior parasite control programmes. The primary goal of treatment should be to eradicate the parasite or disrupt its cycle of transmission.

REFERENCES

[1]   Hide G, Trees AJ. Transmission cycles in parasites. Parasitology 2009; 136(14): 1875-6.
        [http://dx.doi.org/10.1017/S0031182009991144] [PMID: 19765344]

[2]   Radostits OM, Blood DC, Gay CC. Veterinary Medicine. 8th ed., London: Balliere- Tindal 1994.

[3]   Gracey FJ, Collins SD. Meat Hygiene. 5th edition, Baillière, Tindall, 24–28 Oval Road, London NW17DX: 1992; pp. 413-20.

[4]   Dorny P, Praet N. Taenia saginata in Europe. Vet Parasitol 2007; 149(1-2): 22-4.
        [http://dx.doi.org/10.1016/j.vetpar.2007.07.004] [PMID: 17706360]

[5]   Schantz PM. Tapeworms (cestodiasis). Gastroenterol Clin North Am 1996; 25(3): 637-53.
        [http://dx.doi.org/10.1016/S0889-8553(05)70267-3] [PMID: 8863044]

[6]   Kebede N. Cysticercosis of slaughtered cattle in northwestern Ethiopia. Res Vet Sci 2008; 85(3): 522-6.
        [http://dx.doi.org/10.1016/j.rvsc.2008.01.009] [PMID: 18321540]

[7]   Abunna F, Tilahun G, Megersa B, Regassa A. Taeniasis and its socio-economic implication in Awassa town and its surroundings, Southern Ethiopia. East Afr J Public Health 2007; 4(2): 73-9.
        [PMID: 18085135]

[8]   Gracey JF, Collins DS. Meat Hygiene. 9th ed., London: Balliere Tindal 1992.

[9]   Wanzala W, Onyango-Abuje JA, Kang'ethe EK, *et al*. Control of *Taenia saginata* by post-mortem examination of carcasses. Afr Health Sci 2003; 3(2): 68-76.
        [PMID: 12913797]

[10]   Anonymous. Opinion of the Scientific Committee on Veterinary measures relating to Public Health on the control of taeniosis/cysticercosis in man and animals [Internet]. European Commission, Health and Consumer Protection Directorate-General, Directorate C-Scientific opinions, C3-Management of Scientific Committees II, Scientific co-operation and networks 2000. Available from: http://ec.europa.eu/food/fs/sc/scv/out21_en.pdf

[11]   Castoldi F. *Cisticercosi bovina* – Unaparassitosiancora di attualità. Summa (Milano) 1994; 11: 57-60.

[12]   Tappe D, Abdullah S, Heo CC, Kannan Kutty M, Latif B. Human and animal invasive muscular sarcocystosis in Malaysia--recent cases, review and hypotheses. Trop Biomed 2013; 30(3): 355-66.
        [PMID: 24189667]

[13]   Prakas P, Butkauskas D. Protozoan parasites from genus *Sarcocystis* and their investigations in Lithuania. Ekologija (Liet Moksl Akad) 2012; 58(1): 45-58.
        [http://dx.doi.org/10.6001/ekologija.v58i1.2349]

[14]   Matuschka FR, Bannert B. Cannibalism and autotomy as predator-prey relationship for monoxenous *Sarcosporidia*. Z Parasitenkd 1987; 74(1): 88-93.
        [http://dx.doi.org/10.1007/BF00534938] [PMID: 3125543]

[15]   Pathmanathan R, Kan S P. Three cases of human *Sarcocystis* infection with a review of human muscular sarcocystosis in Malaysia. Tropical Geographical Medicine 1992; 44(1- 2): 102-8.

[16]   Dubey JP. A review of toxoplasmosis in cattle. Vet Parasitol 1986; 22(3-4): 177-202.
        [http://dx.doi.org/10.1016/0304-4017(86)90106-8] [PMID: 3551316]

[17]   Esteban-Redondo I, Innes EA. *Toxoplasma gondii* infection in sheep and cattle. Comp Immunol Microbiol Infect Dis 1997; 20(2): 191-6.
        [http://dx.doi.org/10.1016/S0147-9571(96)00039-2] [PMID: 9208205]

[18]   Desmonts G, Couvreur J, Alison F, Baudelot J, Gerbeaux J, Lelong M. Étudeépidémiologiquesur la toxoplasmose: de l'influence de la cuisson des viandes de boucheriesur la fréquence de l'infectionhumaine. Rev Française d'Etudes Clin et Biol, Paris 1965; 10: 95-958.

[19]   Motarjemi Y, Moy G, Todd E. Encyclopedia of food safety. Amsterdam: Academic Press 2014.

[20]   Swierzy IJ, Muhammad M, Kroll J, Abelmann A, Tenter AM, Lüder CGK. *Toxoplasma gondii* within skeletal muscle cells: a critical interplay for food-borne parasite transmission. Int J Parasitol 2014; 44(2): 91-8.
        [http://dx.doi.org/10.1016/j.ijpara.2013.10.001] [PMID: 24184158]

[21]   Hosein S, Limon G, Dadios N, Guitian J, Blake DP. *Toxoplasma gondii* detection in cattle: A slaughterhouse survey. Vet Parasitol 2016; 228: 126-9.
        [http://dx.doi.org/10.1016/j.vetpar.2016.09.001] [PMID: 27692313]

[22]   Anvari D, Saadati D, Nabavi R, Alipour Eskandani M. Epidemiology and Molecular Prevalence of *Toxoplasma gondii* in Cattle Slaughtered in Zahedan and Zabol Districts, South East of Iran. Iran J Parasitol 2018; 13(1): 114-9.
        [PMID: 29963093]

[23]   Craig PS, McManus DP, Lightowlers MW, *et al*. Prevention and control of cystic echinococcosis. Lancet Infect Dis 2007; 7(6): 385-94.
        [http://dx.doi.org/10.1016/S1473-3099(07)70134-2] [PMID: 17521591]

[24]   Cringoli G, Rinaldi L, Musella V, *et al.* Geo-referencing livestock farms as tool for studying cystic echinococcosis epidemiology in cattle and water buffaloes from southern Italy. Geospat Health 2007; 2(1): 105-11.
[http://dx.doi.org/10.4081/gh.2007.259] [PMID: 18686260]

[25]   Khuroo MS. Hydatid disease: current status and recent advances. Ann Saudi Med 2002; 22(1-2): 56-64.
[http://dx.doi.org/10.5144/0256-4947.2002.56] [PMID: 17259768]

[26]   Zhang W, Li J, McManus DP. Concepts in immunology and diagnosis of hydatid disease. Clin Microbiol Rev 2003; 16(1): 18-36.
[http://dx.doi.org/10.1128/CMR.16.1.18-36.2003] [PMID: 12525423]

[27]   Thompson RCA, McManus DP. Aetiology: Parasites and Life Cycles. WHO/OIE manual in echinococcosis in humans and animals WHO/OIE, Paris. 2002; pp. 1-19.

[28]   Muller R. Worms and Human Disease. Oxon, UK: CAB International 2001; pp. 85-6.

[29]   McMANUS DP, Thompson RCA. Molecular epidemiology of cystic echinococcosis. Parasitology 2003; 127(S1) (Suppl.): S37-51.
[http://dx.doi.org/10.1017/S0031182003003524] [PMID: 15042999]

[30]   Schantz PM, Kern P, Brunetti E. Echinococcosis. In: Guerrant R, Walker DH, Weller PF, Eds. Tropical Infectious Diseases: Principles, Pathogens and Practice 2nd. Philadelphia, PA: WB Saunders 2006; pp. 1104-326.

[31]   Gemmell MA, Lawson JR. Epidemiology and control of hydatid disease. In: Thompson RCA, Ed. The Biology of Echinococcous and Hydatid Disease. London: George Allen and Unwin 1986; pp. 189-216.

[32]   Kulesh R, Vareshva R, Verma R, Suman A. Occurrence of hydatid cyst in cattle of Mandla district of Madhya Pradesh. Pharma Innovation Journal 2022; 11(2): 1904-6.

[33]   Kebede N, Gebre-Egziabher Z, Tilahun G, Wossene A. Prevalence and financial effects of hydatidosis in cattle slaughtered in Birre-Sheleko and Dangila Abattoirs, Northwestern Ethiopia. Zoonoses Public Health 2011; 58(1): 41-6.
[http://dx.doi.org/10.1111/j.1863-2378.2009.01250.x] [PMID: 19638161]

[34]   Arkun R, Mete B. Musculoskeletal hydatid disease. Semin Musculoskelet Radiol 2011; 15(5): 527-40.
[http://dx.doi.org/10.1055/s-0031-1293498] [PMID: 22081287]

[35]   Sharif S, Jacquiet P, Prevot F, *et al. Stomoxys calcitrans*, mechanical vector of virulent *Besnoitia besnoiti* from chronically infected cattle to susceptible rabbit. Med Vet Entomol 2019; 33(2): 247-55.
[http://dx.doi.org/10.1111/mve.12356] [PMID: 30666684]

[36]   Di Blasio A, Dondo A, Varello K, *et al.* Bovine besnoitiosis: A case in a native animal in North-West Italy. J Comp Pathol 2020; 174: 172.
[http://dx.doi.org/10.1016/j.jcpa.2019.10.107]

[37]   Diezma-Díaz C, Ferre I, Re M, *et al.* A model for chronic bovine besnoitiosis: Parasite stage and inoculation route are key factors. Transbound Emerg Dis 2020; 67(1): 234-49.
[http://dx.doi.org/10.1111/tbed.13345] [PMID: 31483955]

[38]   Basson PA, McCully RM, Bigalke RD. Observations on the pathogenesis of bovine and antelope strains of Besnoitia besnoiti (Marotel, 1912) infection in cattle and rabbits. Onderstepoort J Vet Res 1970; 37(2): 105-26.
[PMID: 5005082]

[39]   González-Barrio D, Diezma-Díaz C, Tabanera E, *et al.* Vascular wall injury and inflammation are key pathogenic mechanisms responsible for early testicular degeneration during acute besnoitiosis in bulls. Parasit Vectors 2020; 13(1): 113.
[http://dx.doi.org/10.1186/s13071-020-3959-9] [PMID: 32122380]

[40]   Grau-Roma L, Martínez J, Esteban-Gil A, *et al.* Pathological findings in genital organs of bulls

naturally infected with *Besnoitia besnoiti*. Parasitol Res 2020; 119(7): 2257-62.
[http://dx.doi.org/10.1007/s00436-020-06695-3] [PMID: 32458115]

[41]   Villa L, Gazzonis AL, Zanzani SA, Perlotti C, Sironi G, Manfredi MT. Bovine besnoitiosis in an endemically infected dairy cattle herd in Italy: serological and clinical observations, risk factors, and effects on reproductive and productive performances. Parasitol Res 2019; 118(12): 3459-68.
[http://dx.doi.org/10.1007/s00436-019-06501-9] [PMID: 31659452]

[42]   Dubey JP, Shkap V, Pipano E, Fish L, Fritz DL. Ultrastructure of *Besnoitia besnoiti* tissue cysts and bradyzoites. J Eukaryot Microbiol 2003; 50(4): 240-4.
[http://dx.doi.org/10.1111/j.1550-7408.2003.tb00127.x] [PMID: 15132166]

[43]   González-Barrio D, Diezma-Díaz C, Gutiérrez-Expósito D, *et al.* Identification of molecular biomarkers associated with disease progression in the testis of bulls infected with *Besnoitia besnoiti*. Vet Res 2021; 52(1): 106.
[http://dx.doi.org/10.1186/s13567-021-00974-2] [PMID: 34294155]

[44]   Jiménez-Meléndez A, Ramakrishnan C, Hehl AB, Russo G, Álvarez-García G. RNA-Seq Analyses Reveal That Endothelial Activation and Fibrosis Are Induced Early and Progressively by *Besnoitia besnoiti* Host Cell Invasion and Proliferation. Front Cell Infect Microbiol 2020; 10: 218.
[http://dx.doi.org/10.3389/fcimb.2020.00218] [PMID: 32500038]

[45]   Fernández-García A, Álvarez-García G, Risco-Castillo V, *et al.* Development and use of an indirect ELISA in an outbreak of bovine besnoitiosis in Spain. Vet Rec 2010; 166(26): 818-22.
[http://dx.doi.org/10.1136/vr.b4874] [PMID: 20581359]

[46]   Cortes H C, Reis Y, Waap H, *et al.* Isolation of Besnoitia besnoiti from infected cattle in Portugal. Veterinary parasitology 2006; 141(3- 4): 226-33.
[http://dx.doi.org/10.1016/j.vetpar.2006.05.022]

[47]   2015. Waap H. Epidemiologia e diagnóstico da besnoitiose bovina em Portugal (Epidemiology and diagnosis of bovine besnoitiosis in Portugal) [dissertation]. Lisbon: Faculty of Veterinary Medicine, University of Lisbon 2015.

[48]   Frey CF, Gutiérrez-Expósito D, Ortega-Mora LM, *et al.* Chronic bovine besnoitiosis: Intra-organ parasite distribution, parasite loads and parasite-associated lesions in subclinical cases. Vet Parasitol 2013; 197(1-2): 95-103.
[http://dx.doi.org/10.1016/j.vetpar.2013.04.023] [PMID: 23680543]

[49]   Salehi N, Haddadzadeh H, Shayan P, Koohi MK. Isolation of *Neospora caninum* from an aborted fetus of seropositive cattle in Iran. Vet Arh 2012; 82: 545-53.

[50]   Dubey JP, Schares G. Neosporosis in animals—The last five years. Vet Parasitol 2011; 180(1-2): 90-108.
[http://dx.doi.org/10.1016/j.vetpar.2011.05.031] [PMID: 21704458]

[51]   McAllister MM, Dubey JP, Lindsay DS, Jolley WR, Wills RA, McGuire AM. Dogs are definitive hosts of *Neospora caninum.* Int J Parasitol 1998; 28(9): 1473-8.
[http://dx.doi.org/10.1016/S0020-7519(98)00138-6] [PMID: 9770635]

[52]   Lindsay DS, Dubey JP, Duncan RB. Confirmation that the dog is a definitive host for *Neospora caninum.* Vet Parasitol 1999; 82(4): 327-33. a
[http://dx.doi.org/10.1016/S0304-4017(99)00054-0] [PMID: 10384909]

[53]   Dijkstra T, Eysker M, Schares G, Conraths FJ, Wouda W, Barkema HW. Dogs shed *Neospora caninum* oocysts after ingestion of naturally infected bovine placenta but not after ingestion of colostrum spiked with *Neospora caninum* tachyzoites. Int J Parasitol 2001; 31(8): 747-52.
[http://dx.doi.org/10.1016/S0020-7519(01)00230-2] [PMID: 11403764]

[54]   Schares G, Heydorn A, Cüppers A, Conraths F, Mehlhorn H. Hammondia heydorni -like oocysts shed by a naturally infected dog and *Neospora caninum* NC-1 cannot be distinguished. Parasitol Res 2001; 87(10): 808-16.

[http://dx.doi.org/10.1007/s004360100445] [PMID: 11688886]

[55]   Gondim L F P, Gao L, McAllister MM. Improved production of *Neospora caninum* oocysts, cyclical oral transmission between dogs and cattle, and *in vitro* isolation from oocysts. J Parasitol 2002; 88(6): 1159-63.
        [http://dx.doi.org/10.1645/0022-3395(2002)088[1159:IPONCO]2.0.CO;2] [PMID: 12537111]

[56]   Dubey JP, Lindsay DS, Adams DS, *et al.* Serologic responses of cattle and other animals infected with *Neospora caninum.* Am J Vet Res 1996; 57(3): 329-36.
        [http://dx.doi.org/10.2460/ajvr.1996.57.03.329] [PMID: 8669764]

[57]   Shivaprasad HL, Ely R, Dubey JP. A Neospora-like protozoon found in an aborted bovine placenta. Vet Parasitol 1989; 34(1-2): 145-8.
        [http://dx.doi.org/10.1016/0304-4017(89)90174-X] [PMID: 2588466]

[58]   Paré J, Thurmond MC, Hietala SK. Congenital *Neospora caninum* infection in dairy cattle and associated calfhood mortality. Can J Vet Res 1996; 60(2): 133-9.
        [PMID: 8785719]

[59]   Anderson ML, Reynolds JP, Rowe JD, *et al.* Evidence of vertical transmission of *Neospora* sp infection in dairy cattle. J Am Vet Med Assoc 1997; 210(8): 1169-72.
        [http://dx.doi.org/10.2460/javma.1997.210.8.1169] [PMID: 9108925]

[60]   Schares G, Peters M, Wurm R, Bärwald A, Conraths FJ. The efficiency of vertical transmission of *Neospora caninum* in dairy cattle analysed by serological techniques. Vet Parasitol 1998; 80(2): 87-98.
        [http://dx.doi.org/10.1016/S0304-4017(98)00195-2] [PMID: 9870361]

[61]   Davison HC, French NP, Trees AJ. Herd-specific and age-specific scroprevalence of *Neospora caninum* in 14 British dairy herds. Vet Rec 1999; 144(20): 547-50.
        [http://dx.doi.org/10.1136/vr.144.20.547] [PMID: 10371011]

[62]   Anderson ML, Blanchard PC, Barr BC, Dubey JP, Hoffman RL, Conrad PA. *Neospora*-like protozoan infection as a major cause of abortion in California dairy cattle. J Am Vet Med Assoc 1991; 198(2): 241-4.
        [http://dx.doi.org/10.2460/javma.1991.198.02.241] [PMID: 2004983]

[63]   Barr BC, Anderson ML, Dubey JP, Conrad PA. *Neospora*-like protozoal infections associated with bovine abortions. Vet Pathol 1991; 28(2): 110-6. a
        [http://dx.doi.org/10.1177/030098589102800202] [PMID: 2063512]

[64]   Wouda W, Dubey JP, Jenkins MC. Serological diagnosis of bovine fetal neosporosis. J Parasitol 1997; 83(3): 545-7.
        [http://dx.doi.org/10.2307/3284431] [PMID: 9194848]

[65]   Wouda W, Bartels CJM, Moen AR. Characteristics of neospora caninum-associated abortion storms in dairy herds in The Netherlands (1995 to1997). Theriogenology 1999; 52(2): 233-45.
        [http://dx.doi.org/10.1016/S0093-691X(99)00125-9] [PMID: 10734391]

[66]   Anderson ML, Palmer CW, Thurmond MC, *et al.* Evaluation of abortions in cattle attributable to neosporosis in selected dairy herds in California. J Am Vet Med Assoc 1995; 207(9): 1206-10.
        [http://dx.doi.org/10.2460/javma.1995.207.09.1206] [PMID: 7559072]

[67]   Canada N, Meireles CS, Rocha A, *et al.* First Portuguese isolate of *Neospora caninum* from an aborted fetus from a dairy herd with endemic neosporosis. Vet Parasitol 2002; 110(1-2): 11-5.
        [http://dx.doi.org/10.1016/S0304-4017(02)00333-3] [PMID: 12446085]

[68]   Miller CMD, Quinn HE, Windsor PA, Ellis JT. Characterisation of the first Australian isolate of *Neospora caninum* from cattle. Aust Vet J 2002; 80(10): 620-5.
        [http://dx.doi.org/10.1111/j.1751-0813.2002.tb10967.x] [PMID: 12465814]

[69]   Dubey JP, Buxton D, Wouda W. Pathogenesis of bovine neosporosis. J Comp Pathol 2006; May; 134(4): 267-89.
        [http://dx.doi.org/10.1016/j.jcpa.2005.11.004]

[70]   McAllister MM. Diagnosis and Control of Bovine Neosporosis. Vet Clin North Am Food Anim Pract 2016; Jul; 32(2): 443-63.

[71]   Anderson ML, Barr BC, Conrad PA. Protozoal causes of reproductive failure in domestic ruminants. Vet Clin North Am Food Anim Pract 1994; 10(3): 439-61.
[http://dx.doi.org/10.1016/S0749-0720(15)30531-4] [PMID: 7728629]

[72]   Moen AR, Wouda W, Mul MF, Graat EAM, van Werven T. Increased risk of abortion following *neospora caninum* abortion outbreaks: a retrospective and prospective cohort study in four dairy herds. Theriogenology 1998; 49(7): 1301-9.
[http://dx.doi.org/10.1016/S0093-691X(98)00077-6] [PMID: 10732067]

[73]   Thurmond MC, Hietala SK. Effect of congenitally acquired *Neospora caninum* infection on risk of abortion and subsequent abortions in dairy cattle. Am J Vet Res 1997; 58(12): 1381-5. a
[http://dx.doi.org/10.2460/ajvr.1997.58.12.1381] [PMID: 9401685]

[74]   Scholl PJ. Biology and control of cattle grubs. Annu Rev Entomol 1993; 38(1): 53-70.
[http://dx.doi.org/10.1146/annurev.en.38.010193.000413] [PMID: 8424627]

[75]   Hassan M, Khan MN, Abubakar M, Waheed HM, Iqbal Z, Hussain M. Bovine hypodermosis—a global aspect. Trop Anim Health Prod 2010; 42(8): 1615-25.
[http://dx.doi.org/10.1007/s11250-010-9634-y] [PMID: 20607401]

[76]   Urquhart GM, Amour J, Duncan JL, Dunn AM, Jennings FW. Veterinary parasitology. 1st ed. Scotland: Longman Scientific and Technical Publisher Co. 1991; pp. 157-8.

[77]   Andrews A. Warble fly: the life cycle, distribution, economic losses and control. Vet Rec 1978; 103(16): 348-53.
[http://dx.doi.org/10.1136/vr.103.16.348] [PMID: 366859]

[78]   Hall M, Wall R. Myiasis of humans and domestic animals. Adv Parasitol 1995; 35: 257-334.
[http://dx.doi.org/10.1016/S0065-308X(08)60073-1] [PMID: 7709854]

[79]   Macchioni G. Economic aspects of control of bovine hypodermosis in Italy. A symposium on warble fly control in Europe/Brussels, September 1984; 16-7.

[80]   Gingrich RE. Acquired resistance to *Hypoderma lineatum*: Comparative immune response of resistant and susceptible cattle. Vet Parasitol 1982; 9(3-4): 253-60.
[http://dx.doi.org/10.1016/0304-4017(82)90069-3] [PMID: 7046206]

[81]   Baron RW, Weintruab J. Immunization of cattle against hypodermatosis (*Hypoderma lineatum* (Devill.) and *H. Bovis* (L.)) using *H. Lineatum* antigens. Vet Parasitol 1986; 21(1): 43-50.
[http://dx.doi.org/10.1016/0304-4017(86)90142-1] [PMID: 3727345]

[82]   Pruett JH, Kunz SE. Thermal requirements for *Hypoderma lineatum* (Diptera:Oestridae) egg development. J Med Entomol 1996; 33(6): 976-8.
[http://dx.doi.org/10.1093/jmedent/33.6.976] [PMID: 8961649]

[83]   Colwell DD. Stage specific mortality and humoral immune responses during pulse and trickle infestations of the common cattle grub, *Hypoderma lineatum* (Diptera: Oestridae). Vet Parasitol 2001; 99(3): 231-9.
[http://dx.doi.org/10.1016/S0304-4017(01)00459-9] [PMID: 11502370]

[84]   Woodbury MR, Copeland S, Wagner B, Fernando C, Hill JE, Clemence C. *Toxocara vitulorum* in a bison (Bison bison) herd from western Canada. Can Vet J 2012; 53(7): 791-4.
[PMID: 23277649]

[85]   Craig TM. CHAPTER 22-Helminth Parasites of the Ruminant Gastrointestinal Tract. In: Rings DM, Ed. Food Animal Practice. Anderson, DE 2009.
[http://dx.doi.org/10.1016/B978-141603591-6.10022-3]

[86]   Borella LE, Adams JG, Malone MH. The role of histamine in acute experimental ascariasis. J Parasitol 1966; 52(2): 295-302.

[http://dx.doi.org/10.2307/3276488]

[87]   Fitzgerald PR. The pathogenesis of Ascaris lumbricoides var. suum in lambs. Am J Vet Res 1962; 23: 731-6.
[PMID: 13893361]

[88]   Johnston AA. Ascarids in sheep. N Z Vet J 1963; 11(3): 69-70.
[http://dx.doi.org/10.1080/00480169.1963.33497]

[89]   Aitken MM, Sanford J. Experimentally induced anaphylaxis in cattle. Vet Rec 1968; 82: 418-9.

[90]   Taylor EL. Grassland management and parasitism. B.V.A. Publication 1952; 23: 112-26.

[91]   Roepstorff A. *Ascaris suum* in pigs: population, biology and epidemiology. Doctoral Thesis. Copenhagen: The Royal Veterinary and Agricultural University 2003; 112.

[92]   Allen GW. Acute atypical bovine pneumonia caused by *Ascaris lumbricoides*. Can J Comp Med Vet Sci 1962; 26(10): 241-3.
[PMID: 17649400]

[93]   McCraw BM, Lautenslager JP. Pneumonia in calves associated with migrating *Ascaris suum* larvae. Can Vet J 1971; 12(4): 87-90.
[PMID: 5104934]

[94]   McLennan MW, Humphris RB, Rac R. *Ascaris suum* pneumonia in cattle. Aust Vet J 1974; 50(6): 266-8.
[http://dx.doi.org/10.1111/j.1751-0813.1974.tb05294.x] [PMID: 4412090]

[95]   Borgsteede F H M, Deleeuw W A, Dijkstra T, Alsma G, de Vries W. *Ascaris suum* infections causing clinical problems in cattle. Tijdschrift Voor Diergeneeskunde 1992; 117(10): 296e8.

CHAPTER 11

Faecal Examination for Diagnosis of Parasitic Diseases

Joken Bam[1,*], Pallabi Pathak[2], Nitika Sharma[3] and **Doni Jini[1]**

[1] *ICAR-Research Complex for North-eastern Hill Region Arunachal Pradesh Centre, Basar, India*

[2] *Lakhimpur College of Veterinary Science, Assam Agricultural University, Joyhing, Lakhimpur, Assam, India*

[3] *ICAR-Centre Institute for Research on Goat, Makhdoom, Mathura, Uttar Pradesh, India*

Abstract: In veterinary medicine, faecal examination is an important technique for detecting parasite infections. It is a basic marker for the parasitic infection in cattle. It is an affordable and non-invasive method that helps detect parasites across different body systems. Parasites residing in the digestive tract release eggs, larvae, or cysts in faeces, while adult helminth parasites may be visible during enteritis. Additionally, parasites such as worms, eggs, or larvae can be expelled from the respiratory system through coughing and subsequently swallowed, appearing in faeces. Mange or scab mites may be ingested through licking or nibbling, also manifesting in faeces. Various parasite forms with distinct morphological features can be identified in faeces, serving as diagnostic markers for specific species. However, some parasites may produce similar eggs or oocysts, making species-level detection challenging. Overall, faecal examination is a fundamental diagnostic tool for identifying parasitic eggs.

Keywords: Anthelmintic, Cattle, Control, Diagnosis, Economic impact, Faecal examination, Gastrointestinal parasites, Management.

INTRODUCTION

Parasites are a common concern in cattle production and endoparasites are a leading cause of economic loss due to reduced productivity, poor growth, and sometimes death of the affected animals. The most widely used tool for diagnosing parasitic diseases in cattle is faecal examination. The primary objective of a faecal examination is to detect and identify the eggs, larvae, or cysts of parasites [1]. It is most appropriate for parasites that live in the gastrointestinal tract, bile duct, mesenteric artery, portal vein, *etc.* as their eggs, trophozoite, cysts or oocysts are found in the faecal matter. Knowledge of the type of parasite and

* **Corresponding author Joken Bam:** ICAR-Research Complex for North-eastern Hill Region Arunachal Pradesh Centre, Basar, India; E-mail: jode.vet@gmail.com

Tanmoy Rana (Ed.)

the severity of infection is crucial to effective treatment, control and management. Though it is quick, inexpensive and a relatively easy method of diagnosis, it has certain limitations. A correct faecal exam merely detects parasitic forms in the dung, however their excretion is dependent on many factors. This chapter includes diagnostic techniques for parasitic diseases of cattle by faecal examinations, methods of sampling and points to be considered for making correct diagnosis.

FAECAL SAMPLING, PRESERVATION AND TRANSPORTATION TO LABORATORY

Faecal samples should always be collected fresh either directly from the rectum or freshly voided using examination gloves. Old samples can get dehydrated and can make it hard to form a uniform suspension. In old samples, the helminth eggs and coccidian oocysts may undergo further development making it difficult for correct identification or adult parasites may disintegrate to an extent that diagnosis is virtually impossible.

About 20-30 gm of faecal matter is collected in a sterile plastic bag/jar and adequately labelled for identification. The sample container is closed, packed in a cooling box for maintaining a cold chain and transported to the laboratory for examination at the earliest to prevent further development of the parasitic stages. It is best to examine the samples right away but properly sealed faecal samples could be stored in the refrigerator for several days.

The faecal parasite egg output is connected to a variety of host and parasite-related factors. The host-related factors include the natural rhythm of faecal voiding, age, host immune status, effect of recent anthelmintic administration and host's hormonal status. The parasite-related factors are infection load, different developmental stages, predilection site and response to the environment. Some parasites show diurnal fluctuations in egg shedding in cattle, like *Fasciola hepatica* [2]. Dorsman, 1956 recorded a gradual rise in *F. hepatica* egg count during the morning hours and then fell gradually in the afternoon after reaching a peak at 12:30 pm. In general, early morning spontaneous faecal voids are preferred and recommended for the diagnosis of parasitic infections. For sending a sample to a reference laboratory, about 20-30 gm of freshly voided faecal samples packed in a sterile leak-proof container with appropriate labelling and a letter describing the content is to be promptly sent through the mail. In cases when the laboratory is situated at a distant location and the transportation is anticipated to take a few days, 10% formalin may be added to the samples and sent to the laboratory with a clear mention of the preservative in the labels.

METHODS OF FAECAL EXAMINATION

A faecal exam begins with a gross examination of the sample. Samples should be looked for consistency, colour and odour of the faecal matter, presence of mucous, blood, live or dead worms or segments of tapeworms. The observations are recorded to be correlated with the findings of the microscopic examination and clinical findings for correct diagnosis.

A microscopic examination of faeces is performed to detect and identify parasite eggs, larvae, or cysts that suggest an active infection. There are several methods of faecal examination, each with its own set of benefits and drawbacks. They are broadly categorised into qualitative and quantitative methods. The direct smear, floatation and sedimentation techniques are examples of qualitative approaches that are frequently employed in clinical diagnostics to determine if parasite eggs or oocysts are present or absent in faecal samples. On the other hand, the quantitative method involves determining the number of eggs or oocysts per unit weight of faeces [3]. The quantitative approach greatly aids in assessing the effectiveness of antiparasitic drugs and they are frequently used in research of anthelmintic resistance and antiparasitic efficacy of herbal products. Commonly detected parasite eggs in cattle faeces are presented in Fig. (**1**).

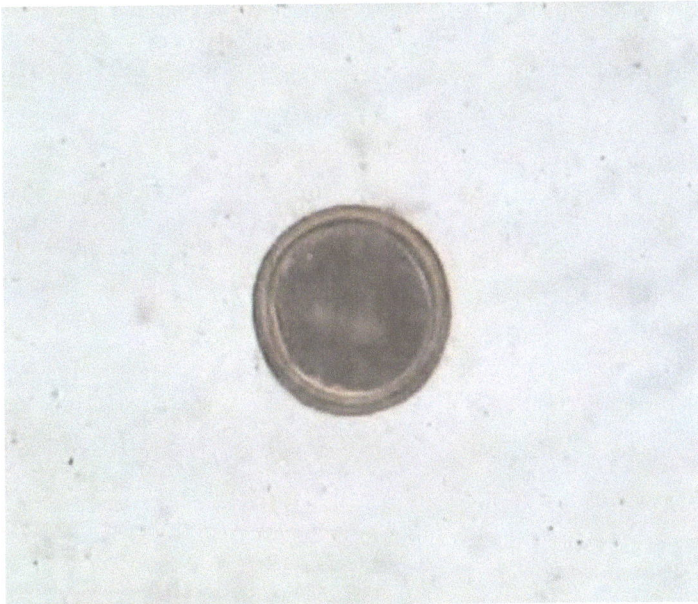

Fig. (1a). *Toxocara vitulorum* egg.

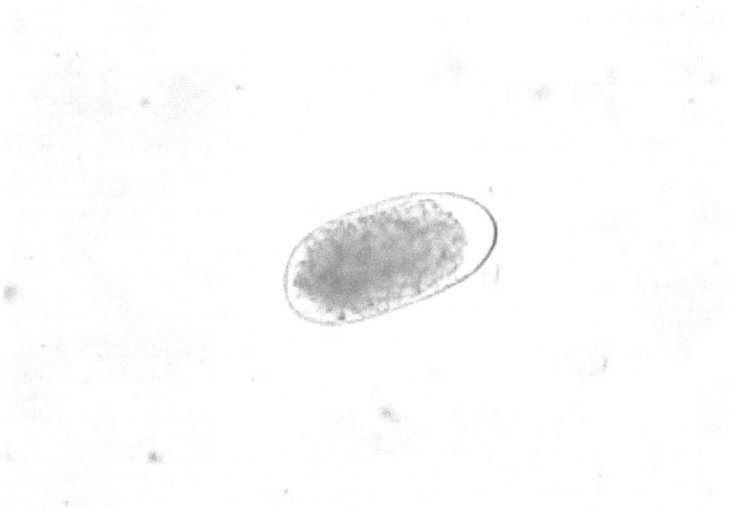

Fig. (1b). Strongyle egg.

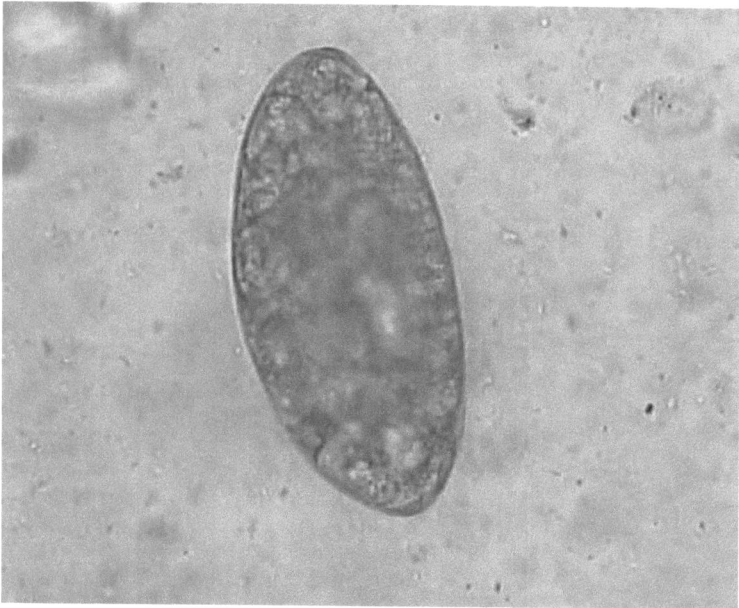

Fig. (1c). *Fasciola spp.* egg.

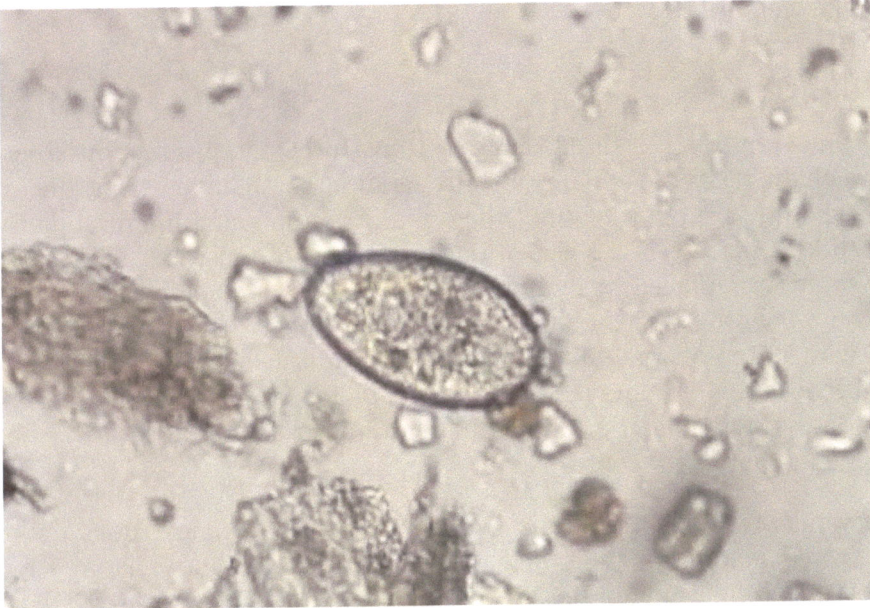

Fig. (1d). *Paramphistome* egg.

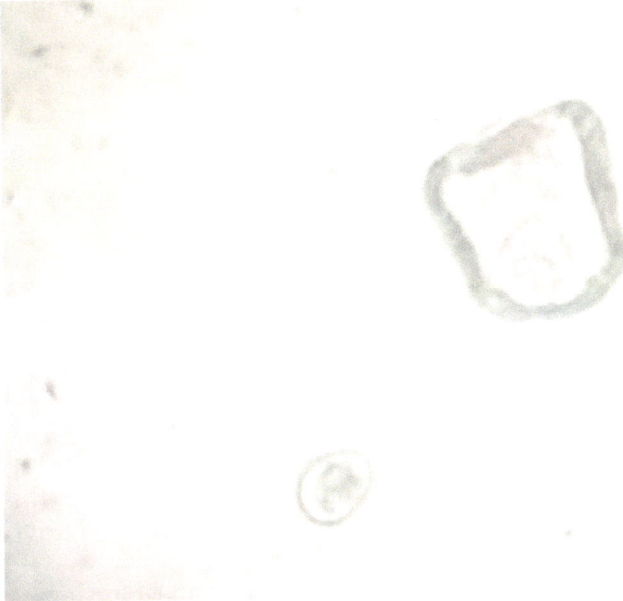

Fig. (1e). *Moniezia* egg and *Eimerian* oocyst.

Qualitative Method

Direct Method

As the name implies, it is direct and easy to perform, and just requires a few basic items, including a micro slide, coverslip, toothpick or bamboo stick, fine forceps, tap water or physiological saline solution and a compound microscope. A clean micro slide is placed on a sheet of paper. A drop of tap water or physiological saline solution is placed in the middle of the slide and some faecal material is added onto the drop with a bamboo stick or toothpick. The sample is thoroughly mixed with a drop of water or saline until a cloudy suspension is formed and any large faecal debris is removed using a pair of fine forceps. A coverslip is then placed on the sample and examined under a microscope in low power objective and then high power for confirmation.

The advantage of this technique is that it is simple, quick, does not require sophisticated laboratory tools and is useful for evaluating a large number of samples under field conditions. It is suitable for the detection of all types of helminth eggs. The demerits of the technique are that it fails to detect low grades of infection and chances of false negative results due to overlapping of undigested faecal matter over helminth eggs.

Concentration Method

Concentrating the parasitic eggs, cysts, or oocysts is the basic premise underlying this method and it is achieved either through the use of floatation fluids or sedimentation technique.

Floatation Method

The principle of this method is the separation of parasite eggs or oocysts from faecal debris through their differential densities. In this method, the faecal sample is mixed with a floatation solution that has a specific gravity greater than most of the parasitic ova, cyst or oocyst, resulting in the floating of ova, cyst or oocyst to the surface of the floatation fluid. The commonly used floatation fluids are presented in Table **1**.

The procedure involves taking 2-3 gm of faecal sample in a fresh pestle and mortar to which a small quantity of floatation fluid is added to help triturate the sample. To this, add 10 to 15 ml of floatation fluid and mix thoroughly. The mixture is then strained and transferred into a clean centrifuge tube and allowed to stand undisturbed. After about 10-15 minutes, using a wire loop, a drop from the top of the suspension is transferred to a micro-slide. After this, place a coverslip over the sample and look for parasite ova, cysts, or oocysts using a compound microscope. This is a passive way of floatation. The alternate method is centrifugal flotation which involves triturating 2-3 gm of faecal samples in a pestle and mortar with water or physiological saline solution and centrifuging the strained suspension at 1500 rpm for 5 mins. The supernatant is discarded and the sediment is mixed with flotation fluid till it forms a meniscus in a centrifuge tube and a coverslip is placed directly on it and centrifuged again for 1500 rpm for 5 mins. The coverslip is carefully removed and placed onto a clean micro-slide and examined under a microscope [4].

Table 1. Different Types of Floatation Fluids.

Floatation Fluids	Composition	Specific gravity
Saturated Salt solution	Saturated solution of Sodium Chloride	1.20
Sheather's Sugar Solution	Table Sugar (Sucrose) - 500 gm Distilled water - 320 ml Phenol - 685 gm	1.12-1.30
Sodium Nitrate Solution	Sodium Nitrate - 400 gm Distilled water - 1000 ml	1.18
Zinc Sulphate Solution	Zinc Sulphate - 386 gm Distilled water - 1000 ml	1.18
Magnesium Sulphate Solution	Magnesium Sulphate - 400 gm Distilled water - 1000 ml	1.28

It overcomes the drawbacks of the direct method by making the detection of light-grade infection possible. The technique is effective for nematode and cestode eggs but with the exception of zinc sulphate, it cannot float the heavy eggs of trematodes.

Sedimentation Method

This method is particularly used for heavier trematode eggs. A small quantity of faecal matter is emulsified in a small quantity of water. The suspension is then strained into a tube and allowed to stand for 10-15 minutes. The supernatant is decanted carefully without disturbing the sediment and fresh water is added to the tube and allowed to stand again. The process is repeated 2-3 times until the turbidity of the suspension is clear. The supernatant is carefully discarded and the sediment is then transferred onto a petri dish and observed under a microscope.

A variation of the method is centrifugal sedimentation, where faecal suspension prepared in water is transferred to a centrifuge tube and centrifuged at 1500 rpm for 5-10 minutes. The resulting supernatant is removed, and freshwater is added to the tube. This process is repeated until the supernatant becomes clear. The sediment is transferred onto a micro-slide, a coverslip is placed and examined under a microscope.

Despite being a reliable method for trematode eggs, sedimentation has several drawbacks. Because it involves a lot of manual processing, the accuracy depends on who is conducting the test and it is time-consuming [5].

Quantitative Method

Modified McMaster Test

This is the most straightforward quantitative method of faecal examination using unique reusable counting slides. The sensitivity of the test is typically set at 25 or 50 eggs per gram (epg) of faeces, as determined by the commonly employed modified McMaster chamber.

For cattle, 4 grams of faecal matter is combined and emulsified with a flotation solution (Saturated Sodium Chloride Solution) to reach a total volume of 60 ml. Alternatively, if only a small amount of faecal sample is available, the test can be conducted using 2 grams of sample and approximately 28 ml of flotation solution, resulting in a total volume of 30 ml. The mixture is strained through a tea strainer and immediately a small volume is filled into each chamber of the McMaster slide (Fig. **2**) using a pipette or syringe. If significant air bubbles are visible, fluid should be removed and refilled. The slide is left undisturbed for about five minutes to allow the flotation process to occur before examining the sample under a 10X microscope. The number of eggs or oocysts on each lane of the two chambers is counted and the total is multiplied by 50 to get the faecal egg count per gram of faeces *i.e.* each egg seen corresponds to 50 eggs in the total count.

Fig. (2). Diagram of a McMaster slide.

Modified Stoll Test

Similar to the Modified McMaster test, the modified Stoll egg-counting method relies on counting the number of eggs within a sample prepared in a mixture of flotation solution.

The process begins with thoroughly mixing 5 g of faeces with 20 ml of water in a container. One ml of mixture is then transferred to a 15 ml centrifuge tube and flotation solution is added until a little meniscus forms. Carefully, a coverslip is positioned on top without causing any overflow, and the tube is centrifuged for 10 minutes at 300-650 × g. Afterwards, the coverslip is gently picked and placed onto a microscope slide and parasite eggs are counted under a 10X objective lens. The tally of eggs observed is then multiplied by 5 to determine the total number of eggs per gram of faeces [4].

Cornell-Wisconsin Egg-counting Test

Also referred to as the double centrifugation flotation test, this method stands out as the most sensitive, capable of detecting every egg present in the faecal sample. It proves particularly valuable when expecting a low number of eggs. This method is especially useful when a low number of eggs are anticipated. Any flotation solution could be used for this method. For this method, 1-5 g faeces are combined with 12-15 ml of water in a cup. The mixture is strained into a fresh cup, following a rinse of the initial cup with 2 to 3 ml of water to ensure no residue remains. The entire suspension is then transferred into a 15 ml centrifuge tube and centrifuged at 300-650 g for 5 to 10 minutes. Following centrifugation, the supernatant is discarded, and the sediment pellet is resuspended in a flotation solution forming a meniscus. Now, as with the centrifugal flotation method, the tube can be spun with a coverslip in place or let it continue to incubate after spinning. Carefully take off the coverslip, set it down on a glass slide and count the eggs under a 10X objective lens. To avoid missing any eggs or counting them twice, caution must be taken to view each microscope field only once. The method enables quantification of less than 1 egg per gram of faeces.

Also referred to as the double centrifugation flotation test, this method stands out as the most sensitive, capable of detecting every egg present in the faecal sample. It proves particularly valuable when expecting a low number of eggs.

Formol-Ether technique

This method is very useful in those circumstances when the preservation of faecal sample is required and in cases where the floatation method is not very so effective due to the presence of fat in the sample and fatty acid. The technique is very effective in light infection of *Giardia* and *Entamoeba,* which may be easily missed by floatation or direct smear method [3].

In a pestle and mortar, combine 1-2 g of faeces with 15 ml of water. The mixture is then strained into a 15 ml centrifuge tube and spun for 2 minutes at 2000 rpm. The step is repeated after decanting the supernatant until the supernatant is clear. To the sediment, 10 ml of Formalin is added and allowed to stand for about 10 mins. The tube is then filled with 4 ml of ether, sealed with a rubber stopper, and shaken vigorously. The tube is then centrifuged for 2 minutes at 2000 rpm. A plug of faecal debris forms between the ether (top) and formalin (middle), leaving the sediment at the bottom. The plug is gently loosened with a pipette, and the supernatant and plug are discarded. A drop of the sediment is placed in a clean micro-slide, along with a drop of 2% iodine solution, and examined under a microscope.

FAECAL CULTURE TECHNIQUES

Cattle commonly harbour a range of strongyle nematodes, whose eggs are challenging to differentiate. Since the majority of broad-spectrum anthelmintics target the entire nematode group rather than specific species, it is typically not required to identify individual species for treatment in veterinary field practice. When identifying the strongyle genera, the most convenient way is to identify the third larval stage, and faecal culture is employed to obtain the third-stage larvae.

Faecal samples directly collected from the rectum are preferred to avoid contamination with free-living nematodes in the culture. The sample is taken in a plastic tub or large Petri dish and using a gloved hand broken into a uniform loose mass. For samples that are dry may need to be moistened by mixing with water. Sawdust, peat moss, or vermiculite might be added to the sample to extremely soft or liquidy sample to create a suitable consistency. Faecal samples should not be too wet or too dry, they should just be moist since larvae do not thrive well in excessively dry or wet environments. Since larvae can not thrive in extremely wet environments, faeces should just be moist, not excessively wet or too dry. The mixed faecal matter could be filled in a jar or a spoutless beaker and a cover that does not obstruct airflow should be placed loosely over the container to prevent desiccation and flies. The culture could be allowed to stand for 10–20 days at room temperature or kept in a BOD incubated for 7 days at 27°C. To prevent the growth of mould and move oxygen to the growing larvae, the culture may be loosely stirred over a few days intervals. Adding more water is an option if the faeces start to dry out. After the completion of the culture period, larvae could be harvested by either of the two methods mentioned below. In the first method, the culture jar is filled with distilled water to the brim and a Petri dish is placed over it. The Petri dish and jar are then carefully turned upside down without leaking any of the water within. The Petri dish is then partially filled with water and left to stand overnight without disturbance. The next day larvae could be easily retrieved as they migrate out into the water in the Petri dish. The second method is by utilising the Baermann's Test [2].

Baermann Test

The Baermann test is commonly used to separate larvae from faecal or pasture soil samples. It is frequently used in cattle to diagnose lungworm infection (Fig. 3) and detect strongyle larvae contamination of pasture. The method is based on the principle that larvae actively migrate from the faeces into the water before eventually sinking to the bottom of the apparatus, from where they can be conveniently collected for identification. Today, different versions of the original Baermann device are employed, such as wine glasses or a funnel. The original Baermann apparatus was made up of a funnel fixed to a metal stand. The funnel was connected to a short tubing with a clamp at the bottom. The larvae in the faeces that are placed in the funnel migrate out and drop into the tubing or hollow stem above the clamp, where they can be readily collected. The complete process includes putting 10 g or more of the faecal or soil sample in a double layer of cheesecloth, placing it inside the funnel and nicely securing it by tying the sample to a stick or pencil placed on the rims of the funnel. This way the sample responded. Alternatively, the sample could be placed on a tea strainer placed on the funnel or wire mesh that is suspended. After filling the funnel with warm water, leave it for at least 8 hours, preferably overnight. By carefully releasing the clamp on the tubing, collect the first 3-4 drops of the fluid and observe under a light microscope. Alternatively, about 10-15 ml of the fluid could be collected and centrifuged at low speed to collect the larvae [1].

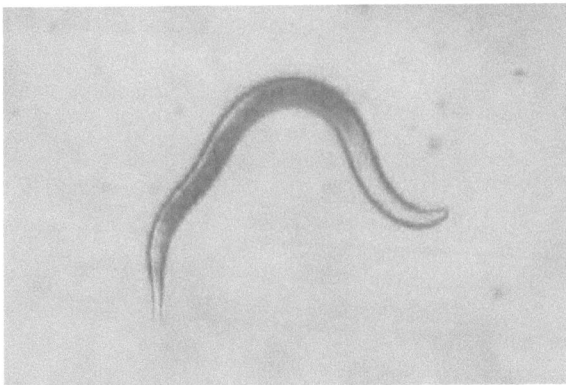

Fig. (3). *Dictyocaulus viviparous* larva.

FAECAL STAINING METHOD FOR DIAGNOSIS OF *Cryptosporidium*

Cryptosporidium infection causes diarrhoea in young calves and is diagnosed by detecting oocysts in faeces using the modified Ziehl Neelsen (MZN) staining method. The procedure begins with the preparation of a thin faecal smeared on a clean glass slide similar to a direct test. The slide is then placed on a staining rack flooded with Carbol fuchsin and allowed to stain for 5 minutes. It is then heated gently with a Bunsen burner from the bottom. After rinsing again with tap water and air drying, the slide is counter-stained with methylene blue for one minute. It is then rinsed once more with tap water, air-dried, and examined under a microscope at high-power and oil immersion magnification. The *Cryptosporidium* oocysts appear as red/pink colour dots against the blue or clear background [5].

CONCLUSION

The faecal examination approach is still a vital diagnostic tool for parasitic diseases despite numerous limitations. False negatives are common in early or low-intensity infections, and because not all parasites continuously shed eggs, cysts, or larvae, hence negative results do not always rule out parasitic infections. When paired with a robust sampling plan that takes into account the parasite's biology, its response to different seasons and management practises, as well as the herd or individual clinical history, it provides different yields . It offers a simple, rapid, and affordable technique to detect a variety of parasites and continues to play a crucial role in parasite diagnosis in the field and research.

REFERENCES

[1]   Boray JC. Experimental Fascioliasis in Australia. Adv Parasitol 1969; 7: 95-210.
        [http://dx.doi.org/10.1016/S0065-308X(08)60435-2] [PMID: 4935272]

[2]   Cable RM. An Illustrated Laboratory Manual of Parasitology. Bombay, India: Allied Pacific Private Limited 1963.

[3]   Dorsman W. Fluctuation within a day in the liver-fluke egg-count of the rectal contents of cattle. Vet Rec 1956; 68(34): 571-4.

[4]   Shams S, Khan S, Khan A, Khan I, Ijaz M, Ullah A. Differential techniques used for detection of *Cryptosporidium* oocysts in stool specimens. J Parasit Dis 2016; 1(1): 1-12.

[5]   Soulsby EJL. Helminths, Arthropods and Protozoa of Domesticated Animals. 7th ed., London: ELBS, Baillier Tindall 1982.

CHAPTER 12

Histopathological Diagnosis of Parasitic Diseases

Paras Saini[1], Sushma Kajal[1], Surbhi Gupta[2] and Snehil Gupta[3],*

[1]*Department of Veterinary Pathology, Lala Lajpat Rai University of Veterinary and Animal Sciences, Hisar, India*

[2]*Department of Veterinary Physiology and Biochemistry, Lala Lajpat Rai University of Veterinary and Animal Sciences, Hisar, India*

[3]*Department of Veterinary Parasitology, Lala Lajpat Rai University of Veterinary and Animal Sciences, Hisar, India*

Abstract: In the bovine industry, histopathological diagnosis plays a crucial role in the identification and characterization of parasitic diseases. Parasites can infect various organs and tissues in the cattle body, causing a wide range of pathological changes. This manuscript aims to provide an overview of the histopathological techniques employed in the diagnosis of parasitic diseases of cattle. It discusses the common parasites encountered, the associated histopathological findings, and the methods used to identify and differentiate these parasites. Understanding the histopathological features of parasitic infections is essential for accurate diagnosis and appropriate management of these diseases.

Keywords: Cattle, Histopathological diagnosis, Microscopic evaluation, Parasitic diseases, Tissues.

INTRODUCTION

Preserving the well-being of animals requires collaborative efforts. An essential component of this process involves the laboratory-based identification of diseases or pathogen(s) responsible for causing the disease that can be of any aetiology such as infectious, neoplastic, parasitic, deficiency disease or intoxication. Parasitic diseases are infectious diseases, which result from infections caused by parasites that sustain themselves by feeding off on their host. One of the laboratory-based tests is histopathological examination of tissues [1]. Before histopathology, diagnosis was made based on macroscopically visible lesions at the time of necropsy. However, based solely on gross examination it was difficult to rule out the actual cause of disease from the other diseases producing similar lesions. Histopathology is a subspecialty of pathology that focuses on the study of

---

*** Corresponding author Snehil Gupta:** Department of Veterinary Parasitology, Lala Lajpat Rai University of Veterinary and Animal Sciences, Hisar, India; E-mail: snehilgupta568@gmail.com

Tanmoy Rana (Ed.)

changes in the cells or tissues caused by a disease. Histopathology offers the benefit of being a versatile diagnostic tool as it is non-specific and can be used for the diagnosis of a broad range of diseases [2]. The majority of the time, parasitic infections go undiagnosed, and superficial diagnosis frequently results in prolonged or even unsuccessful treatment. Histopathological examination makes it feasible to determine the type or species of parasite involved the location of the pathological lesions, any potential bacterial or viral consequences, and the prognosis of the disease [3]. Hence, pathologists can assume a significant role in diagnosing parasitic infections, especially when parasites have not been taken into account by the clinical team and the necessary microbiology tests have not been requested (Boland and Pritt, 2017). Histopathology includes collection and preservation of samples, processing of tissues, tissue sectioning, tissue staining, and microscopic examination to identify the changes. Pathological changes associated with helminth infection in cattle are mechanical obstruction of the lumen of gastrointestinal tract passage and interfering with functions of the organs involved in producing pathogenesis in the host. For instance, schistosomes are responsible for the obstruction of mesenteric blood vessels. Helminth parasite, *Toxocara vitulorum* leads to obstruction of intestinal tracts in young calves. Hydatid cysts in the liver, lung, and brain invade and destroy the cattle tissue and cells. Haemoprotozoan parasites such as *Trypanosoma evansi, Theileria annulata,* and *Babesia* spp. devour blood and cause anaemia in cattle. Parasites such as *T. vitulorum* and *Sarcocystis* secrete certain toxins in the body of the cattle. Among inflammatory cells, eosinophils, basophils, and mast cells played a vital role in host defence against the helminth parasites. In the case of observation of helminth parasites in the tissue section, either solid-bodied acoelomates or tubes within a tube (Pseudocoelomates) are noticed. Nematodes are often filled with organs, eggs, and larvae, whereas, trematodes and cestodes have organs embedded in parenchymatous tissue. Members of the phylum Platyhelminthes have a syncytial tegument, however, nematodes and acanthocephalans secrete acellular cuticles.

There are essentially two sorts of helminth sections during the histopathological examination. In the first case, the section showed parasites with solid bodies (the acoelomates) of trematodes and cestodes. In the second case, there are sections where tubs within a tube plan are observed, for instance, nematodes and acanthocephalans tissue sections. Flatworms tissue section may possess cavities within the different organs, whereas, roundworms and acanthocephalans are generally packed with eggs and larvae. Further, thick acellular cuticles outline the body of nematodes and acanthocephalans, however, syncytial tegument is observed in the case of Platyhelminthes. Fortunately, acanthocephalans are rarely encountered in large ruminants. Common trematode parasites encountered in the cattle tissue section are *Fasciola* spp., *Schistosoma* spp., and *Amphistomes.* Likewise, the Metacestode stage of *Echinococcus granulosus* is most frequently encountered in the lung, liver, and brain tissue section of cattle. Among nematodes, life cycle stage of *Toxocara vitulorum, Strongyloides papillosus, Ostertagia* spp*., Trichostrongylus* spp*., and Bunostomum phlebotomum* are more often seen in tissue sections of cattle.

Histopathological research is critical in the diagnosis of human and animal illnesses. Histopathological alterations detected during specific parasite invasions are very significant for differential diagnosis and frequently establish the presence of parasitic illnesses. Such investigations also enable the identification of the disease's root cause. Many pathogenic organisms induce inflammatory lesions, and microscopic findings can help with aetiological identification. However, histological lesions are restricted in terms of various biological agents that might cause tissue injury. The most common histologic feature of parasite infections is granulomatous inflammation [4]. It is distinguished by a concentrated infiltration of macrophages and epithelioid cells. There are several large cells, lymphocytes, plasma cells, fibroblasts, and granulocytes. Helminths and parasites that multiply intracellularly are among the agents that cause granulomas. In histopathology, several unique stains are used, such as Giemsa's stain, which is beneficial in identifying *Leishmania*. Immunohistochemical approaches give an aetiological diagnosis by using particular antibodies. Tissue damage can sometimes be immune-mediated, dependent on the presence of circulating immune complexes or the participation of T-lymphocytes, rather than caused by direct parasite harm. In general, the lesions seen include vasculitis and inflammatory responses mostly constituted of mononuclear cells, as seen in many viral or bacterial infections. In some circumstances, *in situ* PCR improves aetiological diagnosis. To identify parasites in tissues under the microscope, the observer must have preliminary information on the gross and internal morphological details of the parasite, which are expected to be detected in the tissue under consideration and in that particular host. Parasite localization can result in hyperplastic-neoplastic lesions. Many parasites have been linked to the emergence of various types of neoplasms, but the processes involved remain unknown. Chronic inflammation and/or immune suppression appear to promote tumor growth [5].

Numerous animal parasites, protozoans, metazoans, and, in particular, helminths, can produce granulomatous lesions in humans. The study of two instances, *Ieishmania granuloma* and *Schistosomia granuloma*, would appear to imply that interactions between the host and the parasite at different phases of development are based on facilitation or rejection events involving both humoral and cellular processes. Thus, the emergence of the granuloma is determined by the host's reactional capabilities. The lesions found in these granulomas may be associated with a number of fundamental processes, including necrosis, fibrosis, specific or non-specific responses, and allergic reactions, all of which are present in various aetiological conditions.

Trematodes

Estimating the total size and looking at the location of the sex organs, the types of suckers, the size and branching of the gut, and the excretory system are all necessary for identifying the family and genus of a trematode. Eggs, if present, can be very helpful once the operculum's size, form, type, and developmental stage (with or without a miracidium) have been determined. For an accurate diagnosis, the quantity, shape, and location of spines on the body's surface must all be thoroughly examined. Trematodes lack cavities and possess a solid, spongy body that is not separated into the cortex and medulla. Certain characteristic features for the differentiation of trematodes in a tissue section are as follows:

1. Solid parenchymatous and spongy body with few cavities.

2. Bifurcating intestine ending into bling caeca.

3. Syncytial spiny tegument.

4. Outer circular, middle longitudinal and inner diagonal muscle layer.

5. Presence of 2 suckers, of which, the oral sucker is connected with gut.

6. Larvae are less frequently encountered and are without any reproductive characters.

7. Presence of both testes and ovaries within the same parasites.

8. The taxonomic significance of vitelline gland distribution and sex organ arrangement lies in their ability to identify trematodes.

9. Eggs are often operculated with typical shells and golden-brown shells.

Fasciola hepatica and F. gigantica

Tissue section of bile duct and liver shows the presence of medium to large sized leaf-like organisms with muscular pharynx and intestinal tissue. Adult flukes present in the bile duct are responsible for chronic cholangitis in ruminants. Pipe-stem liver due to chronic cholangitis is peculiar to *Fasciola* infection in cattle. The histopathology of migratory tracks is represented by the presence of fibrous connective tissue juvenile flukes in sections, and infiltration of multinucleated cells such as macrophages, epithelioid cells, and giant cells. Extensive hemorrhages and coagulative necrosis are observed in liver tissue. The uterine section of fluke shows the presence of large-sized eggs at the different stages of embryonic development. Only oral suckers are connected to the gut. It is noted that the gallbladder and bile ducts have adenocarcinomas and adenomas. Vitelline glands are distributed in both dorsal and ventral aspects of the gut. Larval stages are sometimes observed during histopathological examination of the liver, especially, in case of heavy and continuous infection that can lead to cirrhosis. However, their body is poorly defined and only a parenchymatous body with outer syncytial tegument can be appreciated. In the case of *Dicrocoelium dendriticum*, multiple lancet-shaped adult worms are seen in the bile duct showing adenomatous hyperplasia. Further, white migratory tracks are seen on the liver surface.

Schistosomiasis

The tissue section of the mesenteric vein showed a dioecious parenchymatous worm in which a slender female is enclosed in the gynaecophoric canal of the thick and stout male partner. Further, granulomatous inflammatory reactions are seen around the eggs laid by the adult worm in the liver and intestinal tissue.

Amphistomiasis

Ulceration and necrosis are observed at the tips of the ruminal papillae due to adult worms. The lamina propria is infiltrated by eosinophils, macrophages, and lymphocytes. Flukes that are adults can be found beneath the keratinized layer. The serosa has hemorrhage patches and the duodenum's mucosa is swollen and coated in blood-stained mucus. The duodenum contains a large number of juvenile flukes with a flask-shaped appearance. The bile ducts and biliary passages are observed to have embedded paramphistomes, which cause the ducts to dilate, thicken, and fibrose.

Cestodes

Cattle are frequently discovered to have cestoid infection in their intestine. With the exception of severe infestations that cause catarrhal enteritis and eosinophil infiltration, these worms mostly live in the intestine, obstruct digestion and absorption of simplified food material, and appear to have a little influence on health. Common species reported are *Taenia metacestodes, Moniezia benedeni, M. expansa, Stilesia hepatica* (found within the bile ducts), and *Avitellina* species. The holdfast organ of tapeworms is called the scolex, and it can either be radiated (having two longitudinal holdfast grooves) or acetabular (having four suckers).

1. Like trematodes, subcuticular muscles in the tissue sections are situated directly beneath the cuticle (s) in tapeworms.

2. Additionally, tapeworms have longitudinal muscles within the parenchyma, followed by circular muscles, which split the parenchyma into an outer cortical zone and an inner tube that houses the reproductive organs.

3. In the terminal proglottid, excretory channels open.

4. In histological sections, suckers appear as muscular circles due to radial striations of the muscle fibers.

5. Internal organs are embedded into a loose parenchymatous matrix.

6. Outer longitudinal and inner transverse non-striated muscle fibres are divided by body parenchyma into cortex and medulla.

7. The intestine is completely absent.

8. The presence of calcareous corpuscles is an exclusive character of cestode tissues.

9. The larval stage is more commonly observed.

10. Syncytial microvilli are present on the inner side of the tissue section.

11. The presence of suckers and other holdfast organs is typical of cestode tissue.

12. The tegument that protects tapeworms is made up of cytoplasmic protrusions from epidermal cells, and it is visible in histological sections as a thick, homogenous, non-cellular exterior layer that is held up by a basal membrane.

Cysticercus bovis and hydatid cysts are the most frequently observed cestode larvae during histopathological examination of cattle tissue.

1. Unlike other taenidia species metacestodes, *C. bovis* in various cattle tissues cannot be identified based on the shape and measurement of hooks on the scolex due to the absence of hooks in the scolex.

2. In the wall folds, there is more parenchyma with characteristic calcareous corpuscles.

3. The bladder cavity entirely encloses the parenchymatous component of the larva in cysticerci that is seen in the muscles.

4. Only a fibrous tissue (receptaculum) with elongated cells, organized in parallel lines, forms the surface of the parenchymatous region that faces the bladder cavity.

Hydatid cysts develop in the liver, lung, and brain of cattle due to the ingestion of *Echinococcus granulosus, E. multilocularis, E. oligarthus,* and *E. vogeli* eggs.

Hydatid cysts can be identified in tissue section by following characteristic features:

1. It has thick laminated membranes, which separate the germinative layer from the surrounding connective tissue.

2. In sterile hydatid cysts, laminated membranes are the only diagnostic characteristic.

3. In a fertile cyst, germinative membranes bear several sessile small scolices, which are termed protoscolices or brood capsules.

4. On the other hand, the laminated membrane is thin and the development pattern of alveolar hydatid cysts, which are caused by the metacestode of *Echinococcus multilocularis,* is invasive rather than expansive.

Nematodes

Roundworms mainly occupy the gastrointestinal tract and lungs (*Dictyocaulus viviparous*) of cattle. They possess a pseudocoelom and a cylindrical body, which is circular in cross-section (*e.g. Trichuris, Haemonchus, Trichostrongylus, Mecistocirrus, Chaberia, Giageria* and *Oesophagostomum*). Because of the circular cross-section, they are known as roundworms. The digestive tract of a nematode consists of an oral opening, mouth (buccal) capsule, muscular pharynx, esophagus (high variation and varied shape), intestine, and rectum (position of the anus is variable). The fluid-filled within the body cavity provides a hydrostatic skeleton to support the motility of the parasite. On the longitudinal section, nematodes showed several characteristic features, such as acellular external cuticle, thin cellular hypodermis, and somatic musculature. In several species, the multi-layered cuticle has ridges and ornamentation. When a nematode is carefully sectioned, cuticular ornamentations, or cuticular bosses, can be seen around the mouth in *Gongylonema pulchrum*. Lateral chords, which are hypodermis extensions, can also extend deep into the pseudocoelom in a number of nematodes. Nematodes have coelomyarian or platymyarian body muscles, which are made up of dense contractile components and pale sarcoplasm. The cross-section of the central esophagus (oe) has a characteristic tri-radiate (y-shaped) lumen. The cross-section of coelomyarian muscle cells has a U shape, and they can protrude far into the pseudo coelom, hiding the body cavity. The cells that make up platymyarian muscles are typically big and few, lying flat on the hypodermis with very little protrusion into the pseudocoelom.

Identification can be aided by the histological characteristics of the nematode's digestive system. Nematode groups may be distinguished thanks to the type of epithelial cells that make up the gut. Cell types vary from cuboidal to tall columnar, from extremely big multinucleate cells to cuboidal cells. Identification of nematodes can also be aided by features such as the height of the microvillar layer, the presence or lack of microvilli around the intestinal lumen, and the size and position of the intestinal epithelial cell nuclei.

Histological sections of nematodes may reveal their genital tracts. In the majority of nematodes, the sexes are distinct, with females being bigger than males. Male adults have a single genital tract made up of the testis, which generates sperm, and the vas deferens, which house the sperm. H&E-stained nematode sperm has an oval, tiny, eosinophilic nucleus and a basophilic appearance. One or more genital tracts, made up of ovaries that give rise to oviducts that discharge into the uterus, may be present in female nematodes. The uterus houses growing eggs or embryos, while the seminal receptacles and the distal portion of the uterus, may hold sperm from earlier copulations. While some species of nematodes are viviparous, others are oviparous and release eggs with distinct morphology. Lungworm larvae and *Trichuris* eggs can be easily identified in stained tissue sections (Table **1**).

Nematode muscle cells are located beneath the cuticle and hypodermal layer, along the length of their bodies. The long axis of muscle cells runs parallel to the worm's length, and various nematodes have variable numbers and shapes of these cells. Instead of receiving nerve endings from ganglia to muscular cells, muscle cells in worms transmit processes to the dorsal as well as the ventral nerve cord (Table **2**).

Table 1. Description of muscle cells according to their number.

Sr. No.	Type of musculature	Details
1.	Meromyarian worm	Helminth parasite in which cross section showed the presence of 3-5 muscle cells per quadrant.
2.	Polymyarian worm	Helminth parasite in which cross section showed the presence of six or more muscle cells per quadrant.

Table 2. Description of muscle cells according to their appearance.

Sr. No.	Type of musculature	Details
1.	Platymyarian	Contractile elements are suppressed towards the hypodermis leaving the vacant upper portion of the cell.
2.	Coelomyarian	Contractile elements extend up the side of the cell body.

Of these, platymyarian cell are often few in number per quadrant, therefore, such tissue is called platymyarian-meromyarian musculature and such arrangement is observed in members of order Rhabditida, Oxyurida and Strongylida of class nematoda. Likewise, if more numerous coelomyarian muscle cells are present in each quadrant, it is termed as polymyarian-coelomyarian musculature and these are often observed in order Ascaridida and Spirurida of class nematoda.

In majority primitive nematodes, the oesophagus is completely muscular, for instance, the members of order Strongylida, Trichostrongylida, Ascaridoids and Oxyuroids. In other groups, such as filarioids and spiruroids, the oesophagus is anteriorly muscular and posteriorly glandular. Therefore, in the tissue section, musculature is observed in the partial section of esophagus, whereas the rest half is densely stained (Table 3).

Table 3. Different types of oesophagus in members of class Nematoda.

S. No.	Type of oesophagus	Characters	Related Orders
1.	Filariform	Simple, tube-like and cylindrical with slightly thickened posteriorly.	Strongylida and Trichostrongylida
2.	Bulb shaped	Simple, tube-like with large posterior swelling.	Ascaridoids
3.	Double-bulb shaped	Simple, tube-like anteriorly and two bulb-shaped swelling posteriorly.	Oxyuroids
4.	Muscular-glandular	Oesophagus is anteriorly muscular and posteriorly glandular.	Filarioids and Spiruroids
5.	Trichuroid	Oesophagus has a capillary form formed by the single layer of cells.	*Trichuris* spp.
6.	Rhabditiform	Slight anterior and posterior swelling in muscular oesophagus.	Pre-parasitic stages of parasitic nematodes and adult stage of free living nematodes

Toxocara vitulorum Identification

In the early stages, the parasite undergoes migration in the liver, kidneys, lungs, heart, brain, spleen, and other body tissues producing several necrotic migratory tracts. Within the tissue section of these organs, extravasated erythrocytes and a small number of leukocytes are seen with parasite larvae lodged in cellular detritus. Additionally, granulomatous nodules made up of giant cells, lymphocytes, macrophages, and eosinophils are seen around the degenerated larvae. Hemorrhages and localized coagulative necrosis are also seen in a few locations. The bronchi, glomeruli, and portal blood arteries all contain the larvae.

Many mature worms in the small intestine cause catarrhal enteritis with eosinophil infiltrations in the later stages. Obstructive jaundice can also result from mature worms obstructing the pancreatic or bile ducts. Another typical finding is pneumonia caused by intestinal wall invasion. In the tissue section, adult worms are rarely encountered. Larval stages undergo tissue migration and are often identified in tissue sections on the basis of small size (< 21 microns in diameter).

1. They characteristically have a thick multi-layered cuticle, club-shaped esophagus, and three simple lips.

2. Muscles that are polymyarian-coelomyarian and have cytoplasmic processes that extend into the body cavity.

3. The intestinal tract has a significant number of columnar epithelial cells, small microvilli, and a single nucleus close to the base of each cell.

4. The shells of uterine eggs are thick, wrinkled, and frequently sculptured.

5. The *T. vitulorum* larvae in the tissue section are characterized by the presence of single lateral alae and paired H-shaped excretory columns.

Strongyle Worm Identification

These worms (*Haemonchus contortus*, *Ostertagia* spp., *Trichostrongylus axei*, *Mecistocirrus digitatus*, *Cooperia* spp., *Nematodirrus* spp.) mainly inhabit the stomach and small intestine of cattle.

1. Adult strongyle cross section is characterized by platymyarian musculature.

2. The intestine is made up of a small number of cells with noticeable nuclei and a microvillous border.

3. Juvenile adults and fourth stage larvae are discovered tucked in between the abomasal mucosa's epithelial cells and the basement membrane.

4. In the case of *Ostertagia*, the dilated gastric glands of the abomasum contain juvenile adults and fourth stage larvae.

Nodular Worm Identification

The larval stages of nodular worms (*Oesophagostomum radiatum, O. columbianum*) produce suppurative nodules in the wall of the large intestine of cattle during repeated infection. Further, adult parasites develop in these nodules. Therefore, in the tissue section, often developing worms are seen inside these nodules.

1. Larvae have noticeable lateral cords and a smooth, moderately thick cuticle.

2. The musculature is composed of platymyarian and meromyarian muscle cells, with comparatively few muscle cells in each quadrant.

3. The presence of a few multinucleate cells with a noticeable microvilli brush border helps identify the gut.

4. Identification of nests of L4 larvae in nodules of the colon of cattle is of diagnostic importance in nodular worm identification.

Lungworm Identification

Lungworms (*Dictyocaulus viviparus*) typically parasitize the bronchi and bronchioles of cattle. First-stage larvae of size around 300-360 microns are seen threaded in lung parenchyma. The intestinal cells of the larvae contain numerous chromatin granules.

1. In the tissue section, the cuticle is exceptionally thin.

2. The musculature is polymyarian-coelomyarian type.

3. In the gut, microvilli are comparatively less prominent.

4. The uterus is filled with embryonated eggs or larvae. Sometimes, larvae are found embedded in a cyst formed at the lung parenchyma, however, the cuticle is without any anterior protuberance.

Hookworm Identification

Hookworms (*Bunostomum phlebotomum*; *Agriostomum vryburghi*) are recorded in the small intestine as well as tissue sections (skeletal muscle) of cattle.

1. The presence of double lateral alae and small-sized (14-16 micron), deeply stained body are characteristic of hookworm larvae in tissue section.

2. The musculature is of platymyarian type.

3. Intestinal cells form syncytium.

Gongylonema Identification

The adult worms (*G. pulchrum, G. verrucosum*) are found mainly threaded in the forestomach (esophagus/rumen/reticulum/omasum) of cattle and have several distinctive morphological features. The front muscular and posterior strongly pigmented glandular portions of the esophagus are separated. The musculature is of polymyarian-coelomyarian type.

1. Small, thick-shelled embryonated eggs or intensely stained larvae are seen in the uterine section of female worms.

2. Unequal large lateral chords project into the body cavity.

3. Thick cuticular bosses and plagues along with massive cervical alae cover the anterior end.

Onchocerca Identification

The life cycle of this helminth parasite is typically filarioid (*Onchocerca gutturosa*, *O. gibsoni*, *O. ochengi*), with the exception that the larval stage (microfilariae) is found embedded in the tissue space of skin and migrate in the subdermal connective tissue. Even mature worms can be seen firmly coiled, entrenched in thick connective tissue, and occasionally forming separate fibrous nodules. Diagnosis is mainly based on the identification of larvae in skin biopsy samples. The tissue section determines whether the anteriorly located muscular and posteriorly present glandular regions of the esophagus are visible [7].

1. Adult female worms are long, and slender in shape, with distinct external cuticular ridges and striation in the inner cuticular layers.

2. The number of striations within these ridges is helpful in distinguishing various species in this genera.

3. There is a noticeable quantity of hypodermal tissue located beneath the muscle cells, which are feeble and poorly formed.

Parafilaria bovicola Identification

The adult worms are found in the small inflammatory and hemorrhagic nodules in the subcutaneous tissue and skin of the upper body region of cattle. Embryonated eggs, eosinophilia, and microfilariae can be identified by screening skin biopsy samples of bleeding points generated by gravid females while laying their eggs in bright sunlight.

1. Numerous papillae and cuticular ridges are observed in the cross-section of the anterior end of the worm. Oesophagus is divided as in other spiruroids and filariasis worms.

2. In case of a cross-section of the female worm, the vulva is also located near the mouth opening.

3. The musculature is coelomyrian-polymyrian type.

4. Fully embryonated eggs and microfilaria are found filled in the uterus.

Trichuris Identification

These helminth parasites (*T. globulosa*, *T.discolor*) are found embedded in the mucosa of the large intestine of cattle. The diameter of immature worms is homogeneous and they are entirely encased in the mucosa; in contrast, the adult worm's stout section sits free in the lumen while its thin anterior portion is threaded through the large intestine's epithelium. A characteristic feature is the presence of a stichosome oesophagus in which a small cylindrical oesophagus is surrounded by a layer of individual cells known as stichocytes.

1. Secondly, a single bacillary band is present in the oesophageal region, which is composed of specialized hypodermal gland cells embedded in a section of cuticle and hypodermis.

2. In the cross-section, a single tube of the female reproductive system is observed.

3. Muscles are coelomyrian-polymyrian type.

4. Eggs are characteristically large-sized, barrel-shaped, single-celled, un-embryonated stage with bipolar prominences.

5. Anus is only observed in case the terminal area of the worm is observed in the tissue section.

Specific Histopathological Diagnostic Features of Commonly Found Cattle Arthropods

Mange, maggot-infested wounds, and tick bites are common arthropod-borne manifestations on the body of cattle. The majority of these can be screened by gross and skin scraping examination. In a few cases, such as sarcoptic mange, where a single mite excretory-secretory products are capable of inducing immediate hypersensitivity, histopathological diagnosis can be exercised. In the tissue section, arthropods can be identified based on the chitinous exoskeleton, jointed appendages, true coelom, metameric segmentation, a racemose tracheal system, striated musculature attached to the exoskeleton, and darkly stained fat bodies. Larvae of *Hypoderma bovis* and *H. lineatum* are more frequently encountered in endemic areas with characteristic spiracular plates in the musculature of cattle. The presence of sarcoptic mange in the tissue section is identified based on the hyperkeratosis of skin, the presence of globular shape, segmented legs, round mouth parts, hairs, egg development, reproductive organs, and triangular spines on the chitinous exoskeleton. Mites are found in the tunnels formed in the skin up to the stratum germinativum and dermis. In the case of psoroptic mange, lesions are restricted in the stratum corneum and hyperkeratosis, and various life cycle stages are seen in the superficial skin layers. The presence of psoroptic mange in the tissue section can be identified based on the presence of the oval-shaped body, segmented legs, pointed mouth parts, egg development, reproductive appendages such as copulatory tubercles, and absence of spines on the chitinous exoskeleton. Cases of demodicosis are although less common in cattle but cannot be excluded. In the tissue section, *Demodex* mites can be identified based on the presence of cigar-shaped organisms in the hair follicle and associated superficial sebaceous glands. Rarely, a nodular form of demodicosis is noticed in cattle, which can be easily diagnosed in the tissue section by visualization of myriads of cigar-shaped bodies in between the hyperkeratinized tissue.

Specific Histopathological Diagnostic Features of Commonly found Pentastomids Parasites in Cattle

The adult of *Linguatula serrata*, tongue worm, is commonly found in the respiratory tract of dogs and other carnivorous animals. However, the nymphal stage is frequently encysted in the tissue of lymph nodes of cattle. Histopathologically, the nymphal stage can be identified based on the presence of pseudo-segmentation, striated musculature in the subcuticular region, spherical to the oval-shaped body, thick cuticle with sclerotized stomata, complete digestive system in which the intestine is surrounded by acidophilic glands.

Specific Histopathological Diagnostic Features of Commonly Found Protozoan Parasites in Cattle

Ciliates are commensal parasites in the rumen of the ruminants. However, sometimes ciliates are also observed in the lung, hepatic vessels, and intestine and may lead to pneumonia and inflammatory changes in the tissue. In case of severe enteritis, these pleomorphic ciliates may penetrate up to the submucosa.

Identifying coccidian parasites in tissue sections typically involves a combination of histopathological techniques and staining methods. Coccidian parasites belong to the phylum Apicomplexa and include organisms like *Cryptosporidium* and *Eimeria* species in cattle. Coccidian parasites may not always be visible with H&E staining alone. Modified Acid-Fast staining helps in visualizing oocysts of certain coccidian parasites like *Cryptosporidium* in fecal samples. Immunohistochemistry (IHC) can provide specific identification of coccidian parasites within tissue sections. It involves using specific antibodies that bind to coccidian antigens, allowing for their visualization under a microscope. Fluorescent dyes can be used to label specific parasite structures or components, enhancing their visibility and aiding in identification. Depending on the coccidian species, various stages of the parasite's life cycle, such as trophozoites, schizonts, and merozoites, might be visible within host cells or tissues. Coccidian oocysts typically have the following distinct morphological features.

a. **Oocyst Shape:** Coccidian oocysts can be spherical, oval, or ellipsoidal.

b. **Wall Structure:** They have a characteristic double-layered wall.

c. **Internal Contents:** Depending on the developmental stage of the coccidian, the internal contents might include sporozoites, sporocysts, or other structures.

There are several *Eimeria* species, which infect the cattle. The trophozoite and schizont stages can be observed in the intestinal epithelial cells of cattle. Trophozoites usually have a distinct nucleus, which appears as a darker or more prominent spot within the cell. The cytoplasm of trophozoites might be granular and less defined compared to other stages. Their size and shape can vary depending on the *Eimeria* species and the specific host. Schizonts are larger than trophozoites and often more irregular in shape due to the multiple nuclei within. Schizonts have a characteristic "mulberry-like" appearance. The nuclei might be visible as distinct dark spots within the cell. Schizonts may also exhibit some granularity in the cytoplasm, similar to trophozoites. Inside the developing oocyst, the sporozoites might appear as small, elongated structures within the oocyst. Depending on the stage of development, sporozoites might have distinct nuclei or organelles becoming visible. Sometimes, the wall-forming bodies (large spherical eosinophilic granules) are also observed in newly developing oocysts, which later combine to develop the oocyst wall. In the case of *Cryptosporidium* infection, minute basophilic granules may appear at the luminal side of the epithelial cells lining the gastrointestinal tract. The parasite is intracellular extracytoplasmic in location. All stages, *viz.* schizont, gamont, and oocyst are found underneath the host cell membrane [8].

Histopathological Techniques for Parasitic Diagnosis

1. **Collection and preservation of samples**

Tissue samples should be collected in 10% formalin for histopathology from organs/tissues suspected of having parasitic infection at the time of necropsy. For proper fixation, tissue samples should be of approximately 5 mm thickness. The formalin volume should be 20 times that of the tissue to be fixed, and ensure the specimen does not touch the container walls [9].

2. Processing of samples for Histopathology

The fundamental goal of tissue processing is to impart the necessary stiffness to the tissue, enabling it to be sliced into very thin sections suitable for microscopic analysis. The media most used for this purpose is paraffin. However, paraffin is not miscible with water so it is essential to dehydrate the tissues first and then put the tissues in the clearing solutions which are miscible in paraffin. The basic steps of tissue processing are as follows:

a. Overnight washing of formalin-containing tissues – To remove most of the formalin from within the cells.

b. Dehydration – In a series of increasing alcohol concentrations, to replace the water content of the tissues/cells.

c. Clearing - Given the immiscibility of alcohols and paraffins, an intermediary solvent that is miscible with both substances (such as xylene, and benzene) becomes necessary. This solvent displaces the alcohol within the tissue, a stage known as 'clearing.' The term 'clearing' refers to how clearing agents enhance the tissue's optical clarity or transparency by virtue of their higher refractive index.

d. Infiltration - "At this point, the tissue samples are ready for paraffin infiltration. Liquid paraffin permeates the tissues and, upon cooling, solidifies to a texture that enables cutting on a microtome."

3. **Tissue microtome**: Following the embedding of the tissue and the preparation of the block, the subsequent stage involves microtomy. The term "microtomy" has its roots in the Greek language, where "Mikros" translates to small and "Temnein" means to cut. In order to facilitate a successful microscopic examination, it is imperative to obtain thin tissue sections through the process of microtomy. The steps of tissue sectioning are as follows:

a. Trimming of tissue - Trimming of the tissue is necessary to uncover the tissue specimen within the paraffin wax, preparing it for the cutting process.
b. Cooling of blocks on ice - Cooling aids in preserving a consistent texture for both the paraffin and the tissue.
c. Cutting tissue and making ribbons of it –At first microtome is set up for cutting tissue of the expected thickness. Cutting of tissue samples is done by slow, gentle, and smooth strokes. Ribbons like tissue sections are produced by

adequate heat and pressure.

d. Floating of ribbons – Ribbons of tissue are floated in the water bath for flattening and removal of wrinkles from tissue.

e. Picking up the tissue on slide and drying – Picking up of tissue should be gentle and smooth. Drying of slides is done in the hot air oven and the temperature of the oven should be slightly more than the melting point of paraffin.

4. **Tissue staining:** The tissue slice appears transparent due to the fixed proteins sharing a refractive index identical to that of glass. We utilize dyes that selectively bind to various tissue proteins, imparting distinct colors. This approach enhances our comprehension of the tissue's morphology. The staining predominantly involves a chemical interaction between the dye and the tissue. In routine morphological visualization of tissues, Haematoxylin and Eosin stain are used. The steps of staining (H&E) are as follows:

a. Deparaffinization – done with the xylene.

b. Rehydration – descending grades of alcohol.

c. Nuclear stain – for staining of the nucleus, hematoxylin is used.

d. Differentiation – 1% acid alcohol dips are required for differentiation in regressive staining.

e. Counter staining – 1% aqueous Eosin is used.

f. Dehydration – Ascending grades of alcohol are used.

g. Clearing – xylene is used as the clearing agent.

h. Mounting – Mounting is the last procedure after the coloring process. DPX is used routinely. Subsequent to the staining procedure, the specimen is blocked, rendering it incapable of absorbing water or other solutions, resulting in its prolonged preservation.

After staining and mounting of slides, tissue sections were examined under a light microscope. Various parasites in the tissue sections are diagnosed based on histopathological descriptions.

5. **Special staining:** It is performed for the demonstration of the specific parasites/their eggs/their growing stages/part of parasites. There are some stains apart from H&E, which are used for making diagnoses. Boland and Pritt (2013) have mentioned some of the special staining for the demonstration of parasites.

a. PAS staining – For highlighting trophozoites of *Entamoeba histolytica*, for demonstration of a laminated layer of *Echinococcus granulosus*.

b. Ziehl Neelsen - For demonstration of hooklets in case of *E. granulosus*.

c. iGMS - For demonstration of hooklets in case of *E. granulosus*.

6. **Immunohistochemistry:** Traditional diagnosis, in the field of veterinary medicine, has primarily depended on routine staining methods like hematoxylin and eosin. Immunohistochemistry (IHC) is an important ancillary technique in the diagnosis of infections. IHC enables the identification of the antigens within the formalin-fixed, paraffin-embedded (FFPE) tissue sections (Ramos-Vara *et al.*, 2008). IHC is a technique that combines chemical and immunological reactions as it is based on the binding of antibodies and specific target antigens present in the FFPE tissue sections [10] and the interaction between antibodies and antigens can be observed through either chromogenic detection (involving enzymes) or fluorescent detection (using fluorophores. Diagnosis is confirmed through the detection of antibodies specific to the organism, mainly IgG and IgM antibodies. There are various antibodies that are commercially available for the diagnosis of various parasites.

Numerous investigations have been carried out to diagnose *Leishmania* amastigotes using an immunohistochemistry response in paraffin-embedded tissue sections from both humans and dogs. *Leishmania can* also be demonstrated using commercially available anti-*Leishmania* lipophosphoglycan monoclonal antibodies and polyclonal hyperimmune sera [11]. There arc few reports on theileriosis in livestock, parasitic schizonts were detected by immunochemical techniques in formalin-fixed, and paraffin-embedded (FFPE) tissues [3]. There are few studies conducted on the immunohistochemical detection of the *Toxoplasma gondii* (*T. gondii*). Silva *et al.*, [8] demonstrated the *T. gondii* in sheep tissue by the immunohistochemical method.

In a nutshell, there are many zoonotic parasitic diseases, and their diagnosis is required for the treatment and prevention of diseases. Histopathological examination of H&E-stained sections is usually ineffective in identifying different parasite growth phases, especially in organs such as the kidney, lung, and intestines that have modest parasite loads. On the other hand, immunohistochemistry made it simple to see developing phases (*Amastigotes* and schizonts) in several organs. Therefore, the immunohistochemistry method is helpful as an additional tool to confirm the diagnosis based on sections stained with Hematoxylin and Eosin (H&E), especially in organs with low parasite loads [11].

CONCLUSION

Parasitic infection can be a challenge for pathologists due to the uncommonness of these specimens in routine practice. Familiarity with the potential organisms that can infect organs, coupled with their characteristics histological attributes, can assist in accurately identifying the infection. Various histopathological techniques can aid in the confirmatory diagnosis of various parasitic diseases.

REFERENCES

[1] Boland JM, Pritt BS. Histopathology of parasitic infections of the lung. Seminars in Diagnostic Path 2017; 34(6): 550-9. WB Saunders.
[http://dx.doi.org/10.1053/j.semdp.2017.06.004]

[2] Brown C, Torres F, Rech R. A Field Manual for Collection of Specimens to Enhance Diagnosis of Animal Diseases. Boca Publications Group Incorporated 2012.

[3] Clift SJ, Martí-Garcia B, Phaswane RM, *et al.* Polyclonal antibody–based immunohistochemical detection of intraleukocytic *Theileria* parasites in roan and sable antelopes. J Vet Diagn Invest 2021; 33(6): 1079-88.
[http://dx.doi.org/10.1177/10406387211033272] [PMID: 34333997]

[4] Dey P. Basic and advanced laboratory techniques in histopathology and cytology. 2nd ed., Springer Singapore 2023.
[http://dx.doi.org/10.1007/978-981-10-8252-8]

[5] Rahsan Y, Nihat Y, Bestami Y, Adnan A, Nuran A. Histopathological, immunohistochemical, and parasitological studies on pathogenesis of in sheep. J Vet Res (Pulawy) 2018; 62(1): 35-41.
[http://dx.doi.org/10.2478/jvetres-2018-0005] [PMID: 29978125]

[6] Ramos-Vara JA. Technical aspects of immunohistochemistry. Vet Pathol 2005; 42(4): 405-26.
[http://dx.doi.org/10.1354/vp.42-4-405] [PMID: 16006601]

[7] Ramos-Vara JA, Kiupel M, Baszler T, *et al.* Suggested guidelines for immunohistochemical techniques in veterinary diagnostic laboratories. J Vet Diagn Invest 2008; 20(4): 393-413.
[http://dx.doi.org/10.1177/104063870802000401]

[8] Silva AF, Oliveira FCR, Leite JS, *et al.* Immunohistochemical identification of *Toxoplasma gondii* in tissues from Modified Agglutination Test positive sheep. Vet Parasitol 2013; 191(3-4): 347-52.
[http://dx.doi.org/10.1016/j.vetpar.2012.09.022] [PMID: 23062690]

[9] Šlais J. Morphology of Cysticercus cellulosae and Cysticercus bovis. The Morphology and Pathogenicity of the Bladder Worms. Dordrecht: Springer 1970.
[http://dx.doi.org/10.1007/978-94-011-6466-5_5]

[10] Slais J. The morphology and pathogenicity of the bladder worms: Cysticercus cellulosae and Cysticercus bovis. Springer Science & Business Media 2013.
[http://dx.doi.org/10.1007/978-94-011-6466-5]

[11] Tafuri WL, Santos RL, Arantes RME, *et al.* An alternative immunohistochemical method for detecting Leishmania amastigotes in paraffin-embedded canine tissues. J Immunol Methods 2004; 292(1-2): 17-23.
[http://dx.doi.org/10.1016/j.jim.2004.05.009] [PMID: 15350508]

CHAPTER 13

Anti-parasitic Drugs

Muhammad Asmat Ullah Saleem[1], Muhammad Asif Wisal[2], Muhammad Waqas[3], Muhammad Mohsin[4] and Muhammad Tahir Aleem[5,6,*]

[1] *College of Veterinary Medicine, Northeast Agricultural University, Harbin 150030, P.R. China*

[2] *College of Animal Sciences and Technology, Jilin Agricultural University, Changchun, China*

[3] *Ondokuz Mayıs University, Samsun, Turkey*

[4] *Shantou University Medical College, Shantou, Guangdong, 515045,China*

[5] *MOE Joint International Research Laboratory of Animal Health and Food Safety, College of Veterinary Medicine, Nanjing Agricultural University, Nanjing 210095, China*

[6] *Center for Gene Regulation in Health and Disease, Department of Biological, Geological, and Environmental Sciences, College of Sciences and Health Professions, Cleveland State University, Cleveland, OH 44115, USA*

Abstract: Gastrointestinal parasites pose a significant threat to cattle health, welfare as well as productivity throughout the globe. This chapter describes the major gastrointestinal parasites that affect cattle, their impact on the industry, proper management strategies, and also potential future directions for effective control and preventive measures. The economic upliftment of parasite infections in cattle production systems is generally explored, highlighting the major need for integrated approaches to combat these potential parasites. Key and major aspects including grazing management, proper anthelmintic treatment, genetic selection criteria as well as emerging research, are elaborately discussed in the context of sustainable parasite control strategies. The chapter magnifies the importance of continued updated research with major collaboration to mitigate the impact of gastrointestinal parasites on cattle populations.

Keywords: Anthelmintics, Cattle, Control, Eeconomic impact, Gastrointestinal parasites, Management.

INTRODUCTION

The increased population of humans in the world also increased the demand for milk and meat therefore, the productivity of farm animals must be at an optimum

---

* **Corresponding author Muhammad Tahir Aleem:** MOE Joint International Research Laboratory of Animal Health and Food Safety, College of Veterinary Medicine, Nanjing Agricultural University, Nanjing 210095, China; Center for Gene Regulation in Health and Disease, Department of Biological, Geological, and Environmental Sciences, College of Sciences and Health Professions, Cleveland State University, Cleveland, OH 44115, USA;
E-mail: dr.tahir1990@gmail.com

level to fulfill such increasing demands. Their productivity could be affected by the presence of internal and external parasites such as gastrointestinal nematodes *Haemonchus, Cooperia, Oesophagostomum,* and *Trichostrongylus*, as well as *Rhipicephalus microplus* ticks and *Haematobia irritans* flies. These parasites lower the productivity of livestock in countries situated in tropical and subtropical regions of the world [1]. The parasitic problem among livestock could be controlled by synthetic drugs having antiparasitic activities such as *endodectocidal* drugs, ectoparasiticide, and endoparasiticide. Endoparasiticide specifically targets internal parasites while ectoparasiticides are used against ectoparasites. The third category is endodectocidal, which is equally effective against both external and internal parasites and is most widely used in animals for the control of parasites such as gastrointestinal nematodes, ticks, mites, flies, lice, and myiasis. However, the extensive and irrational use of *edodectocidal* drugs leads to the emergence of drug-resistant strains of parasites in animals, which are difficult to control [2]. Regarding the susceptibility of animals to parasites, the Indian breed of cattle (*Bos taurus indicus*) demonstrates greater resistance and resilience to ticks and gastrointestinal nematodes respectively. On the other hand, the taurine breed (*Bos taurus taurus*) is more susceptible to these parasites. However, the productivity of the Indian breed is less as compared to the taurine breed [3].

The world population of large ruminants is increasing to get surplus food of animal origin for humans. According to the Food and Agriculture Organization of the United Nations (FAO), worldwide the number of cattle and buffalo has increased from approximately 1.03 billion head combined (942.15 million cattle and 88.32 million buffalo) in 1961 to approximately 1.72 billion head combined (1.52 billion cattle and 203.93 million buffalo) in 2021. The production of meat has increased by approximately 28.75 million tons (Mt) combined (27.68Mt cattle meat and 1.07Mt buffalo meat) in 1961 to approximately 76.76 Mt combined (72.44Mt cattle meat and 4.32Mt buffalo meat) in 2021. Similarly, the production of milk from animal origin has increased from approximately 331.47 Mt combined (313.62Mt cattle milk and 17.85Mt buffalo milk) in 1961 to approximately 883.81 Mt combined (746.05Mt cattle milk and 137.76Mt buffalo milk) in 2021 [4]. An increase in trends is given in Figs. (**1-3**). As there is an increase in the food of animal origin, people's interest in disease-free food is increasing [5]. Therefore, the health of the animals is important and could be maintained by controlling infection *via* chemotherapy and prevention.

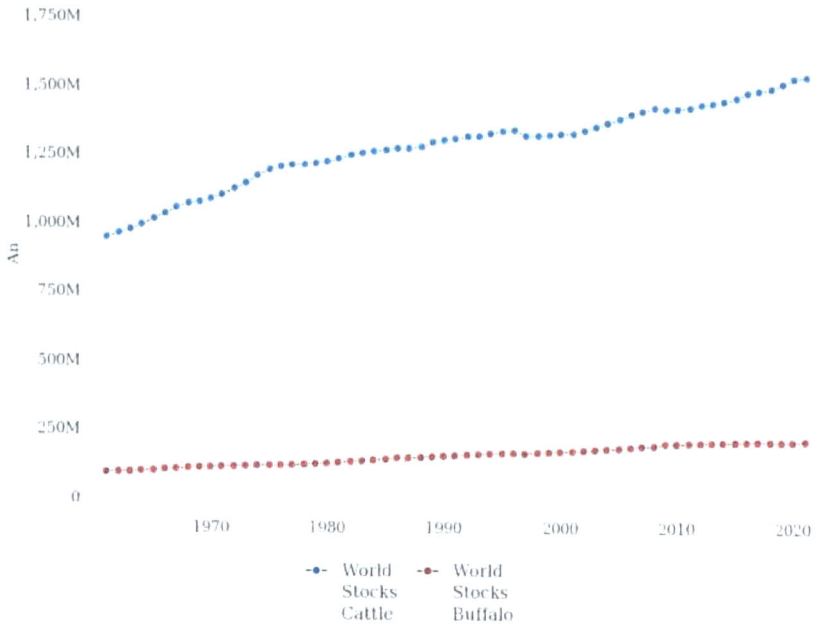

Fig. (1). A trend in increased production of cattle and buffalo from 1961 to 2021.

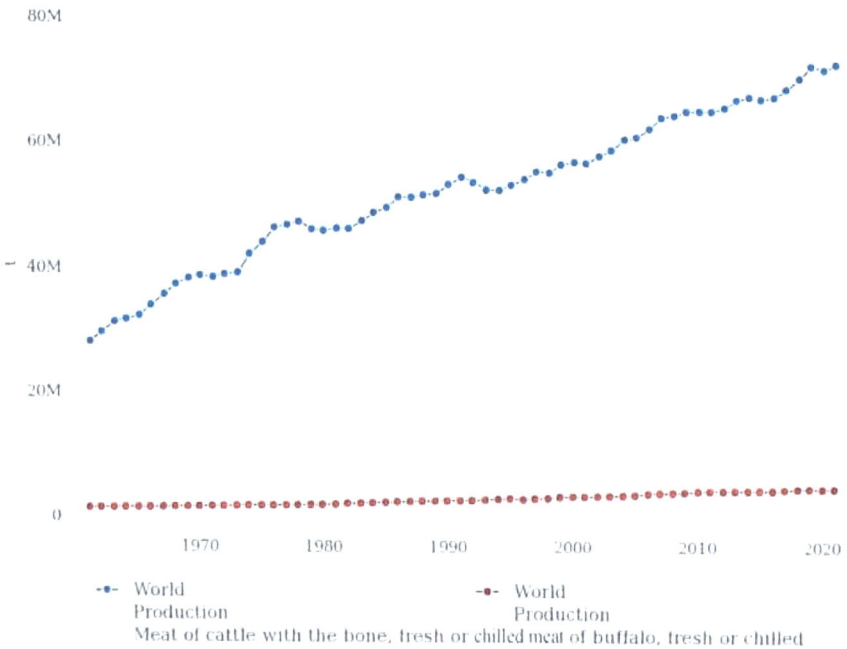

Fig. (2). A trend in increased production of cattle and buffalo meat from 1961 to 2021.

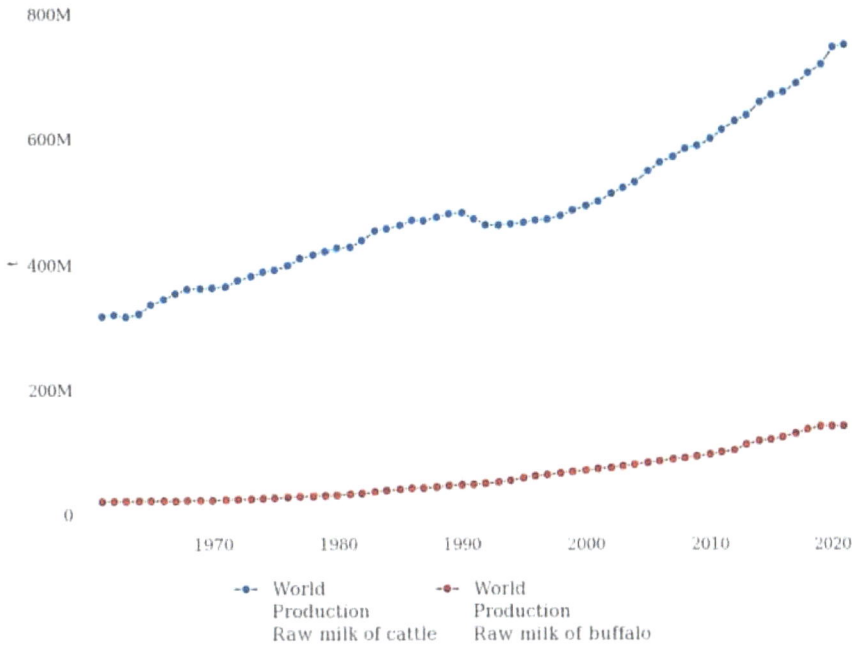

Fig. (3). A trend in increased production of cattle and buffalo milk from 1961 to 2021.

For the development of antiparasitic drugs, there are many stages by passing through which drugs reach the market. First compounds are screened for the activity of anthelmintic or insecticidal. The screening procedure in the case of anthelmintics requires *in vitro* activity as well as *in vivo* activity against the parasites [6]. *In vitro* assays give rapid results in screening potential candidates for antiparasitic activity. The advantage of preliminary screening tests in the development of drugs is that these studies reduce the list of compounds having no antiparasitic activity [7]. Moreover, the response of these compounds varies with the species and strain of parasites as well as the host. For example, piperazines are effective against ascarids but show quite refractory results against hookworms. Most breeds of cattle can tolerate organophosphate insecticides whereas the Brahman breed of cattle is unable to tolerate such treatments and becomes fatally intoxicated [8].

The Food and Drug Administration (FDA) deals with the safety, efficacy, and all other necessary information associated with the development of new drugs [9]. When a New Animal Drug Application is filed by a commercial manufacturer, the FDA requires information about the chemistry of the compound, manufacturing process, and bioassay methods. When a drug is intended to be used for animals, it should also be accustomed to data about the specific route, metabolism, excretion rate, and tissue residues of parent compounds and their metabolites. Moreover, toxicity experiments in mice and rats are also required [10]. Similarly, the data about the impact of drugs on the environment, fish, the animals in which it will be administered, and workers is also required by the Environment Protection Agency. Moreover, before the approval of any antiparasitic drug, well-controlled experiments involving the sacrifice of animals [11]. Many independent laboratories also conduct confirmatory experiments to ensure the safety of the compound. The remaining procedures include the preparation of package labels, assigning the code for identification, and giving the generic name. One anthelmintic compound may have more than one brand name (a name given by pharmaceutical companies) [12].

There are many classes of parasites and not every drug is effective against all of them. Therefore, in this chapter, antiparasitic drugs are classified into three categories such as antiprotozoal drugs, anthelmintic drugs, and ectoparasitic drugs. This chapter highlights the three main categories as well as the mechanism of development of drug resistance against infectious parasites and their management.

ANTI-PROTOZOAL DRUGS

Protozoa are ubiquitous unicellular organisms. There are over 65,000 species of protozoa so far described out of which many occur as harmless commensal or free living. In the gastrointestinal tract of cattle, a large number of protozoa are present, which are harmless. However, there are many protozoa that have the potential to cause disease and have significant zoonotic importance. Some of the species of protozoa that cause diseases in cattle include, *Eimeria* species which cause coccidiosis, *Cryptosporidium parvum,* which causes cryptosporidiosis, *Giardia* responsible for giardiasis, *Babesia,* which causes babesiosis, as well as *Theileria, Trypanosoma, Toxoplasma,* and *Tritrichomonas* [13]. Therefore, to control the infections caused by protozoa, chemotherapy along with proper management is necessary. Some of the drugs used for the treatment of infections caused by protozoa are discussed below in Fig. (**4**).

Non-sulfonamides

Amprolium

It is a coccidiostat drug administered for the treatment of coccidiosis in animals. It mimics thiamine and competes with parasites for the absorption of thiamine because of its structural similarities with thiamine. It shows maximum activity against the first stage in the life cycle of *Eimeria* species *i.e.,* schizonts, therefore it is more useful as a preventive medicine rather than treatment. It is intended for use in cattle and poultry for the treatment and control of coccidiosis. The effect of amprolium could be minimized by feeding excessive thiamine to the animals. In cattle, the coccidiosis is mainly caused by *E. bovis* and *E. zuernii*. Amprolium is formulated for cattle as a 9.6% drenching solution [14]. Depending on the severity of the infection, the dosage varies. In cattle, amprolium at a dose rate of 10 mg/kg for 5-21 consecutive days is administered for the treatment of coccidiosis. On the other hand, a dose of 5 mg/kg for 21 days daily amprolium is administered for the prevention of coccidiosis in livestock. It is also effective against other species of *Eimeria* however, the drug labels claim its efficacy only against *E. bovis* and *E. zuernii* [15]. Animals must not be slaughtered before the completion of the withdrawal period.

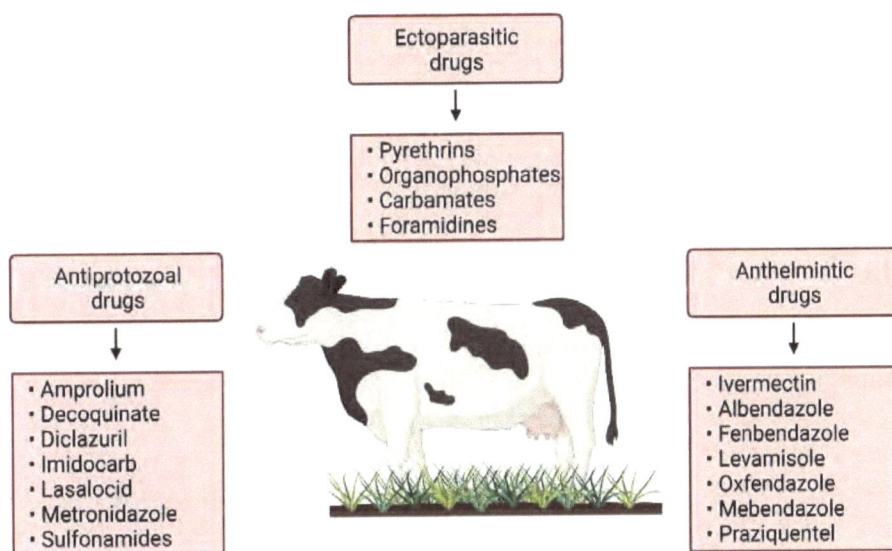

Ectoparasitic drugs
- Pyrethrins
- Organophosphates
- Carbamates
- Foramidines

Antiprotozoal drugs
- Amprolium
- Decoquinate
- Diclazuril
- Imidocarb
- Lasalocid
- Metronidazole
- Sulfonamides

Anthelmintic drugs
- Ivermectin
- Albendazole
- Fenbendazole
- Levamisole
- Oxfendazole
- Mebendazole
- Praziquentel

Fig. (4). Antiparasitic drugs used in cattle.

Decoquinate

Decoquinate is also a coccidiostat approved for the treatment of coccidiosis in ruminants. It shows its anticoccidial activity by killing the sporozoite stage of the *Eimeria* species. Moreover, it also interrupts the transport of electrons in the cytochrome system of the mitochondria of the parasites. It is useful for the prevention of coccidiosis in animals rather than treatment [16]. For cattle, it could be added to their feed as a supplement as well as in the milk of calves for the prevention of coccidiosis. The dose rate for decoquinate is 0.5 mg/kg/day for 28 days. It is also used for the prevention of coccidial infections in calves. In this case, it is applied at a dose rate of 1.25 mg/kg/day for 8 days after and 30 days before the parturition [17].

Diclazuril

Diclazuril is an antiprotozoal drug that belongs to the class of triazine, which primarily targets the plastid body of protozoa. The Plastid body is an organelle that occurs in members of the Apicomplexa phylum [18]. It is also used as a coccidiostat for the prevention of coccidial infection in animals. It has a wide range of safety and does not cause abnormalities in cattle when a 60 times overdose of the drug is administered. The dose rate of diclazuril is 1 mg/kg for the prevention and treatment of coccidiosis in calves [19].

Imidocarb

Imidocarb is an antiprotozoal drug used for the treatment of babesiosis in animals. It is an aromatic diamidine that inhibits nucleic acid metabolism in the parasites. It causes oncogenesis in rats. It is available in the form of imidocarb dipropionate as a sterile solution administered subcutaneously or intramuscularly. Its dose rate in cattle is 1-3 mg/kg [20].

Lasalocid

Lasalocid is an ionophore in relation to monensin produced by *Streptomycete*. It acts against the parasites by forming complexes with potassium and sodium ions. This makes the membranes of parasites permeable to ions and inhibits the functions of mitochondria. It is approved for the control of coccidiosis in cattle and shows the highest activity in the trophozoites stage of the *Eimeria* species [21]. It is given to animals with their feed and can also be mixed with milk replacers for young calves. Therefore, it is available in the form of liquid or dry feed additives with a particular dose rate of 1 mg/kg/day [22].

Metronidazole

Metronidazole is an antibiotic that belongs to the class nitroimidazole, which is very useful and has a broad spectrum of activity against amoeba, *Giardia*, *Trichomonas*, *Entamoeba*, cocci, and bacillus species. The other drugs that belong to the class nitroimidazole include dimetridazole, ipronidazole, ronidazole, tinidazole, ornidazole, dimetridazole, benznidazole, and Carnidazole [23]. These drugs are not approved to be used in food-producing animals because of their harmful effects such as the production of tumors in rats. From the gastrointestinal tract, it is absorbed well, has a low capacity with protein binding, thoroughly distributed throughout the body. It acts against the parasites by interacting with the DNA of protozoa and breaking its helical structure. The metabolism of the drug occurs in the liver [24]. The co-administration of metronidazole with phenobarbital or cimetidine requires dose adjustment because of their interaction [25].

Sulfonamides

Sulfonamides are one of the oldest groups having antimicrobial properties initially derived from prontosil. These drugs are the treatment of choice for coccidiosis in large animals such as cattle. They have a synergistic effect when combined with ormetoprim or trimethoprim resulting in greater and broad-spectrum antimicrobial activity. The mechanism of action of sulfa drugs includes they act by impairing metabolism, synthesis of protein, and pathogen growth. These are the structural analogs of PABA (para-aminobenzoic acid), therefore, dihydropteroate synthetase is competitively inhibited by folic acid synthesis [26]. There are many sulfa drugs discovered so far and the important differences among them include solubility, duration, and activity against the pathogen. Sulfa drugs except sulfaquinoxaline are very weak acids therefore absorbed from the gastrointestinal tract of the animals. Therefore half-life is high because of their affinity of binding with the serum proteins. They are metabolized in the liver and thereby excreted from the kidney with urine. Moreover, sulfa drugs also have idiosyncratic and toxic effects on animals because of crystallization [27]. The adverse effects associated with sulfa drugs in animals include crystalluria, hypersensitivity, keratoconjunctivitis sicca, glomerulopathy, fever, hepatotoxicity, anemia, and thyroid metabolic disorders [28]. The sulfonamides used for the treatment of animals are discussed below.

Sulfadimethoxine

Sulfadimethoxine is used for the treatment of coccidiosis in animals. It is a long-acting drug because of its affinity with the serum proteins and is rapidly absorbed through the gastrointestinal tract of the animals. Its safety margin is high in animals, however, when administered, it must be accompanied by an adequate intake of water to prevent adverse reactions such as crystalluria and dehydration [29]. It is available in the form of oral solutions, bolus, powders, as well as injectables. In cattle, its dose rate is 55 mg/kg intravenous (IV) or per oral (PO) for the first day. The subsequent dose rate is 27.5 mg/kg/day IV or PO for not more than five days. The residue of the drugs appears in milk for about 60 hours, therefore, we discard milk during the treatment and completion of the withdrawal period. Likewise, animals must not be slaughtered within 7 days after the end of the treatment [30]. The withdrawal period varies depending on the different formulations of different pharmaceutical companies [31].

Sulfamethazine

Sulfamethazine is also used for the treatment of coccidiosis in animals. It could be administered orally as an oral bolus or by mixing with water. Its dose rate for the first and subsequent days include 237-247 mg/kg and 123 mg/kg respectively [32]. The total days of treatment are 5. After this, its administration must be stopped. Its slow-release formulations (Bolus) are also available for cattle which deliver 32.1 g of drug over a period of 3 days. One bolus is for 200 pounds of the animal's weight. The consumption of milk and meat is done after the withdrawal period [33].

Sulfaquinoxaline

Sulfaquinoxaline is intended for use in cattle for the treatment and control of coccidiosis [34]. Its absorption through the gastrointestinal tract is not well. It is given to animals with water at a dose rate of 6 mg/pound/day. Caution must be taken for its use in animals. It must not be used in veal calves and lactating dairy cattle [35]. Before slaughtering the animals, the withdrawal period must be completed as their residues appear in the meat of animals [36].

ANTHELMINTICS

The most significant helminth species that parasitize cattle are gastrointestinal nematodes (GIN), lungworms, and liver flukes. These parasites are among the most significant production-limiting parasites of grazing ruminants because they can cause serious illness, reduce productivity in livestock, and cause severe sickness. In a grass-based production system, virtually all herds and flocks are impacted [37]. The main economic impact of GIN and liver fluke infections is related to subclinical infections that impair growth, milk output, and fertility. These infections are more persistent. Lungworm infections are more severe and can suddenly place a heavy economic burden on a farm due to fatalities and significant drops in milk production [38]. Drugs are frequently prescribed by practicing veterinarians to treat and prevent helminth infections in animals. The common anthelmintics used in veterinary practice will be discussed in this section.

Ivermectin

The first commercially available macrolide was ivermectin, discovered by Merck for animal use in 1981, just six years after avermectins were discovered. The *Streptomyces avermitilis* fermentation broth was used to isolate the avermectins. After mice were infected with *Nematospiroides dubius* and were given actinomycetic broth, anthelmintic activity was found. Because of ivermectin's economic success, other businesses have created analogs such as milbemycin oxime, moxidectin, doramectin, eprinomectin, abamectin, and selamectin [39]. Ivermectin works well against a wide variety of nematodes and arthropods. Although it has a little effect on adult heartworms, it is particularly effective against *Dirofilaria immitis*, an immature heartworm. Ivermectin only caused teratism in fetuses when given to pregnant rats, mice, and rabbits at or near maximally lethal levels [40]. When ivermectin was given to pregnant animals at a dose that was four times the advised level, there was no evidence of teratogenesis in cattle [41].

Ivermectin was once thought to disrupt GABA-mediated neurotransmission, but it is now understood that its effects are actually caused by its strong propensity for binding to glutamate-gated chloride channels, which results in chloride influx, hyperpolarization, paralysis, and death. Ivermectin blocks signal transmission at neuromuscular junctions in arthropods by a similar method. Both nematodes and arthropods experience death as a result of paralysis [42].

Ivermectin is procurable as an active component in two formulations for cattle: a 1% (10 mg/mL) liquid for subcutaneous injection (IVOMEC 1%) and a pour-on 5-mg/mL solution (IVOMEC) [43]. These formulations are offered in products with essentially identical package inserts and are created by a variety of different manufacturers [44]. Ivermectin administered subcutaneously persistently protects cattle from re-infection [45]. Ivermectin's effectiveness in treating biting lice is unpredictable. Ivermectin injection has shown good efficacy against the eyeworm and *Parafilaria bovicola*, which causes summer bleeding [46].

Albendazole

Strong broad-spectrum anthelmintic action is exhibited by albendazole. When used as directed on the label, it offers a large margin of safety for cattle. In farm animals, albendazole has been shown to have a wide range of anthelmintic efficacy against gastrointestinal nematodes, and lung nematodes [47] In other countries, albendazole (Zentel) is used to treat human cysticercosis, hydatid disease, and intestinal helminth infections. Cattle can be treated with albendazole 11.36% suspension (113.6 mg/mL). The dosage for cattle is 10 mg/kg [48]. The removal and control of liver flukes, tapeworms, stomach worms (including fourth-stage inhibited larvae of *Ostertagia ostertagi*), intestinal worms, and lungworms in cattle are all made easier to control. When administered early in pregnancy to rats, rabbits, and sheep, albendazole has been linked to teratogenic and embryotoxic consequences in these species [49]. Although it was recognized as an oncogenic in 1984, later research was unable to show any evidence of its carcinogenic potential. Albendazole may result in GI, hepatic, and infrequently, aplastic anemia malfunction.

For the removal and control of internal parasites in cattle, albendazole is orally administered at a dose level of 10 mg/kg [50]. In healthy and parasitized cattle, the safety of albendazole in single and repeated treatments was assessed. 75 mg/kg of body weight administered once had a good effect against parasites. When given to cows between the first seven and seventeen days of pregnancy at a dosage rate of 25 mg/kg, albendazole proved embryotoxic. All treated cows gave birth to healthy calves, and the conception rate was comparable to that of control cows after the twenty-first day of gestation [51].

Fenbendazole

A popular benzimidazole used in domestic animals is fenbendazole. Rats and mice have oral LDs of greater than 10,000 mg/kg. Rats, sheep, and cattle are not affected by the teratogenic or embryotoxic effects of fenbendazole. Fenbendazole was teratogenic but not fetotoxic in the rabbit [52]. It is the medication of choice for treating *Giardia* spp. in pregnant animals. It is widely regarded for pregnant animals. Lifetime studies on rats and mice revealed no evidence of carcinogenesis. A dose of fenbendazole up to 100 times the normal dosage is tolerated. Oxfendazole sulfoxide and oxfendazole sulfone are at least two active metabolites that are produced from absorbed fenbendazole. It is known to go through the enterohepatic cycle in ruminants, which prolongs the effective blood levels [53]. Fenbendazole is not entirely absorbed when used orally. Fenbendazole is offered as a premix, top dress pellets, granules, suspension, paste, blocks, and a free-choice mineral supplement, among many more designed items. These medications are intended to be given orally at a rate of 5 mg/kg for the control of intestinal worms such as *Bunostomum phlebotomum, Nematodirus helvetianus, Cooperia punctata, Cooperia encephora, Trichostrongylus colubriformis*, and *Oesophagestemum radiatum* [54].

Levamisole

Levamisole is sold for the application of cattle all over the world. Levamisole is produced as an injectable solution for cattle in the United States, as well as a bolus or oral drench for cattle. It has no activity against flukes, protozoa, and tapeworms, it is used to control gastrointestinal and lung nematodes. Levamisole has antinematodal properties in addition to stimulating the immune system in canines and felines. For use in cattle, levamisole hydrochloride is produced as a drench, bolus, or injectable solution [55]. The dosage for cattle is 6 mg/kg of phosphate salt administered subcutaneously and 8 mg/kg orally. The injectable medication has a label indicating its effectiveness against *Chabertia* spp. Early fourth-stage larvae of *Ostertagia* species that have been arrested are resistant to levamisole [56].

There might be muzzle foam, but it should go away in a few hours. Levamisole phosphate injection site swelling is possible but should go away in 7 to 14 days. The label for the injectable medicine warns that using it during stressful conditions and while also taking cholinesterase inhibitors increases the risk. In the edible tissues of cattle, a limit of 0.1 ppm has been determined for minute residues [57]. Within 7 days of an injection or 2 days after taking an oral medicine, cattle should not be slaughtered. To prevent medication residues in milk, levamisole should not be administered to dairy animals that are at breeding age.

ECTOPARASITIC DRUGS

The majority of 1.49 billion head of cattle in the world are vulnerable to infestation by various ectoparasites. The direct impact of severe infestations on health and food output makes arthropods, primarily insects, mites, and ticks, the most economically important group of bovine ectoparasites. Arthropods are also carriers of various zoonotic infections that cause illnesses in cattle. Additionally, a number of illnesses are directly brought on by ectoparasites or the pathogens they spread to cattle [58]. Ectoparasites have been managed or eliminated using veterinary medicines, and mechanical/environmental, biological, and genetic techniques alone or in combination. Practitioners and producers frequently utilize ectoparasiticide-containing veterinary medications to treat or prevent ectoparasites and lessen exposure to infections carried by vectors. Ectoparasite populations exposed to ectoparasiticides on a regular basis due to their heavy use in some regions of the world have chosen to develop resistance [59]. In order to address public concerns about the widespread application of ectoparasiticides in the context of food safety, global change, animal welfare, and environmental health, strategies integrating various techniques for sustainable cow ectoparasite management are required.

Pyrethrins

Six closely related insecticidal compounds known as pyrethrins are found in the flower heads of the pyrethrum plant, *Chrysanthemum cinerariifolium*. These compounds include pyrethrin I and II, cinerin I and II, and jasmolin I and II. Pyrethrins are quickly biodegradable and rapidly degradable in the presence of moisture, air, and light. They have a high kerosene solubility but are insoluble in water. Although pyrethrins are not thought to be cutaneous irritants, they do stimulate the activity of the hepatic microsome and result in tumor development in rats and mice [60]. Pyrethrins may cause some inhalation issues in rats, however regular aerosol applications to domestic animals should not cause any negative effects. Pyrethrin aerosols should not be applied next to fish tanks because they are hazardous to fish [61].

By interfering with sodium and potassium ion transport in nerve membranes and interrupting neurotransmission along the axon and at the synapse, pyrethrins quickly knock down, paralyze, and thereby kill arthropods. Pyrethrin residues can occasionally be repellant. Pyrethrins are typically coupled with a synergist like N-octyl bicycloheptene dicarboximide or piperonyl butoxide. The mixed function oxidases, which detoxify pesticides in the insect, are poisoned by synergists [62]. Pyrethrins are approved for use on cattle (beef and lactating dairy), in a number of locations, including bovine quarters such as milk houses, dairy barns, and milk parlors. Since they are not long-lasting insecticides, frequent and repeated applications are required. Examples of pyrethroids include cypermethrin, deltamethrin, tetramethrin, and cyfluthrin, *etc* [63].

Carbamates and Organophosphates

The two most widely used pesticides are carbamates and organophosphates. Because they prevent acetylcholinesterase (AChE), a vital enzyme in the nervous system that deactivates synaptic acetylcholine, these insecticides arc poisonous. The pesticides with organophosphates bind to and permanently inactivate AChE. Contrarily, carbamates are reversible inhibitors of AChE. Carbamates are broken down over the course of many hours, and AChE inhibition stops. The end outcome of both organophosphates and carbamates is the same: because AChE is dysfunctional, acetylcholine builds up at the neuronal synapse. Acetylcholine must be eliminated for nerve stimulation to stop [64].

As acetylcholine builds up in the body, anorexia, salivation, vomiting, lacrimation, diarrhea, dyspnea, miosis or mydriasis, frequent urination, and tachycardia or bradycardia are the main symptoms of acute poisoning. Along with extreme weakness and paralysis, it can also result in the twitching of rapid involuntary muscles and dispersed fasciculation at the neuromuscular junction. DUMBBELS (diarrhea, urination, miosis, bronchospasm, bradycardia, emesis, salivation, lacrimation) and SLUD (salivation, lacrimation, urination, defecation) are mnemonic acronyms for the clinical symptoms [65]. Numerous organophosphate insecticides cause long axons in the spinal cord and peripheral nerves (such as the sciatic nerve) to degenerate, resulting in a pattern of persistent neurotoxicity. Organophosphate exposure has also been linked to pancreatitis [66]. Their examples include propoxur, dichlorvos, coumaphos, tetrachlorvinphos, *etc.*

Foramidines

The only formamidine that has been authorized for use on animals in the United States is amitraz, which is given to pigs, cattle, and dogs. Amitraz is a monamine oxidase (MAO) inhibitor in mammals and an octopamine receptor agonist in insects. For usage on beef cattle, dairy cattle, and pigs, Amitraz is marketed as a 12.5% emulsifiable concentrate to treat ticks, mange mites, and lice [67]. After mixing, the product must be used within six hours. The chemical is diluted 760 mL/100 gallon of water and administered as a spray or dip to treat cattle ticks and lice. Since lice treatment does not remove lice eggs, it is advised to repeat the procedure in 10 to 14 days to eradicate newly hatched lice. The solution is diluted 760 mL/50 liters of water and used as a spray or dip to treat lice as well as scabies and mange mites in cattle. After 7 to 10 days, a second treatment for scabies is required [68]. Cattle are not required to be withheld for slaughter, and dairy cattle are not obliged to be withheld for milk (Fig. **5**).

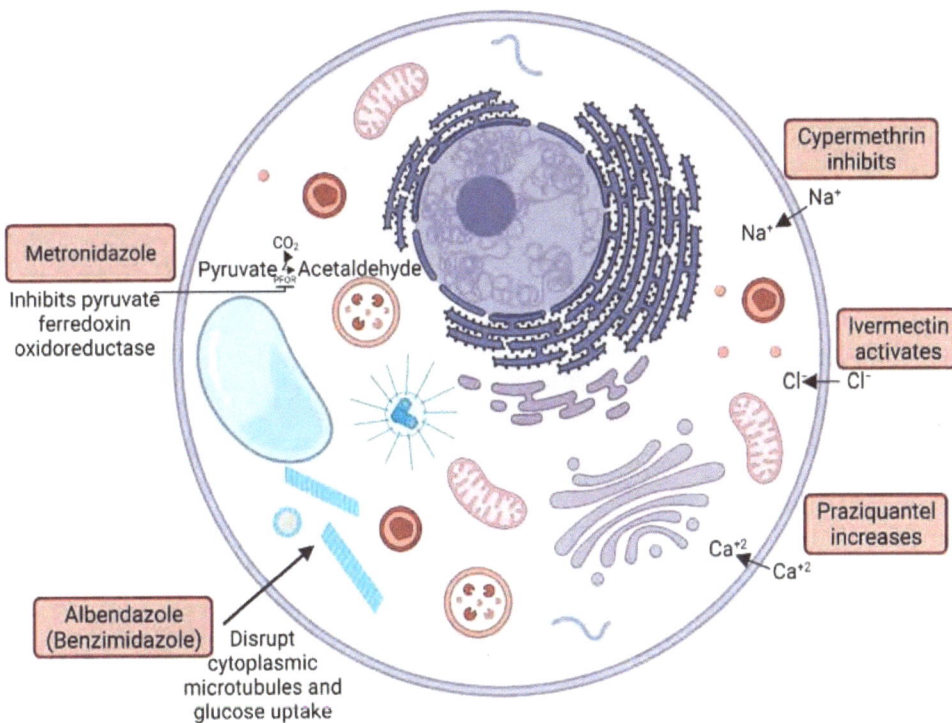

Fig. (5). General mechanisms of antiparasitic drugs.

RESISTANCE TO ANTIPARASITIC DRUGS

The biggest obstacle to controlling numerous parasite species, including protozoa, helminths, and arthropods that infect both humans and animals, is drug resistance. As a result, resistance affects the majority of animal and health parasitology subfields. Regular administration of antiparasitic medications to parasite populations frequently causes the selection of resistance phenotypes, which leads to the formation of resistant parasite populations. Eventually, the medication that was once effective stops working and needs to be changed with another. Unfortunately, if the resistant strain is a chemical congener of the original, the replacement may likewise fail to combat it. This has occurred frequently enough to warrant a warning. Instead of slamming them with one poison after another, we need to find more effective strategies to control parasites (Table **1**). In general, the optimal product to use in each unique circumstance should be determined using the principles of evidence-based medicine [69].

Table 1. Antiparasitic drug, category, mode of action, and target species/disease.

Antiparasitic Drug	Category	Mode of Action	Target Species/Disease	References
Amprolium	Antiprotozoal	Thiamine antagonist	*E. bovis* and *E. zuernii*	[15]
Decoquinate	Antiprotozoal	Interrupts the transport of electrons in the cytochrome system of the mitochondria of the parasites.	*Eimeria* species	[16]
Diclazuril	Antiprotozoal	Interfere with the mitochondrial transmembrane potential of the parasite.	Coccidiosis	[18]
Imidocarb	Antiprotozoal	Interfere with polyamine production or prevent inositol into parasite-containing erythrocyte.	Babesiosis, trypanosomiasis	[20]
Lasalocid	Ionophore	Form complexes with sodium and potassium ions, making the membrane permeable to ions and inhibiting mitochondrial function.	*E. bovis* and *E. zuernii*	[21]
Metronidazole	Antimicrobial	Inhibit nucleic acid synthesis.	Protozoa and bacteria	[23]
Sulfonamides	Antimicrobial	Inhibit protein synthesis.	Coccidiosis	[29]
Ivermectin	Antiparasitic	Act by binding with glutamate-gated chloride channel receptors.	Lice, mites, roundworms, lungworms	[41]

(Table 1) cont.....

Antiparasitic Drug	Category	Mode of Action	Target Species/Disease	References
Albendazole	Anthelmintic	Inhibits microtubule synthesis by binding to β-tubulin and inhibits mitochondrial reductase causing reduced glucose transport.	Nematodes, trematodes, and cestodes	[47]
Levamisole	Anthelmintic	Interfere with carbohydrate metabolism and inhibit fumarate reductase.	Effective against *Dictyocaulus, Haemonchus, Ostertagia, Trichostrongylus, Trichostrongylus, Cooperia, Nematodirus, Bunostomum,* and *Oesophagostomum*	[56]
Pyrethrins	Ectoparacidal	By interfering with sodium and potassium ion transport in nerve membranes and interrupting neurotransmission along the axon and at the synapse, pyrethrins quickly knock down, paralyze, and kill arthropods.	Face flies, horse flies, deer flies, horn flies, house flies, stable flies, gnats, moths, bedbugs, mites, mosquitoes, fleas, ticks, lice, and other insects.	[63]
Carbamates and organophosphates	Ectoparacidal	Inhibit acetylcholinesterase.	Ectoparasites	[64]
Amitraz	Ticks, lice, mite	Inhibit monoamine oxidase.	Ectoparasites	[68]

CONCLUSION

Drugs that fight parasites are essential for keeping cattle healthy. These medications are essential tools in the fight against a variety of parasitic illnesses that can negatively impact cattle productivity and general animal welfare. Antiparasitic medications boost growth rates, increase production, and reduce economic losses in the cattle sector by successfully preventing and controlling internal and external parasites. To avoid resistance among parasite populations and to guarantee the safety of animal products for human consumption, these medications must be used carefully. The creation of sustainable antiparasitic approaches will remain essential as long as research and innovation are conducted to address new problems, guarantee the long-term health of cow populations, and reduce environmental effects.

REFERENCES

[1]   Melo LRB, Medeiros MA, Beserra LAF, *et al.* Development and number of generations of *Haematobia irritans* (Diptera: Muscidae) in bovine fecal masses in the semiarid region of Brazil. Vet Parasitol Reg Stud Rep 2020; 20: 100411.
[http://dx.doi.org/10.1016/j.vprsr.2020.100411] [PMID: 32448539]

[2]   Rodriguez-Vivas RI, Jonsson NN, Bhushan C. Strategies for the control of *Rhipicephalus microplus* ticks in a world of conventional acaricide and macrocyclic lactone resistance. Parasitol Res 2018; 117(1): 3-29.
[http://dx.doi.org/10.1007/s00436-017-5677-6] [PMID: 29152691]

[3]   Prajapati BM, Gupta JP, Pandey DP, Parmar GA, Chaudhari JD. Molecular markers for resistance against infectious diseases of economic importance. Vet World 2017; 10(1): 112-20.
[http://dx.doi.org/10.14202/vetworld.2017.112-120] [PMID: 28246455]

[4]   Food and Agriculture Organization of the United Nations. FAOSTAT. 2022. Available from: https://www.fao.org/faostat/en/ #compare

[5]   Sosnowski M, Osek J. Microbiological safety of food of animal origin from organic farms. J Vet Res (Pulawy) 2021; 65(1): 87-92.
[http://dx.doi.org/10.2478/jvetres-2021-0015] [PMID: 33817400]

[6]   Kayser O, Olbrich C, Croft SL, Kiderlen AF. Formulation and biopharmaceutical issues in the development of drug delivery systems for antiparasitic drugs. Parasitol Res 2003; 90(0) (Suppl. 2): S63-70.
[http://dx.doi.org/10.1007/s00436-002-0769-2] [PMID: 12937968]

[7]   Gomes TC, Andrade Júnior HF, Lescano SAZ, Amato-Neto V. *In vitro* action of antiparasitic drugs, especially artesunate, against *Toxoplasma gondii*. Rev Soc Bras Med Trop 2012; 45(4): 485-90.
[http://dx.doi.org/10.1590/S0037-86822012000400014] [PMID: 22930046]

[8]   Riviere JE, Papich MG, Eds. Veterinary pharmacology and therapeutics, ed 9, Ames, Lowa,. Wiley-Blackwell, 2009.

[9]   Pathania S, Singh PK. Analyzing FDA-approved drugs for compliance of pharmacokinetic principles: should there be a critical screening parameter in drug designing protocols? Expert Opin Drug Metab Toxicol 2021; 17(4): 351-4.
[http://dx.doi.org/10.1080/17425255.2021.1865309] [PMID: 33320017]

[10]   Rick Turner J. FDA's New Guidance for Industry Addressing Evaluation of the Safety of New Drugs for Improving Glycemic Control: A Case Study in Regulatory Science. Ther Innov Regul Sci 2021; 55(1): 1-5.
[http://dx.doi.org/10.1007/s43441-020-00211-6] [PMID: 33085070]

[11]   de Moraes J, Geary TG. FDA-Approved Antiparasitic Drugs in the 21st Century: A Success for Helminthiasis? Trends Parasitol 2020; 36(7): 573-5.
[http://dx.doi.org/10.1016/j.pt.2020.04.005] [PMID: 32387059]

[12]   Geary TG. *Haemonchus contortus*. Adv Parasitol 2016; 93: 429-63.
[http://dx.doi.org/10.1016/bs.apar.2016.02.013] [PMID: 27238010]

[13]   Sadeddine R, Diarra AZ, Laroche M, *et al.* Molecular identification of protozoal and bacterial organisms in domestic animals and their infesting ticks from north-eastern Algeria. Ticks Tick Borne Dis 2020; 11(2): 101330.
[http://dx.doi.org/10.1016/j.ttbdis.2019.101330] [PMID: 31786146]

[14]   Davis JL, Gookin JL. Antiprotozoan drugs, In Riviere JE, Papich MG, eds: Veterinary pharmacology and therapeutics, ed 9, Ames, Lowa,. Wiley-Blackwell, 2009.

[15]   Plumb DC. Plums veterinary drug hand book, ed 7, Ames, lowa,. Blackwell publishing, 2011.

[16]   Souza TS, Moreira DRM, Marcelino HR. Chemical and Pharmacological Properties of Decoquinate:

A Review of Its Pharmaceutical Potential and Future Perspectives. Pharmaceutics 2022; 14(7): 1383.
[http://dx.doi.org/10.3390/pharmaceutics14071383] [PMID: 35890280]

[17]   Heinrichs AJ, Bush GJ. Evaluation of decoquinate or lasalocid against coccidiosis from natural exposure in neonatal dairy calves. J Dairy Sci 1991; 74(9): 3223-7.
[http://dx.doi.org/10.3168/jds.S0022-0302(91)78508-1] [PMID: 1779071]

[18]   Dirikolu L, Lehner AF, Tobin T. Plasma concentrations of diclazuril following oral administration of diclazuril and diclazuril sodium salt to cattle. J Vet Pharmacol Ther 2022; 45(4): 392-401.
[http://dx.doi.org/10.1111/jvp.13062] [PMID: 35488857]

[19]   Zechner G, Bauer C, Jacobs J, Goossens L, Vertenten G, Taylor MA. Efficacy of diclazuril and toltrazuril in the prevention of coccidiosis in dairy calves under field conditions. Vet Rec 2015; 176(5): 126.
[http://dx.doi.org/10.1136/vr.102237] [PMID: 25371497]

[20]   Sarli M, Novoa MB, Mazzucco MN, *et al.* Efficacy of long-acting oxytetracycline and imidocarb dipropionate for the chemosterilization of *Anaplasma marginale* in experimentally infected carrier cattle in Argentina. Vet Parasitol Reg Stud Rep 2021; 23: 100513.
[http://dx.doi.org/10.1016/j.vprsr.2020.100513] [PMID: 33678368]

[21]   Waggoner JK, Cecava MJ, Kazacos KR. Efficacy of lasalocid and decoquinate against coccidiosis in naturally infected dairy calves. J Dairy Sci 1994; 77(1): 349-53.
[http://dx.doi.org/10.3168/jds.S0022-0302(94)76961-7] [PMID: 8120204]

[22]   Stromberg BE, Schlotthauer JC, Armstrong BD, Brandt WE, Liss C. Efficacy of lasalocid sodium against coccidiosis (Eimeria zuernii and Eimeria bovis) in calves. Am J Vet Res 1982; 43(4): 583-5.
[PMID: 7073077]

[23]   Love D, Fajt VR, Hairgrove T, Jones M, Thompson JA. Metronidazole for the treatment of *Tritrichomonas foetus* in bulls. BMC Vet Res 2017; 13(1): 107.
[http://dx.doi.org/10.1186/s12917-017-0999-2] [PMID: 28410582]

[24]   Kather EJ, Marks SL, Kass PH. Determination of the *in vitro* susceptibility of feline trichomonas foetus to 5 antimicrobial agents. J Vet Intern Med 2007; 21(5): 966-70.
[http://dx.doi.org/10.1111/j.1939-1676.2007.tb03050.x] [PMID: 17939550]

[25]   Gupte S. Phenobarbital and metabolism of metronidazole. N Engl J Med 1983; 308(9): 529.
[http://dx.doi.org/10.1056/NEJM198303033080922] [PMID: 6823276]

[26]   Carta F, Scozzafava A, Supuran CT. Sulfonamides: a patent review (2008 - 2012). Expert Opin Ther Pat 2012; 22(7): 747-58.
[http://dx.doi.org/10.1517/13543776.2012.698264]

[27]   Azevedo-Barbosa H, Dias DF, Franco LL, Hawkes JA, Carvalho DT. From Antibacterial to Antitumour Agents: A Brief Review on The Chemical and Medicinal Aspects of Sulfonamides. Mini Rev Med Chem 2020; 20(19): 2052-66.
[http://dx.doi.org/10.2174/1389557520666200905125738] [PMID: 32888265]

[28]   Vicente D, Pérez-Trallero E. Tetraciclinas, sulfamidas y metronidazol [Tetracyclines, sulfonamides, and metronidazole]. Enferm Infecc Microbiol Clin 2010; 28(2): 122-30. Spanish.
[http://dx.doi.org/10.1016/j.eimc.2009.10.002]

[29]   Fayer R. Activity of sulfadimethoxine against cryptosporidiosis in dairy calves. J Parasitol 1992; 78(3): 534-7.
[http://dx.doi.org/10.2307/3283662] [PMID: 1597803]

[30]   Bourne DWA, Bialer M, Dittert LW, *et al.* Disposition of sulfadimethoxine in cattle: inclusion of protein binding factors in a pharmacokinetic model. J Pharm Sci 1981; 70(9): 1068-72.
[http://dx.doi.org/10.1002/jps.2600700926] [PMID: 6101158]

[31]   Tolika EP, Samanidou VF, Papadoyannis IN. Development and validation of an HPLC method for the determination of ten sulfonamide residues in milk according to 2002/657/EC. J Sep Sci 2011; 34(14):

1627-35.
[http://dx.doi.org/10.1002/jssc.201100171] [PMID: 21644254]

[32]   Waldner CL, Parker S, Gow S, Wilson DJ, Campbell JR. Antimicrobial usage in western Canadian cow-calf herds. Can Vet J 2019; 60(3): 255-67.
[PMID: 30872848]

[33]   Constable PD. Antimicrobial use in the treatment of calf diarrhea. J Vet Intern Med 2004; 18(1): 8-17.
[http://dx.doi.org/10.1111/j.1939-1676.2004.tb00129.x] [PMID: 14765726]

[34]   Chapman MP. The use of sulfaquinoxaline in the control of liver coccidiosis in domestic rabbits. Vet Med 1948; 43(9): 375-9.
[PMID: 18880526]

[35]   Campbell WC. History of the discovery of sulfaquinoxaline as a coccidiostat. J Parasitol 2008; 94(4): 934-45.
[http://dx.doi.org/10.1645/GE-1413.1] [PMID: 18837573]

[36]   Jank L, Martins MT, Arsand JB, *et al.* An LC–ESI–MS/MS method for residues of fluoroquinolones, sulfonamides, tetracyclines and trimethoprim in feedingstuffs: validation and surveillance. Food Addit Contam Part A Chem Anal Control Expo Risk Assess 2018; 35(10): 1975-89.
[http://dx.doi.org/10.1080/19440049.2018.1508895] [PMID: 30141745]

[37]   Charlier J, De Waele V, Ducheyne E, van der Voort M, Vande Velde F, Claerebout E. Decision making on helminths in cattle: diagnostics, economics and human behaviour. Ir Vet J 2015; 69(1): 14.
[http://dx.doi.org/10.1186/s13620-016-0073-6] [PMID: 27708771]

[38]   Charlier J, van der Voort M, Kenyon F, Skuce P, Vercruysse J. Chasing helminths and their economic impact on farmed ruminants. Trends Parasitol 2014; 30(7): 361-7.
[http://dx.doi.org/10.1016/j.pt.2014.04.009] [PMID: 24888669]

[39]   Laing R, Gillan V, Devaney E. Ivermectin – Old Drug, New Tricks? Trends Parasitol 2017; 33(6): 463-72.
[http://dx.doi.org/10.1016/j.pt.2017.02.004] [PMID: 28285851]

[40]   Molyneux DH, Ward SA. Reflections on the Nobel Prize for Medicine 2015 – The Public Health Legacy and Impact of Avermectin and Artemisinin. Trends Parasitol 2015; 31(12): 605-7.
[http://dx.doi.org/10.1016/j.pt.2015.10.008] [PMID: 26552892]

[41]   Crump A. Ivermectin: enigmatic multifaceted 'wonder' drug continues to surprise and exceed expectations. J Antibiot (Tokyo) 2017; 70(5): 495-505.
[http://dx.doi.org/10.1038/ja.2017.11] [PMID: 28196978]

[42]   Johnson-Arbor K. Ivermectin: a mini-review. Clin Toxicol (Phila) 2022; 60(5): 571-5.
[http://dx.doi.org/10.1080/15563650.2022.2043338] [PMID: 35225114]

[43]   Baumans V, Havenaar R, Van Herck H, Rooymans TP. The effectiveness of Ivomec and Neguvon in the control of murine mites. Lab Anim 1988; 22(3): 243-5.
[http://dx.doi.org/10.1258/002367788780746368] [PMID: 3172705]

[44]   Sunderkötter C, Wohlrab J, Hamm H. Scabies: epidemiology, diagnosis, and treatment. Dtsch Arztebl Int 2021; 118(41): 695-704.
[http://dx.doi.org/10.3238/arztebl.m2021.0296] [PMID: 34615594]

[45]   Bushra M, Shahardar RA, Allaie IM, Wani ZA. Efficacy of closantel, fenbendazole and ivermectin against GI helminths of cattle in central Kashmir. J Parasit Dis 2019; 43(2): 289-93.
[http://dx.doi.org/10.1007/s12639-019-01091-w] [PMID: 31263335]

[46]   Swan GE, Soll MD, Gross SJ. Efficacy of ivermectin against *Parafilaria bovicola* and lesion resolution in cattle. Vet Parasitol 1991; 40(3-4): 267-72.
[http://dx.doi.org/10.1016/0304-4017(91)90106-6] [PMID: 1788933]

[47]   Movahedi F, Li L, Gu W, Xu ZP. Nanoformulations of albendazole as effective anticancer and

antiparasite agents. Nanomedicine (Lond) 2017; 12(20): 2555-74.
[http://dx.doi.org/10.2217/nnm-2017-0102] [PMID: 28954575]

[48] Williams JC, DeRosa A, Nakamura Y, Loyacano AF. Comparative efficacy of ivermectin pour-on, albendazole, oxfendazole and fenbendazole against *Ostertagia ostertagi* inhibited larvae, other gastrointestinal nematodes and lungworm of cattle. Vet Parasitol 1997; 73(1-2): 73-82.
[http://dx.doi.org/10.1016/S0304-4017(97)00066-6] [PMID: 9477494]

[49] Eckardt K, Kaltenhäuser J, Kilb C, Seiler A, Stahlmann R. Relative potency of albendazole and its sulfoxide metabolite in two *in vitro* tests for developmental toxicity: The rat whole embryo culture and the mouse embryonic stem cell test. Reprod Toxicol 2012; 34(3): 378-84.
[http://dx.doi.org/10.1016/j.reprotox.2012.05.037] [PMID: 22652462]

[50] Bloemhoff Y, Danaher M, Andrew Forbes , *et al.* Parasite control practices on pasture-based dairy farms in the Republic of Ireland. Vet Parasitol 2014; 204(3-4): 352-63.
[http://dx.doi.org/10.1016/j.vetpar.2014.05.029] [PMID: 24924698]

[51] Theodorides VJ, Carakostas MC, Colaianne JJ, Freeman JF, Page SW. Safety of albendazole in developing bovine fetuses. Am J Vet Res 1993; 54(12): 2171-4.
[http://dx.doi.org/10.2460/ajvr.1993.54.12.2171] [PMID: 8116955]

[52] Cray C, Altman NH. An Update on the Biologic Effects of Fenbendazole. Comp Med 2022; 72(4): 215-9.
[http://dx.doi.org/10.30802/AALAS-CM-22-000006] [PMID: 35764389]

[53] Capece BPS, Virkel GL, Lanusse CE. Enantiomeric behaviour of albendazole and fenbendazole sulfoxides in domestic animals: Pharmacological implications. Vet J 2009; 181(3): 241-50.
[http://dx.doi.org/10.1016/j.tvjl.2008.11.010] [PMID: 19124257]

[54] Kouam MK, Fokom GT, Luogbou DDN, Kantzoura V. Gastro-intestinal parasitism and control practices in dairy cattle in North-west Cameroon (Central Africa). Acta Parasitol 2021; 66(3): 947-53.
[http://dx.doi.org/10.1007/s11686-021-00343-1] [PMID: 33721185]

[55] Becerra-Nava R, Alonso-Díaz MA, Fernández-Salas A, Quiroz RH. First report of cattle farms with gastrointestinal nematodes resistant to levamisole in Mexico. Vet Parasitol 2014; 204(3-4): 285-90.
[http://dx.doi.org/10.1016/j.vetpar.2014.04.019] [PMID: 24867275]

[56] Prichard RK. Anthelmintics for Cattle. Vet Clin North Am Food Anim Pract 1986; 2(2): 489-501.
[http://dx.doi.org/10.1016/S0749-0720(15)31259-7] [PMID: 3488116]

[57] Idika IK, Okonkwo EA, Onah DN, Ezeh IO, Iheagwam CN, Nwosu CO. Efficacy of levamisole and ivermectin in the control of bovine parasitic gastroenteritis in the sub-humid savanna zone of southeastern Nigeria. Parasitol Res 2012; 111(4): 1683-7.
[http://dx.doi.org/10.1007/s00436-012-3007-6] [PMID: 22760239]

[58] Pérez de León AA, Mitchell RD III, Watson DW. Ectoparasites of Cattle. Vet Clin North Am Food Anim Pract 2020; 36(1): 173-85.
[http://dx.doi.org/10.1016/j.cvfa.2019.12.004] [PMID: 32029183]

[59] Cortinas R, Jones CJ. Ectoparasites of cattle and small ruminants. Vet Clin North Am Food Anim Pract 2006; 22(3): 673-93.
[http://dx.doi.org/10.1016/j.cvfa.2006.06.003] [PMID: 17071359]

[60] Matsuo N. Discovery and development of pyrethroid insecticides. Proc Jpn Acad, Ser B, Phys Biol Sci 2019; 95(7): 378-400.
[http://dx.doi.org/10.2183/pjab.95.027] [PMID: 31406060]

[61] Dara D, Drabovich AP. Assessment of risks, implications, and opportunities of waterborne neurotoxic pesticides. J Environ Sci (China) 2023; 125: 735-41.
[http://dx.doi.org/10.1016/j.jes.2022.03.033] [PMID: 36375955]

[62] Anadón A, Martínez-Larrañaga MR, Martínez MA. Use and abuse of pyrethrins and synthetic pyrethroids in veterinary medicine. Vet J 2009; 182(1): 7-20.

[http://dx.doi.org/10.1016/j.tvjl.2008.04.008] [PMID: 18539058]

[63]   Chen M, Du Y, Zhu G, *et al.* Action of six pyrethrins purified from the botanical insecticide pyrethrum on cockroach sodium channels expressed in Xenopus oocytes. Pestic Biochem Physiol 2018; 151: 82-9.
[http://dx.doi.org/10.1016/j.pestbp.2018.05.002] [PMID: 30704718]

[64]   King AM, Aaron CK. Organophosphate and carbamate poisoning. Emerg Med Clin North Am 2015; 33(1): 133-51.
[http://dx.doi.org/10.1016/j.emc.2014.09.010] [PMID: 25455666]

[65]   Jokanović M. Medical treatment of acute poisoning with organophosphorus and carbamate pesticides. Toxicol Lett 2009; 190(2): 107-15.
[http://dx.doi.org/10.1016/j.toxlet.2009.07.025] [PMID: 19651196]

[66]   Barelli A, Soave PM, Del Vicario M, Barelli R. New experimental Oximes in the management of organophosphorus pesticides poisoning. Minerva Anestesiol 2011; 77(12): 1197-203.
[PMID: 21799476]

[67]   Dhooria S, Agarwal R. Amitraz, an underrecognized poison: A systematic review. Indian J Med Res 2016; 144(3): 348-58.
[http://dx.doi.org/10.4103/0971-5916.198723] [PMID: 28139533]

[68]   Jonsson NN, Klafke G, Corley SW, Tidwell J, Berry CM, Koh-Tan HC. Molecular biology of amitraz resistance in cattle ticks of the genus Rhipicephalus. Front Biosci 2018; 23(2): 796-810.
[http://dx.doi.org/10.2741/4617] [PMID: 28930573]

[69]   Kornele M, O'Brien A, Phillippi-Taylor A, Marchiondo AA. Preface. Vet Parasitol 2014; 204(1-2): 1-2.
[http://dx.doi.org/10.1016/j.vetpar.2014.04.010] [PMID: 24854214]

CHAPTER 14

Host Resistance to Parasitic Diseases

Farhat Bano[1], Muhammad Ahsan[2], Muhammad Asmat Ullah Saleem[1], Muhammad Mohsin[3] and Muhammad Tahir Aleem[4,5,*]

[1] *College of Veterinary Medicine, Northeast Agricultural University, Harbin150030, P.R. China*

[2] *Faculty of Veterinary Sciences, University of Agriculture, Faisalabad, Pakistan*

[3] *Shantou University Medical College, Shantou, Guangdong, 515045, China*

[4] *MOE Joint International Research Laboratory of Animal Health and Food Safety, College of Veterinary Medicine, Nanjing Agricultural University, Nanjing 210095, China*

[5] *Center for Gene Regulation in Health and Disease, Department of Biological, Geological, and Environmental Sciences, College of Sciences and Health Professions, Cleveland State University, Cleveland, OH 44115, USA*

Abstract: Resistance to parasitic infections falls under two main domains. The first is known as innate resistance, it comprises age resistance, breed resistance, and in some situations, species resistance which does not have an immunological basis. The second category is termed as acquired resistance and it depends on humoral and cell response. However, for reasons elaborated in this chapter, parasitic diseases can be countered by a few vaccines. The main role of protecting animals against infections and modulating the spread of parasitic diseases is contributed by the natural expression of acquired resistance. Host-parasite relationships are mostly perceived as a defense race, where parasites are continuously trying to take over host machinery. A common source of parasite spread is herbivory, which constitutes the most prevalent challenge to mammalian growth and reproduction. Factors affecting the immune response against infection include (a) genetics, (b) host status at the time of exposure comprising age, disease, and underlying illness, and (c) transmission and population of parasite loading dose.). The immune system works in the same fashion against parasites as for other pathogens, but there are some major changes depending upon the nature of the response. Different antigens show up as a parasite develops through certain stages of its life cycle. This results in the occurrence of many antibodies dependent and independent responses. The immune system of the host becomes confused in certain infections, progressing to conditions where the host is targeted rather than supported.

Keywords: Evolution, Host, Infection, Interaction, Immunity, Parasite, Strategy.

* **Corresponding author Muhammad Tahir Aleem:** MOE Joint International Research Laboratory of Animal Health and Food Safety, College of Veterinary Medicine, Nanjing Agricultural University, Nanjing 210095, China; Center for Gene Regulation in Health and Disease, Department of Biological, Geological, and Environmental Sciences, College of Sciences and Health Professions, Cleveland State University, Cleveland, OH 44115, USA;
E-mail: dr.tahir1990@gmail.com

INTRODUCTION

Understanding the host-parasite coevolution is a time-honored goal of evolutionary biology. There is a well-established conceptual framework to explain the host-parasite relationship under the inference of two-species relatedness, that can lead to defense race kinetics or persistent genotype variations [1, 2]. Although a lot of hosts depend on symbionts for countering the parasitic attacks. The potential significance of defensive symbionts against disease control is greatly recognized, but there is still much confusion about how symbionts regulate and play a role in host-parasite coevolution [3, 4]. Theoretical and empirical studies help us address these questions by synthesizing information from available data. Firstly, we generate theories on how mutual defensive approaches originated from host-parasite interactions. All important determinants of evolutionary dynamics are influenced by defensive symbionts [5]. The underlying mechanism of defense influences parasitic virulence [6]. Many mechanisms are involved in parasitic infestation which are likely to be regulated by certain complex factors. Many of the processes of host immunity and their regulating factors have been recognized, however much is left to be elaborated. The diversity in protective mechanism against tick infestation is mostly noticeable in *Bos taurus* and *Bos indicus* cattle, there are five to ten times more tick attacks in taurine cattle as compared to indicine given the same exposure. Parasitic infection is manifested by attaching larvae, which struggle to feed and infect the host. The main responses against parasitic attack are innate and adaptive responses and their relative significance differs in taurine and indicine cattle. The role of humoral immunity against infection has conflicting evidence, the latest research tells that a significant IgG response against parasitic attack is not effective. T-cell response mounted by indicine cattle against larval stages is more protective. The role of innate resistance is critical against parasitic infections, while adaptive immunity mainly plays a role in long-term or chronic infections [2].

Early studies focused on the mechanical and physical qualities of indicine and taurine skin. Further studies concerning innate responses to infection and the potential role of the physical qualities of skin against parasitic infestation have been conducted [4].

Resistance against parasites in cattle is manifested in decreased tick population feeding to get engorged, less egg production, and less viability of eggs. Various animal species react differently to parasitic infections. Some breeds have innate resistance to pathogenic consequences of infection and there is no decline in their productivity and growth. Some breeds exhibit more rapid and documented responses against infection [3].

The most common route of transmission is the gastrointestinal tract, which later spreads *via* the bloodstream and lymphatics. The parasite can also spread by the ingestion of oocytes that are present in the fecal matter of acutely infected animals or by transplacental infection from mother to fetus. Consecutive pregnancies act as a source of continuous transmission through the placenta. This consistent transmission is seen in cattle that are naturally infected, and it indicates that it is a significant challenge to exhibit a resistance strategy [1].

The main characteristics of parasites that make them difficult to control are the size of the parasite, life cycle, and antigenic complexity. Parasites escape the host immune response in several ways: (a) They prefer to be at such body locations that are comparatively safe from an immune response. (b) Certain changes in surface antigens. (c) Different processes alter immunity [5].

Evolution of Resistance

Many breeds of cattle belonging to endemic disease areas have developed strategies to adapt them to co-exist with parasites. Genes responsible for resistance and tolerance can offer new mechanisms of health improvement and livestock welfare. The Sahiwal express a low level of pathology as compared to Holstein and can survive an infection [7]. To develop effective eradication programs, understanding the process of resistance to nematodes is essential. Most animals are categorized for their immunity nematodes [8]. Ruminants have a natural genetic variation that effectively avoids gastrointestinal parasites without using anthelmintics [9].

The heterogeneity of the ecosystem is believed to have direct implications for the evolution of the host and parasite [10]. The geographical distribution of the genetic variation is formed by various phenomena that interrelate with each other and affect the adaptive traits' selection. The magnitude of such processes can be understood by analyzing the population patterns of the genetic framework and it is helpful in forming an assumption about the evolution of traits [11].

The parasites affecting the mating system and transmission processes have variations in their life cycle which can lead to variations in the genetic structure of the population because the rate of gene flow is influenced by it [12]. The phenotypic specialties formed by genetic signals have just started to be revealed and important evolutionary clues are expected from reproductive and morphologic traits [13].

An important role in the maintenance and distribution of genetic variability is played by mating systems. Hurdles in adapting standard procedures of secondary deductions about the life cycle of parasites certainly elaborate the present lack of information regarding the mating systems of parasites. The current research focuses on developing a mix of direct and indirect illustration procedures managing such hurdles and particularly explains how such a mix can alter our understanding of the biology of cattle [14].

Phenotypic changes result from both natural evolutionary processes and modern genetic selection, the mechanisms that direct these variations are quite contrasting. Evolution is continuous natural variation in reaction to climatic stress. Genetic selection is independent of climatic stress as it is artificially directed. Genetic selection has been able to enhance direct variation by decreasing climatic stress. The protocols to manage this stress are good quality nutrition and drugs to combat diseases [15]. Parasites evade the effective protective resistance response by mimicking the action of apoptotic bodies. It is a good approach to act like apoptotic bodies from an evolutionary perspective as it can decrease the inflammatory response. Again, there may be a counter mechanism developed by the Sahiwal breed to avoid this type of response [16]. Hosts and parasites struggle to become co-adapted which makes it possible for both types of populations to exist and mate in the presence of each other. The host population develops a new defense strategy after the first encounter with the parasite, which results in tolerance against disease. This can lead to parasites adapting ways to combat their defense. So, host communities face different patterns of fitness levels [17]. Just like all parasites, ticks can be easily transmitted to their hosts. Ticks attach themselves to vertebrates for different periods of time as they are obligate parasites. Ticks are quietly adapted to their transmission mode. They are able to wait several months for a new host (on which they start a new life cycle) to come after the transport stage is complete and they have detached their desired destination. This can result in the formation of a secondary tick population. *Rhipicephalus microplus* and *Amblyomma variegatum* have developed this approach of occupation of friendly zones. *Rhipicephalus microplus* has high specificity for ungulates and it has spread throughout the tropical belt due to cattle movement. It has an origin in South Asia. *Amblyomma variegatum* has its origin in Africa. These two are carriers of lethal diseases of cattle; Babesiosis and Anaplasmosis. Expected environmental variations can alter the geographic distribution of these species of parasites [18].

Host-parasite Relationship

An important phenomenon of host-parasite interaction is the way parasites correlate with the host. There is a continuous interaction between the immune system of the host and the pathogen which has different effects for both groups (Fig. **1**). Disease pathogenesis is contributed by the outcome of immune responses produced by parasite-protective and host-protective mechanisms. It is therefore essential to comprehend the possible outcomes of producing specific responses to the immune system while making vaccines [19]. Countless interactions are involved in every host-parasite relationship that affects parasite transmission. Transmission of almost all kinds of parasites is limited by the host's immune response. Immunity has been seen to have a significant role in controlling the progression of parasitic infections. The individual phenomena are greatly complicated and hard to measure but stress has a well-documented impact on host immunity [20].

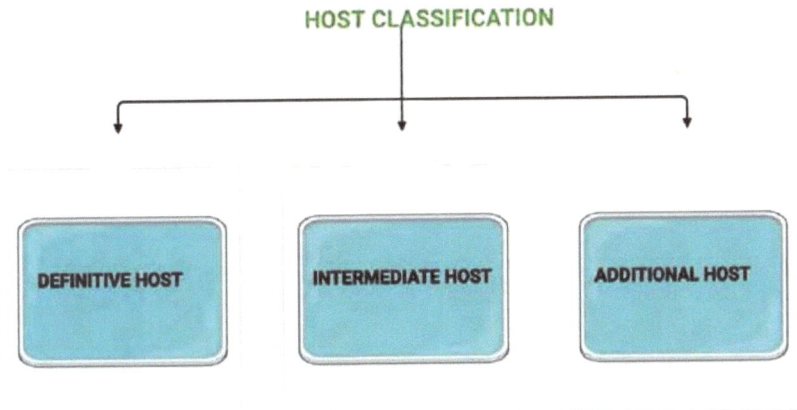

Fig. (1). Classification of host.

Neospora caninum infection with protozoan parasites is considered to be a major reason for reproductive insufficiency in cattle around the globe. Neosporosis is an infection of gestation and the change in the balance between parasite and host that may lead to infection can be understood by studying the fetal and maternal immune response. Gestational age and immune competence of the fetus at the time of infection are other significant components. Death of the fetus may occur due to *N.caninum* infection during periods of early gestation. While congenitally infected or healthy calf may be born if this infection occurs during mid to late pregnancy [21]. Environmental variations are related to an increase in parasitic load [22].

Prevalence, abundance, mode of transmission, and effect of parasites play an important role in determining these interactions and host mortality and magnitude of parasitic defense [23]. Methods of transmission of *N.canium,* which is considered to take place in cattle are 1. Sporulated cyst ingestion; 2. Transmission *via* vertical route (endogenous); 3. Horizontal transmission is followed by vertical (exogenous, transplacental) transmission. The main factor linked to climatic change is increasing temperature although air movement also has an effect on it

[24, 25]. Most of the parasites have advanced their emergence time, those which were active during summer only are now moving throughout the year [26]. The number of parasites per year is increasing due to extended and earlier phases of mating by parasites as parasites with selective benefit are provided by an extended breeding season [27, 28]. Host and parasite characteristics have a genetic basis and coevolution can shape them. Infections calculated in a controlled environment have proved that the atmosphere in which parasites and hosts connect might affect the selection strength [29]. Additionally, the environment changes the various factors of host-parasite interaction (Fig. **2**). A heterogeneous environment serves as a place for most host parasitic relations [30].

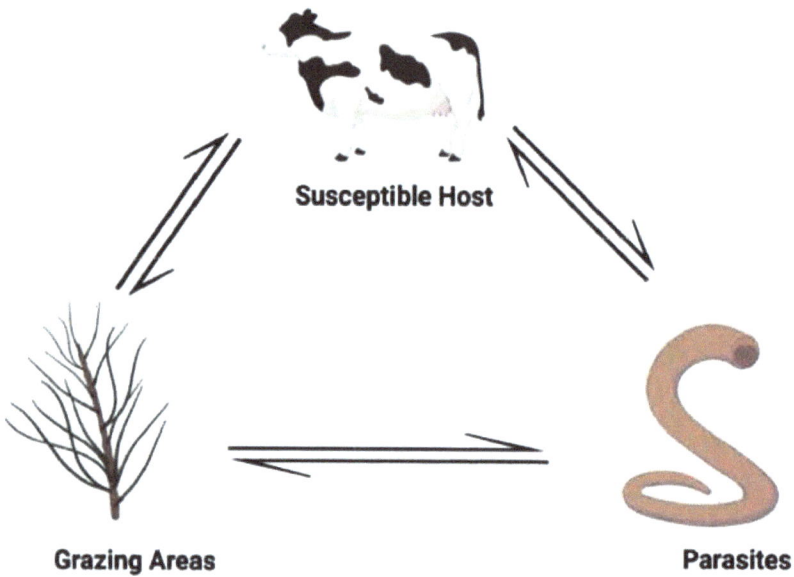

Fig. (2). Host parasitic relationship.

Host susceptibility and parasite resistance have significant outcomes for the development of virulence in parasites, sexual preference, and strategies of biological control. Host susceptibility and parasite virulence need to be genetically different in order to favor host-parasite evolution. Proof regarding natural population is still rare in spite of epidemiological implications of heterogeneities in host-parasite. To review the evidence of inheritance of host susceptibility or immunity to pathogens, we need to focus on better knowledge of genetics [31].

Role of Innate and Acquired Immunity

Most genera of parasites in cattle can incite a sufficient level of immunity in animals after they have been in grazing areas for a longer period. However, the infection by *Ostertagia* can still infect the cattle. Until the animals reach more than 2 years of age, the immune response that minimizes the growth of new larvae is not usually evident. For an extended period of time, the animals remain prone to infection, and an enhanced level of immunity in the herd is the result of a lot of manifestations of immune mechanisms [32]. African trypanosomiasis has the ability to escape immune eradication by changing the immunodominant variant surface glycoprotein coat at the time of infection. Trypanosomes can also manipulate the host immune system by antigenic variation. The relation of these mechanisms can be seen in the host and parasite survival context [33].

Immunologic control of acute infection can lead to a condition of consistent infection for many vector-transmitted parasites. In clinically normal animals, the parasites in the blood can cycle silently. Parasitism is favored by gaining infection, which is persistent in nature. Subsequent transmission is provided by parasite reservoirs that belong to endemically infected animals [34]. Host defense against parasites is divided into two different categories; first is the capacity to decrease parasitic load, which is called resistance, and second is the capacity to reduce the harm induced by parasites. The effects of parasites against the host can be protected by these two mechanisms. The hosts that are good at combating pathogens are not always the healthiest ones [35]. The variation between tolerance and immunity is that immunity prevents the host and tolerance prevents the host from danger without having any declining outcomes on parasites. The ecological outcomes of immunity must differ. The development of immunity should minimize the dominance of parasites in the host population, while tolerance should have a supporting effect on the dominance of parasites [36]. Variation in resistance is contributed by innate immune factors [37].

Immunocompetent animals can protect themselves against infective parasites and pathogens. The ability to save oneself needs a way of surveillance and measures to reduce the danger. Both capacities show up very early in history [38].

Regulation between adaptive and innate immune responses leads to the effective growth of the overall immunity of the host. The proper study of these systems is required to differentiate targets against which a proper reaction is generated [39].

Adaptive tick resistance is a process in which the host induces a resistance response against tick secretory factors after many tick infections. The salivary factors are targeted by potential immune response and animals develop immunity to further tick infestations. When a tick feeds on an unnatural host and not on the natural host, the formation of tick immunity is mostly seen. There is an incomplete understanding of the processes involved in the development of immunity against ticks. New molecular techniques to deal with ticks and hosts are starting to show advanced clues about this phenomenon [40].

The host is exposed to numerous parasitic pathogens but theories about resistance evolution mainly point to single infections. The evolution of resistance is facilitated by multiple parasites under the consideration that pathogens and hosts exist together as an outcome of superinfection [41]. There is a clear relationship of parasites with host which occurs through competition but upon the evolution of immunity against a parasite, the magnitude to which this immunity counters the invading parasites constitutes a less visible relationship among parasites. Thus, there is a complexity regarding the interaction between parasites and modes of resistance evolution [42] (Fig. **3**).

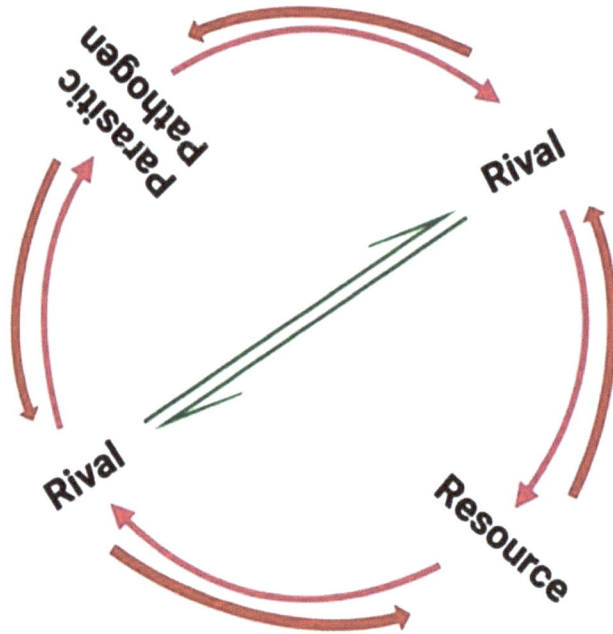

Fig. (3). Parasites and modes of resistance evolution.

Parasites and pathogenic species can endanger the animals that they infect. As an outcome a vast range of innate and acquired defense strategies evolve which may range from developing physical barriers to acquiring behavioral avoidance. Physical barriers against cell-mediated immune systems have also evolved [43]. Although these reactions are very diverse. There is a significant variability among animals in their immune strategies and hosts react to different infections in several possible ways [44]. This is evident in terms of constant resistance memory, which occurs due to different parasitic diseases. The everlasting immune system is far away from the average consequence of healing with incomplete immune memory in response to many infections, like syphilis. In some infections, like many bacterial infections, there is no evidence of immune memory [45]. These results may be regarded as immune system failures, but the studies have shown that both state and kind of immunity are the outcomes of the evolutionary relationships between parasite and host [46]. When protection from infection is costly, this is not just an ideal stage of protection, but the stage of resistance is an important factor of host fitness. Such evolution is also helpful inproducing a dominant variation in defense level with populations of host animals [47].

Resistance against Ecto and Endoparasites

About 1.49 billion cattle around the world are prone to infection with a wide variety of ectoparasites. The most economically important group of ectoparasites consists of mites, insects, and ticks due to the direct impact related to serious impacts on food and the health of animals [48]. Most of the arthropod ectoparasites also work as carriers of pathogens that cause diseases in bovines, few of them are zoonotic in nature [49]. Many infections induced by ectoparasites or by pathogens transmitted by them are documented by WOAH (World Organization for Animal Health) [50]. The evolution of ectoparasites is distinctive. Complex epidemiological aspects and farming systems have an impact on the dominance and occurrence of ectoparasites and vector-born infections in cattle. Mutations of traditional and nontraditional meat or dairy systems around the globe can extend from extensive farming to integrated farming under the supervision of international companies where modern techniques are used to control ectoparasites [51, 52]. So, a veterinarian should use husbandry procedures to deal with infestations properly [53]. Several drugs and biological methods have been used to eliminate the population of ectoparasites. Veterinary items consisting of ectoparasiticides are mostly used by veterinarians to deal with invasion of ectoparasites [54]. Deadly parasitic infections can reduce the production of cattle and in serious situations, it can lead to mortality. This causes major financial losses to farmers around the globe [55]. Several *Diptera* species are ectoparasites in nature as they feed on blood, also known as hematophagous behavior. They also induce irritation in infected animals during their adult life. At immature stages, they cause myiasis, harm soft tissues, or work as biological carriers to transmit pathogens to cattle [56]. There are evident advantages of mounting an immune response for defense against pathogens, so the ideal defense stage relies upon the balance between costs and advantages. The advantages of immune surveillance are well known for their value [57]. In endoparasitism and some other diseases, the infestation can accompany the inability of animals to create a sufficient immune response due to poor nutrition. Poor nutrition is important in two senses; it occurs with considerable impact on humans and livestock and later during low financial situations [58]. Nematodes causing gastrointestinal infection pose serious production losses in animals [59].

Various strategies are used by intracellular parasites to attack host cells, deceive signaling pathways, and obtain a stand to evade the host defense mechanism. Optimum cell invasion, capacity to destroy cell defense mechanisms, and constant attack make the parasites successful pathogens. Most of the parasites get entry through processes mediated by the host but an adhesion-based motility model called gliding is used by apicomplexans to enter the cells efficiently. Parasite movement is facilitated by actin polymerization that makes the dissemination within tissues possible. The optimum invasion strategy has given broad success to this group, which belongs to *Plasmodium, Cryptosporidium,* and *Toxoplasma* [60]. Protozoans are intracellular parasites, and they can be the source of deadly and lethal infections in humans and animals. The defense system has a series of control systems to eliminate infections and has an active locating mechanism that works to find and kill pathogenic factors. It is challenging to overcome host cell barriers imposed by cell membranes. The parasite deploys its potential ways to escape from the host immune system in order to be successful in invasion. Thus, it is important to explain how parasites gain entry into the host cells [61].

A highly efficient method for cells to enter the host cell is used by a vast group of parasites in the Apicomplexa phylum. A parasite's cytoskeleton uses an active method to gain cell entry [62]. Entry of apicomplexan occurs without changing the host actin cytoskeleton [63].

Cellular Response to Parasitic Attack

Calves when infected with tick-borne pathogens do not show serious infection with babesiosis. They rather show constantly reduced parasitemia without showing severely sick results. Not only does the host gain benefits from age-related resistance, but also it further enhances the spread of parasites. In primary infection, both adult animals and calves react to immune responses. The variation in outcome can be elaborated by the timing of the inflammatory response. In adult animals, there is proof that a late and inflammatory response probably enhances the infection. A proper study of the given strategies that underlie this mechanism may result in new methods for immune prophylaxis of the infection [64]. There is proof that the natural immunity of animals against parasitic diseases is dependent upon antibodies because, in primary infection, the antibodies in immune sera show up late long after the pathogens have been removed from the system [65].

Additionally, immune-efficient antigens are directed by early antibodies, these are considered to be originated from the immune evasion by parasites [66]. Early studies suggested that the innate immune response to *B. bovis* was served by low-molecular-weight factors that are independent of the antibodies. These factors are found in the serum of calf, and they can halt the growth of parasites [67]. This finding resulted in the behavior of not using the calf serum for the Babesia species' culture [68]. Normal calf serum does not stop the *B. divergence* growth in culture [69]. Inverse age immune response is a unique behavior, mostly well-considered for bovines (Fig. **4**).

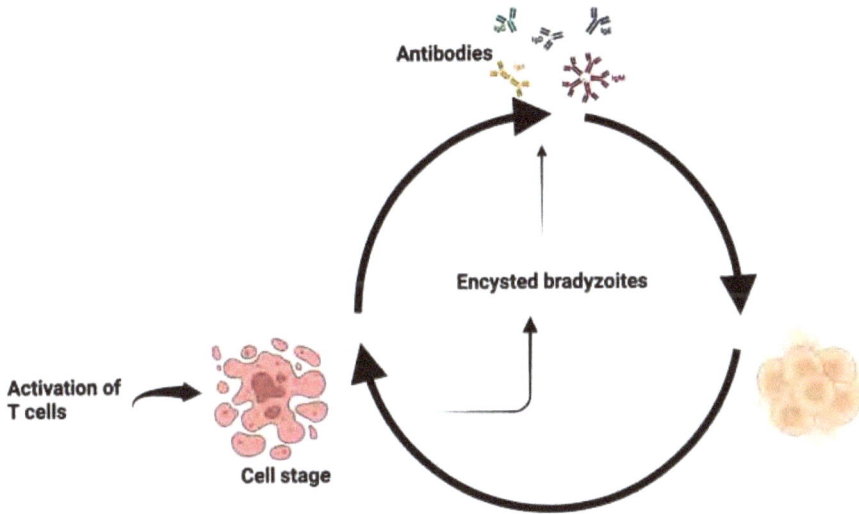

Fig. (4). Cellular response to parasitic attack.

When barriers of enzootic stability are breached, cases of babesiosis happen [70].

It is well accepted that the development of immune response changes the spread and especially the dominance of an infection in the community and this feedback has the ability to produce variation in hosts if the immune response is costly [71].

Immunity comprises methods that either stop parasites from entering or eradicate them when they attempt to attack. Contrarily, tolerance works to reduce the harm that is inflicted by the infection. Allocation of resources is needed by both resistance and tolerance [72]. Mostly, the responses that are induced are thought to be beneficial as they are only used when needed. A strategy is adopted by variability in the growth of parasites that attaches both induced and constitutive immune responses. The selection of both types of immune responses is not necessarily explained by differential costs. Variable parasites are challenged by hosts and this defense is sufficient to elaborate why it is important to use both aspects of innate immune response [73]. A mechanism to understand the various immune factors is essential to animal health. The forms of immune responses are formed by the process of evolution. Selection determines the complexity of an organization [74]. Innate immunity is the main factor of defense for all animal species. It is also important for immune response mediation. There is no adaptive immune response in invertebrates, but their innate immune response is very reliable and more efficient in its functioning [75, 76]. Both invertebrates and vertebrates have an immune response that is innate in nature and is always ready to react to external stimuli. This type of behavior can also be observed in plants where some products take part in defense in reaction to stimuli [77]. The fact that all animals depend upon innate immunity is astonishing that comparatively small studies have observed that is why this mechanism of defense is placed the way it is [78].

The Sources of Variation in Resistance to Parasitic Diseases

Several studies have suggested that variations in immunology exist in the sexes that may underlie elevated levels of parasites in males. Males typically have a lower immune response than females [79]. A double-edged sword is created by enhanced immune levels in females, which is important against parasitic infections, but it has no effect when there is a progression of autoimmune disease [80]. Research shows that susceptibility to infection is increased due to sex differences in immune function [81]. One of the leading causes of increased deaths is increased susceptibility to infection [82]. Genetic factors play a vital role in creating variation in susceptibility to a vast range of parasitic infections. The type of genetic variation will affect scientific and commercial uses. Breed substitution can be used to exploit variation among breeds. Selective breeding can be used to exploit variation within breeds to enhance immunity against diseases. Mechanisms of immune response can be understood by the identification of genes that contribute to variation in resistance, but more efforts are required to evaluate if these genes contribute to variation in resistance [83] (Fig. **5**).

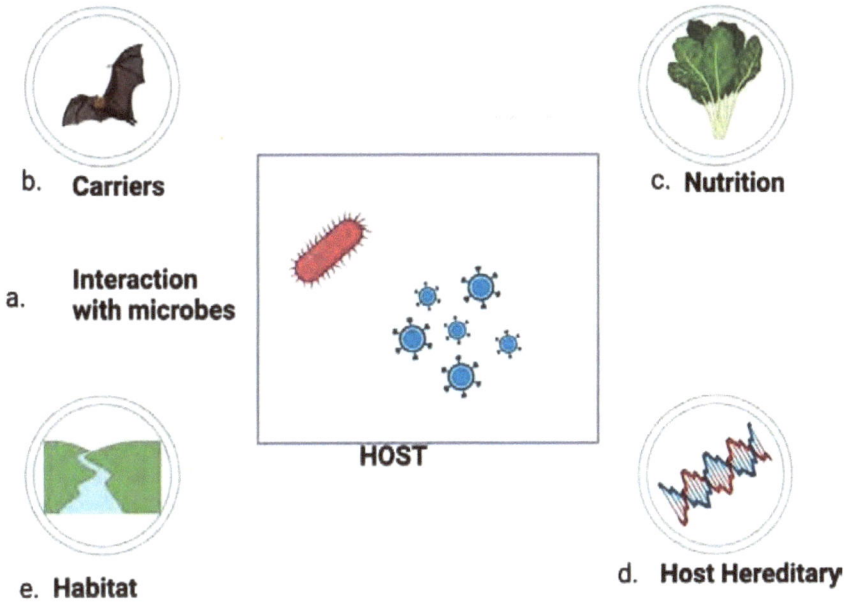

Fig. (5). Parasitic co-infection.

The additive gene effect is the main source of genetic variation. The total mean effects of genes are additive gene effects, and it is calculated from similarity among related animals [84]. The resistance to infections is enhanced by the heritable differences. Resistance to some forms of poisoning has been shown in experimental animals [85]. The application of breeding to develop resistance against disease is mostly used in livestock and is used to deal with a vast range of infections [86]. Genetic selection can be used as a management method. The time interval between the treatments can be increased by the application of genetic selection. The patterns of immunity conform to those of other infections in animal populations [87].

The Process of Parasite Rejection

The processes involved in parasite rejection are not simple, they utilize various aspects of the adaptive immune system to host. Tick immunity can be readily gained by cattle, and it has been widely used to observe bite location [88]. Immune cell infiltration results from repeated infections by parasites [89].

A tick bite can cause an immune response that can result in considerable changes in the skin, which can be beneficial to reduce feeding by ticks. Repeated tick infestation can result in a number of complications [90]. Each tick species appears to develop a preference for the host, which is directed by a combination of ticks, host, and some factors related to ecology. Hosts act as carriers for certain tick infestations and have the capacity to entertain multiple infestations without expressing any resistance response that is harmful to tick feeding. This feature is important to guarantee the accomplishment of the life cycle of the tick [91].

Inherent structural and immunological variations can drive the immune response to tick feeding [92]. It is a well-accepted fact that the vaccine having certain antigens has the capacity to incite a huge immune response to tick infestation. In a small number of situations, this immune response has been imitated by vaccines, containing antigens. The availability of commercially produced vaccines has permitted a lot of evidence showing that the present drugs can serve an important role in a combined approach to eradicate the ticks. The use of the tick vaccine alone seems to need more efficient vaccinations than those available now. The number of antigens that are left to be examined is increasing quickly [93].

In tropical and subtropical places, ticks are an important constraint on the production of livestock. Synthetic acaricides are commonly used in order to control ticks, therefore it is important to maintain the strategies to conserve the efficiency of acaricides currently available [94].

The method of choice for host resistance is genetic selection for non-chemical control of ticks. Previous research has proved that the most susceptible stages to host resistance mechanism are larval stages [95]. Cattle have the ability to survive in environments that present continuous dangers in the form of flies, ticks and worms, and pathogens as a source of contamination in wounds. Animals have evolved many mechanisms that make them enable to combat parasites. These mechanisms include the use of saliva and eating plant-based compounds containing natural medicines. These mechanisms are all specific for each species and show the specific habitat the animal lives in [96]. Many phenomena have been understood about the immunity against parasites [97]. Approaches used for parasitic control in ungulates, include defecation in the form of clumps and avoiding foraging in the neighborhood of fecal matter [98]. The avoidance of feces is believed to be a way to meet nutritional demands and the possibility of the danger of getting parasitic infections from nearby feces [99]. Animals are expected to get a parasitic load in contrast to parasites, a small dose of bacteria and viruses can be the cause of major illness and behavioral defenses are not similar to those used with parasites. Gradual exposure to common pathogens activates the steady state as an immune response. The pathogens are mostly specific to their host and animals can get pathogens in several different ways, possibly by being exposed to bacteria or viruses [100, 101].

How Parasites Escape Host Immune System

Parasites have evolved mechanisms and strategies to escape the host's immune response in order to be successful in their invasion. There is a unique approach adopted by African Trypanosomiasis, it never gains entry into the cells during their growth. They move freely in the host, which is immunologically hostile. During the time of infection, a complicated relationship exists between the survival strategies of the host and the immune system of the host. A strong selection stress is created for African trypanosomiasis due to the continuous interaction with the immune system of the host, which leads to the evolution of special strategies to escape the host killing [102]. Platelets create local plug and clotting during pathogen transmission by arthropods, immediately after vessel laceration. The process of inflammation is very complicated [103].

Some proteins and chemical factors belonging to arthropods are transmitted to host animals during the process of Trypanosomatidae transmission by their carrier. They can intercede with the development of trypanosomatids. There is a difference in the composition of organic matter that is transmitted into the skin of the host. A large amount of salivary gland protein is present in the injected cell-free biological material. In this situation, the invasion by parasites takes place later, *via* wound inflicted by bite [104]. The successful survival of parasites is mainly dependent on their ability to evade the immune system. Their strategies include entering dividing inside the cells and removing their protein coat. Some parasitic products can cause immunosuppression, which includes copying antigens, which is seen in relation to parasitic infection (Fig. **6**). Selective stimulation is one of the most sophisticated mechanisms of evasion [105].

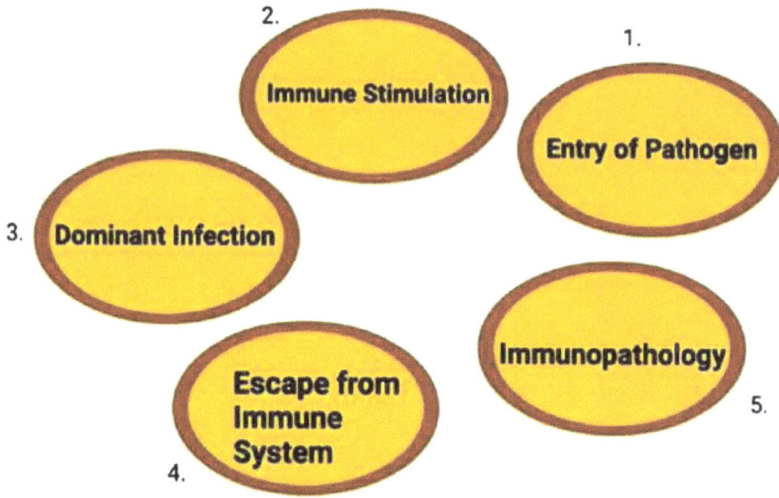

Fig. (6). How parasites escape host immune system.

Hosts can evade parasites or infected habitats through migration. Immune function can also be reduced by the demands of migration, which can result in lethal consequences for the host. There is an urgent need for research on pathogens to estimate the disease risks in the near future for animals [106].

Protozoan parasites have successfully evolved mechanisms to avoid host immunity by exhibiting a highly organized molecular surface coat that mainly works for the protection of plasma membranes from immunological attack. Antigenic variation is possessed by many parasitic species to escape the host defense [107]. Parasites have indirect interactions that they develop with the target host for success in their invasion [108]. Mortality is not directly caused by parasites, so no prominent effect is observed in the density of animal populations. A decreased competition is seen in the trait-mediated effects of the parasites [109]. Several studies believe that parasites are limited to hosts. Immunological dynamics can better help us to understand parasitic behavior towards the host [110]. The consequence of infection is dependent on the relationship between the immune system of the host and the parasite. This is mostly seen in hosts, which are immunocompromised. Resource competition, an ecological process may be superimposed. Many life-related traits like, antigen variation and growth rate are affected by host-parasite interaction [111]. *Leishmania*, an obligate intracellular parasite has the ability to survive the antimicrobial response of host cells to prevent the immune system from activation. A lot of highly rewarding mechanisms are acquired by Leishmania for manipulating the responses, like the generation of oxygen and nitric oxide radicals and the production of cytokines. This is mostly the consequence of relationships between surface molecules of *Leishmania* and less considered surface receptors of macrophages [112].

Parasites have the ability to change the behavior of hosts. They can do this by various methods: (1) Interceding with the immune-neural network of the host, (2) Altering the neural activity by releasing various products, and (3) Creating genome-based alterations in the host brain. Changes in the behavior of the host are limited to specific types, with many other aspects of behavior remaining unchanged. This level of selectivity can be produced by targeting particular areas of the brain. Discrete areas of the brain are not selectively attacked by parasites. Parasites can produce various types of effects on the brain. To maintain the survival of parasites, parasitic influence on the host behavior is observed within the context of influencing the physiological systems of the host. Parasites employ various strategies to influence the behavior of the host [113].

Parasites have evolved many strategies to adapt them to reproduce and survive. The nature of these strategies may be active or passive, or they may cause active interference with the immune regulation of the host [114].

Parasitic Infections in the Compromised Host

An immunocompromised host is defined as one having impairment in both acquired and innate immunity and unable to mount an effective immune response against an invading pathogen and there is an increased risk of infection by microorganisms [129]. An important predisposing factor to infections in the host that is immunocompromised is severe trauma [130]. The severity and manifestation of some parasitic infections can be altered by immune compromise. The use of immunosuppressive therapies, the increasing number of individuals with low immune status, and the long-term survival of these patients have changed the mode of parasitic infection [115]. There is complexity in the life cycle of parasites and these life cycles involve host exposure and a carrier defense mechanism (Fig. 7). Associated vector strategies are not completely defined, the immune response of cattle is believed to be intensely focused and there is a variation in their specificity among individuals [116].

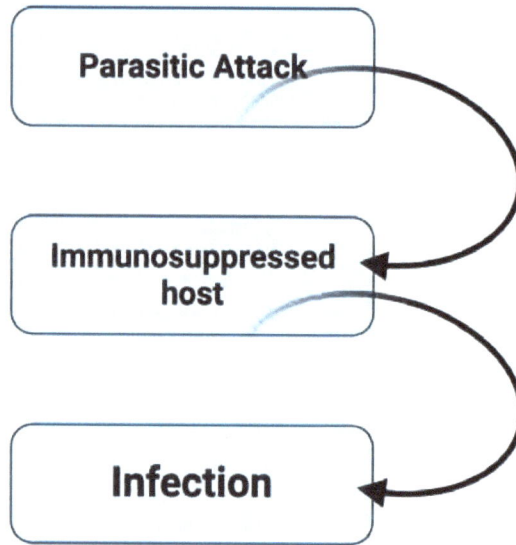

Fig. (7). Parasitic infections in the compromised host.

It has become evident that there exists a co-infection with multiple conspecific strains under natural conditions. Intraspecific infections result from infections with multiple strains, and they may have evolutionary and ecological importance. There is rare intraspecific competition due to hurdles in identifying individual co-infecting strains [117].

A change in selective pressures is driven by any form of interaction. Parasite life history traits like pathogenicity are served by selection. In most theories, virulence has an elaborative response [118]. Adaptive alterations in the host behavior may occur if they fulfill certain requirements: (1) They should be complex, (2) They must exhibit signals of purposive nature, (3) They must be declared to enhance the normality of the host or parasite [119]. Parasitism is broadly seen as the basic cost of pressure on animal communities, yet there is an association between parasitism and the size of the community [120]. Parasites can be found in hosts with high or lower parasite species variation, specific parasites mainly exist in host animals with a greater level of diversity [121]. The relationship between species richness and specificity in parasites is called specialization asymmetry [122].

Either at the humoral or cell level, suppression of the immune system has different outcomes for the host animal, and it will change the access of parasites to which they are susceptible [123]. Chronic parasitosis can occur when there is a situation of immunosuppression [124, 125]. The ability of a parasite to circumvent the immune system of the host is the basis of its success. These mechanisms involve escaping the pathogenic parasite and reducing the infestation [126].

The number of immunosuppressed individuals rises in areas that are endemic for infection of parasites, we can assume that these diseases will have new manifestations that will be discovered in the future [127]. The immune response of the host against the parasite keeps the parasite in its latent stage [128-131].

FUTURE PERSPECTIVES

The type of infection caused by parasites is believed to be a constraint that theories should verify rather than an important consequence of the relationship of parasites with the immune system of the host. Immune system modeling can be the basis of a broad range of considerations, for explaining how host immunity eliminates a parasitic invasion and for an understanding of the evolution of immune response against parasitic pathogens. We summarize by considering new perspectives that are based on combined models and locate future perspectives for infectious disease modeling. Certain factors that can influence the resistance of the host towards parasitic diseases should be taken into consideration. The animals that have lost or reduced immunity against pathogens due to nutritional or pathological causes should be treated accordingly. There is a dire need to build strategies that can enhance the efficiency of the host in dealing with the parasites. An improper immune response of the host can be compensated by the use of various drugs, which may prove beneficial to assist the host in the fight against diseases. Resistance has a genetic and evolutionary basis. The animals living in areas teamed with parasitic species have greater immunity against them and this immunity is also transferred to their offspring. A lack of immune response can prove lethal enough to cause huge economic losses and pose a serious threat to other susceptible populations of animals. One of the important factors to focus on should be the availability of clean and hygienic food and environment so that animals do not fall prey to parasitic diseases.

Another strategy for disease resistance is the selection and breeding of cattle breeds that have a history of greater parasitic resistance. The animals expressing severe immune responses should be considered for breeding to avoid economic losses in the future. Animals having suppressed immune responses should not be on this list of priorities to use for farming.

Some breeds like Brahman have developed greater resistance to parasites over the course of time. Their offspring also exhibit a greater ability to fight against disease and they can survive under stressed environmental conditions. A great barrier to studies in immunology is devising new plans that can enhance immunity against parasitic protozoans and eliminate their infection and related pathologies.

It is important to understand the mechanism involved in the evasion of the immune response. In the future, combined strategies regarding killing and neutralizing parasites are necessary.

CONCLUSION

In comparison to living free, a parasitic life cycle is more attractive. Parasites are the source of problems for animals. There are various mechanisms that the host adopts to respond to infection, like learning how to live with parasites resisting them, or avoiding them by becoming infected first. Parasites invade to feed and cause infection. Hosts react to these parasites by employing various strategies to deal with these parasites. Hosts that are genetically immune to these pathogens do not have to make much effort to eliminate them. Host-parasite relationship plays an important role in deciding the extent of harm. Some parasites mimic various ways to escape the immune strategy of the host and become successful in their attack. The immune system is one of the most complex systems in an organism and gives rise to several antibodies if a pathogen enters the host body. The success of an animal depends on having a proper amount of resistance against parasites. Parasites enhance their fitness by using the host for feeding and survival purposes, which results in the host being weak and sick. Each animal species has its own mechanism and there is a greater diversity by which a parasite is prevented from harming the host. The parasite can find a way into the host body mainly *via* food sources or by contact. The size of the parasitic population is an important factor that poses serious difficulty in mounting an effective immune response.

REFERENCES

[1]   Innes EA, Wright S, Bartley P, *et al.* The host–parasite relationship in bovine neosporosis. Vet Immunol Immunopathol 2005; 108(1-2): 29-36.
[http://dx.doi.org/10.1016/j.vetimm.2005.07.004] [PMID: 16098610]

[2]   Jonsson NN, Piper EK, Constantinoiu CC. Host resistance in cattle to infestation with the cattle tick R *Rhipicephalus microplus.* Parasite Immunol 2014; 36(11): 553-9.
[http://dx.doi.org/10.1111/pim.12140] [PMID: 25313455]

[3]   Wikel SK. Host immunity to ticks. Annu Rev Entomol. 1996;41(1):1-22
[http://dx.doi.org/10.1146/annurev.en.41.010196.000245]

[4]   Porto Neto LR, Jonsson NN, D'Occhio MJ, Barendse W. Molecular genetic approaches for identifying the basis of variation in resistance to tick infestation in cattle. Vet Parasitol 2011; 180(3-4): 165-72.
[http://dx.doi.org/10.1016/j.vetpar.2011.05.048] [PMID: 21700395]

[5]   Davidson RA. Immunology of parasitic infections. Med Clin North Am 1985; 69(4): 751-8.
[http://dx.doi.org/10.1016/S0025-7125(16)31017-3] [PMID: 3903378]

[6]   Vorburger C, Perlman SJ. The role of defensive symbionts in host–parasite coevolution. Biol Rev Camb Philos Soc 2018; 93(4): 1747-64.
[http://dx.doi.org/10.1111/brv.12417] [PMID: 29663622]

[7]   Glass EJ, Crutchley S, Jensen K. Living with the enemy or uninvited guests: Functional genomics approaches to investigating host resistance or tolerance traits to a protozoan parasite, *Theileria*

annulata, in cattle. Vet Immunol Immunopathol 2012; 148(1-2): 178-89.
[http://dx.doi.org/10.1016/j.vetimm.2012.03.006] [PMID: 22482839]

[8] Li RW, Sonstegard TS, Van Tassell CP, Gasbarre LC. Local inflammation as a possible mechanism of resistance to gastrointestinal nematodes in Angus heifers. Vet Parasitol 2007; 145(1-2): 100-7.
[http://dx.doi.org/10.1016/j.vetpar.2006.11.015] [PMID: 17182188]

[9] Sonstegard TS, Gasbarre LC. Genomic tools to improve parasite resistance. Vet Parasitol 2001; 101(3-4): 387-403.
[http://dx.doi.org/10.1016/S0304-4017(01)00563-5] [PMID: 11707308]

[10] Koskella B, Brockhurst MA. Bacteria–phage coevolution as a driver of ecological and evolutionary processes in microbial communities. FEMS Microbiol Rev 2014; 38(5): 916-31.
[http://dx.doi.org/10.1111/1574-6976.12072] [PMID: 24617569]

[11] Criscione CD, Anderson JD, Sudimack D, *et al.* Landscape genetics reveals focal transmission of a human macroparasite. PLoS Negl Trop Dis 2010; 4(4): e665.
[http://dx.doi.org/10.1371/journal.pntd.0000665] [PMID: 20421919]

[12] Mas-Coma S, Valero MA, Bargues MD. Fasciola, Lymnaids and human Fascioliasis with global overview, evolutionary genetics, molecular epidemiology and control. Adv Parasitol 2009; 69: 41-146.
[http://dx.doi.org/10.1016/S0065-308X(09)69002-3] [PMID: 19622408]

[13] Utsunomiya YT, Milanesi M, Fortes MRS, *et al.* Genomic clues of the evolutionary history of *Bos indicus* cattle. Anim Genet 2019; 50(6): 557-68.
[http://dx.doi.org/10.1111/age.12836] [PMID: 31475748]

[14] Chevillon C, Koffi BB, Barré N, Durand P, Arnathau C, de Meeûs T. Direct and indirect inferences on parasite mating and gene transmission patternsPangamy in the cattle tick *Rhipicephalus* (Boophilus) *microplus*. Infect Genet Evol 2007; 7(2): 298-304.
[http://dx.doi.org/10.1016/j.meegid.2006.11.007] [PMID: 17215171]

[15] O'Neill CJ, Swain DL, Kadarmideen HN. Evolutionary process of *Bos taurus* cattle in favourable *versus* unfavourable environments and its implications for genetic selection. Evol Appl 2010; 3(5-6): 422-33.
[http://dx.doi.org/10.1111/j.1752-4571.2010.00151.x] [PMID: 25567936]

[16] Sambo MR, Trovoada MJ, Benchimol C, *et al.* Transforming growth factor beta 2 and heme oxygenase 1 genes are risk factors for the cerebral malaria syndrome in Angolan children. PLoS One 2010; 5(6): e11141.
[http://dx.doi.org/10.1371/journal.pone.0011141] [PMID: 20585394]

[17] Durand PM, Coetzer TL. Hereditary red cell disorders and malaria resistance. Haematologica 2008; 93(7): 961-3.
[http://dx.doi.org/10.3324/haematol.13371] [PMID: 18591619]

[18] Barré N, Uilenberg G. Spread of parasites transported with their hosts: case study of two species of cattle tick. Rev Sci Tech 2010; 29(1): 149-160, 135-147.
[PMID: 20617654]

[19] Innes EA, Bartley PM, Maley SW, Wright SE, Buxton D. Comparative host–parasite relationships in ovine toxoplasmosis and bovine neosporosis and strategies for vaccination. Vaccine 2007; 25(30): 5495-503.
[http://dx.doi.org/10.1016/j.vaccine.2007.02.044] [PMID: 17367899]

[20] Host Factors Affecting Parasite Transmission. Handbook of Equine Parasite Control. 2018; pp. 55-60.
[http://dx.doi.org/10.1002/9781119382829.ch4]

[21] García-Sánchez M, Jiménez-Pelayo L, Horcajo P, Collantes-Fernández E, Ortega-Mora LM, Regidor-Cerrillo J. *Neospora caninum* infection induces an isolate virulence-dependent pro-inflammatory gene expression profile in bovine monocyte-derived macrophages. Parasit Vectors 2020; Jul 25;13(1): 374.

[22] Møller AP, Merino S, Soler JJ, *et al.* Assessing the effects of climate on host-parasite interactions: a

comparative study of European birds and their parasites. PLoS One 2013; 8(12): e82886.
[http://dx.doi.org/10.1371/journal.pone.0082886] [PMID: 24391725]

[23] Combes C. Parasitism: The ecology and evolution of intimate interactions. Chicago: University of Chicago Press 2001.

[24] Calero-Torralbo MA, Václav R, Valera F. Intra-specific variability in life-cycle synchronization of an ectoparasitic fly to its avian host. Oikos 2013; 122(2): 274-84.
[http://dx.doi.org/10.1111/j.1600-0706.2012.20374.x]

[25] Merino S, Møller AP. Host-parasite interactions and climate change. In: Møller AP, Fiedler W, Berthold P, Eds. Birds and climate change. Oxford: Oxford University Press 2010; pp. 213-26.

[26] Mehlhorn H, Al-Rasheid KA, Abdel-Ghaffar F, Klimpel S, Pohle H. Life cycle and attacks of ectoparasites on ruminants during the year in Central Europe: recommendations for treatment with insecticides (*e.g.*, Butox). Parasitol Res 2010; Jul;107(2): 425-31.

[27] Dunn PO, Winkler DW. Effects of climate change on timing of breeding and reproductive success in birds. In: Møller AP, Fiedler W, Berthold P, Eds. Effects of climate change on birds. Oxford: Oxford University Press 2010; pp. 113-28.

[28] Dunn PO, Winkler DW, Møller AP, Fiedler W, Berthold P. Effects of climate change on timing of breeding and reproductive success in birds. In: Møller AP, Fiedler W, Berthold P (eds) Effects of climate change on birds 2010; 113-28.

[29] Goodswen SJ, Kennedy PJ, Ellis JT. A review of the infection, genetics, and evolution of *Neospora caninum*: From the past to the present. Infect Genet Evol 2013; 13: 133-50.
[http://dx.doi.org/10.1016/j.meegid.2012.08.012] [PMID: 22985682]

[30] Wolinska J, King KC. Environment can alter selection in host–parasite interactions. Trends Parasitol 2009; 25(5): 236-44.
[http://dx.doi.org/10.1016/j.pt.2009.02.004] [PMID: 19356982]

[31] Sorci G, Møller AP, Boulinier T. Genetics of host-parasite interactions. Trends Ecol Evol 1997; 12(5): 196-200.
[http://dx.doi.org/10.1016/S0169-5347(97)01056-2] [PMID: 21238038]

[32] Gasbarre LC, Leighton EA, Sonstegard T. Role of the bovine immune system and genome in resistance to gastrointestinal nematodes. Vet Parasitol 2001; 98(1-3): 51-64.
[http://dx.doi.org/10.1016/S0304-4017(01)00423-X] [PMID: 11516579]

[33] Mansfield JM, Paulnock DM. Regulation of innate and acquired immunity in African trypanosomiasis. Parasite Immunol 2005; 27(10-11): 361-71.
[http://dx.doi.org/10.1111/j.1365-3024.2005.00791.x] [PMID: 16179030]

[34] Brown WC. Molecular approaches to elucidating innate and acquired immune responses to *Babesia bovis*, a protozoan parasite that causes persistent infection. Vet Parasitol 2001; 101(3-4): 233-48.
[http://dx.doi.org/10.1016/S0304-4017(01)00569-6] [PMID: 11707299]

[35] Råberg L, Graham AL, Read AF. Decomposing health: tolerance and resistance to parasites in animals. Philos Trans R Soc Lond B Biol Sci 2009; 364(1513): 37-49.
[http://dx.doi.org/10.1098/rstb.2008.0184] [PMID: 18926971]

[36] Boots M. Fight or learn to live with the consequences? Trends Ecol Evol 2008; 23(5): 248-50.
[http://dx.doi.org/10.1016/j.tree.2008.01.006] [PMID: 18374449]

[37] De Castro JJ, Newson RM. Host resistance in cattle tick control. Parasitol Today 1993; Jan;9(1): 13-7.

[38] Bayne CJ. Origins and evolutionary relationships between the innate and adaptive arms of immune systems. Integr Comp Biol 2003; 43(2): 293-9.
[http://dx.doi.org/10.1093/icb/43.2.293] [PMID: 21680436]

[39] Dempsey PW, Vaidya SA, Cheng G. The Art of War: Innate and adaptive immune responses. Cell Mol Life Sci 2003; 60(12): 2604-21.

[http://dx.doi.org/10.1007/s00018-003-3180-y] [PMID: 14685686]

[40] Narasimhan S, Kurokawa C, DeBlasio M, *et al.* Acquired tick resistance: The trail is hot. Parasite Immunol 2021; 43(5): e12808.
[http://dx.doi.org/10.1111/pim.12808] [PMID: 33187012]

[41] Donnelly R, White A, Boots M. Host lifespan and the evolution of resistance to multiple parasites. J Evol Biol 2017; 30(3): 561-70.
[http://dx.doi.org/10.1111/jeb.13025] [PMID: 27983771]

[42] Boots M, Donnelly R, White A. Optimal immune defence in the light of variation in lifespan. Parasite Immunol 2013; 35(11): 331-8.
[http://dx.doi.org/10.1111/pim.12055] [PMID: 23869870]

[43] Previtali MA, Ostfeld RS, Keesing F, Jolles AE, Hanselmann R, Martin LB. Relationship between pace of life and immune responses in wild rodents. Oikos 2012; 121(9): 1483-92.
[http://dx.doi.org/10.1111/j.1600-0706.2012.020215.x]

[44] Tidbury HJ, Pedersen AB, Boots M. Within and transgenerational immune priming in an insect to a DNA virus. Proc Biol Sci. 2011;278(1707):871-6
[http://dx.doi.org/10.1098/rspb.2010.1517]

[45] Best A, White A, Boots M. Resistance is futile but tolerance can explain why parasites do not always castrate their hosts. Evolution 2010; 64(2): 348-57.
[http://dx.doi.org/10.1111/j.1558-5646.2009.00819.x] [PMID: 19686267]

[46] Versteegh MA, Schwabl I, Jaquier S, Tieleman BI. Do immunological, endocrine and metabolic traits fall on a single P ace-of- L ife axis? Covariation and constraints among physiological systems. J Evol Biol 2012; 25(9): 1864-76.
[http://dx.doi.org/10.1111/j.1420-9101.2012.02574.x] [PMID: 22817634]

[47] Boots M. The evolution of resistance to a parasite is determined by resources. Am Nat 2011; 178(2): 214-20.
[http://dx.doi.org/10.1086/660833] [PMID: 21750385]

[48] Wall RL, Shearer D. Veterinary ectoparasites: biology, pathology and control 2008; 15.

[49] Garros C, Bouyer J, Takken W, Smallegange RC, Eds. Pests and vector-borne diseases in the livestock industry. Wageningen Academic Publishers 2018.
[http://dx.doi.org/10.3920/978-90-8686-863-6]

[50] OIE W. OIE-Listed diseases, infections and infestations in force in 2018. World Organ, Anim, Heal. 2018.

[51] Endres MI, Schwartzkopf-Genswein K. Overview of cattle production systems. InAdvances in cattle welfare 2018; 1-26.
[http://dx.doi.org/10.1016/B978-0-08-100938-3.00001-2]

[52] Henrioud AN. Towards sustainable parasite control practices in livestock production with emphasis in Latin America. Vet Parasitol 2011; 180(1-2): 2-11.
[http://dx.doi.org/10.1016/j.vetpar.2011.05.026] [PMID: 21723040]

[53] Wileman BW, Thomson DU, Reinhardt CD, Renter DG. Analysis of modern technologies commonly used in beef cattle production: Conventional beef production *versus* nonconventional production using meta-analysis. J Anim Sci 2009; 87(10): 3418-26.
[http://dx.doi.org/10.2527/jas.2009-1778] [PMID: 19617517]

[54] Meng Q, Sluder AE, Selzer Ectoparasites PM. Selzer Ectoparasites: drug discovery against moving targets Wiley-VCH,. Weinheim (Germany) 2018.

[55] Grisi L, Leite RC, Martins JRS, *et al.* Reassessment of the potential economic impact of cattle parasites in Brazil. Rev Bras Parasitol Vet 2014; 23(2): 150-6.
[http://dx.doi.org/10.1590/S1984-29612014042] [PMID: 25054492]

[56]   Mullen GR, Durden LA, Eds. Medical and veterinary entomology. Academic press 2009.

[57]   Bonneaud C, Mazuc J, Gonzalez G, *et al.* Assessing the cost of mounting an immune response. Am Nat 2003; 161(3): 367-79.
[http://dx.doi.org/10.1086/346134] [PMID: 12703483]

[58]   Calder PC, Field CJ, Gill HS. Nutrition and immune function. CABI 2002.
[http://dx.doi.org/10.1079/9780851995830.0000]

[59]   Cardoso CP, Silva BF, Trinca LA, Amarante AFT. Resistance against gastrointestinal nematodes in *Crioulo Lageano* and crossbred Angus cattle in southern Brazil. Vet Parasitol 2013; 192(1-3): 183-91.
[http://dx.doi.org/10.1016/j.vetpar.2012.10.018] [PMID: 23177359]

[60]   Sibley LD. Intracellular parasite invasion strategies. Science 2004; 304(5668): 248-53.
[http://dx.doi.org/10.1126/science.1094717] [PMID: 15073368]

[61]   Baldauf SL, Roger AJ, Wenk-Siefert I, Doolittle WF. A kingdom-level phylogeny of eukaryotes based on combined protein data. Science 2000; 290(5493): 972-7.
[http://dx.doi.org/10.1126/science.290.5493.972] [PMID: 11062127]

[62]   Dobrowolski JM, Sibley LD. *Toxoplasma* invasion of mammalian cells is powered by the actin cytoskeleton of the parasite. Cell 1996; 84(6): 933-9.
[http://dx.doi.org/10.1016/S0092-8674(00)81071-5] [PMID: 8601316]

[63]   Lovett JL, Marchesini N, Moreno SNJ, Sibley LD. *Toxoplasma gondii* microneme secretion involves intracellular Ca(2+) release from inositol 1,4,5-triphosphate (IP(3))/ryanodine-sensitive stores. J Biol Chem 2002; 277(29): 25870-6.
[http://dx.doi.org/10.1074/jbc.M202553200] [PMID: 12011085]

[64]   Zintl A, Gray JS, Skerrett IIE, Mulcahy G. Possible mechanisms underlying age-related resistance to bovine babesiosis. Parasite Immunol 2005; 27(4): 115-20.
[http://dx.doi.org/10.1111/j.1365-3024.2005.00748.x] [PMID: 15910419]

[65]   Guglielmone AA, Lugaresi CI, Volpogni MM, Anziani OS, Vanzini VR. Babesial antibody dynamics after cattle immunisation with live vaccines, measured with an indirect immunofluorescence test. Vet Parasitol 1997; 70(1-3): 33-9.
[http://dx.doi.org/10.1016/S0304-4017(96)01143-0] [PMID: 9195707]

[66]   Bossaert K, Jacquinet E, Saunders J, Farnir F, Losson B. Cell-mediated immune response in calves to single-dose, trickle, and challenge infections with Fasciola hepatica. Vet Parasitol 2000; Feb 29;88(1-2): 17-34.

[67]   Levy MG, Clabaugh G, Ristic M. Age resistance in bovine babesiosis: role of blood factors in resistance to Babesia bovis. Infect Immun 1982; 37(3): 1127-31.
[http://dx.doi.org/10.1128/iai.37.3.1127-1131.1982] [PMID: 7129632]

[68]   Taylor AE, Baker JR. In vitro methods for parasite cultivation. No Title 1987.

[69]   Zintl A, Skerrett HE, Gray JS, Brophy PO, Mulcahy G. Babesia divergens (Phylum Apicomplexa) *in vitro* growth in the presence of calf serum. Vet Parasitol 2004; 122(2): 127-30.
[http://dx.doi.org/10.1016/j.vetpar.2004.03.014] [PMID: 15177717]

[70]   Bastos RG, Laughery JM, Ozubek S, Alzan HF, Taus NS, Ueti MW and Suarez CE. Identification of novel immune correlates of protection against acute bovine babesiosis by superinfecting cattle with *in vitro* culture attenuated and virulent *Babesia bovis* strains. Front Immunol 2022; 13: 1045608.

[71]   Best A, White A, Kisdi É, Antonovics J, Brockhurst MA, Boots M. The evolution of host-parasite range. Am Nat 2010; 176(1): 63-71.
[http://dx.doi.org/10.1086/653002] [PMID: 20465424]

[72]   Rauw WM. Immune response from a resource allocation perspective. Front Genet 2012; 3: 267.
[http://dx.doi.org/10.3389/fgene.2012.00267] [PMID: 23413205]

[73]   Hamilton R, Siva-Jothy M, Boots M. Two arms are better than one: parasite variation leads to combined inducible and constitutive innate immune responses. Proc Biol Sci 2008; 275(1637): 937-45. [http://dx.doi.org/10.1098/rspb.2007.1574] [PMID: 18230594]

[74]   Frank SA. Immunology and evolution of infectious disease 2002; 31. [http://dx.doi.org/10.1515/9780691220161]

[75]   Jiravanichpaisal P, Lee BL, Söderhäll K. Cell-mediated immunity in arthropods: Hematopoiesis, coagulation, melanization and opsonization. Immunobiology 2006; 211(4): 213-36. [http://dx.doi.org/10.1016/j.imbio.2005.10.015] [PMID: 16697916]

[76]   Kurtz J. Memory in the innate and adaptive immune systems. Microbes Infect 2004; 6(15): 1410-7. [http://dx.doi.org/10.1016/j.micinf.2004.10.002] [PMID: 15596128]

[77]   Claerebout E, Vercruysse J. The immune response and the evaluation of acquired immunity against gastrointestinal nematodes in cattle: a review. Parasitology 2000; 120 Suppl: S25-42.

[78]   Sheldon BC, Verhulst S. Ecological immunology: costly parasite defences and trade-offs in evolutionary ecology. Trends Ecol Evol 1996; 11(8): 317-21. [http://dx.doi.org/10.1016/0169-5347(96)10039-2] [PMID: 21237861]

[79]   Klein SL. The effects of hormones on sex differences in infection: from genes to behavior. Neurosci Biobehav Rev 2000; 24(6): 627-38. [http://dx.doi.org/10.1016/S0149-7634(00)00027-0] [PMID: 10940438]

[80]   Pardue ML, Wizemann TM, Eds. Exploring the biological contributions to human health: does sex matter?.

[81]   Roberts CW, Walker W, Alexander J. Sex-associated hormones and immunity to protozoan parasites. Clin Microbiol Rev 2001; 14(3): 476-88. [http://dx.doi.org/10.1128/CMR.14.3.476-488.2001] [PMID: 11432809]

[82]   Moore SL, Wilson K. Parasites as a viability cost of sexual selection in natural populations of mammals. Science 2002; 297(5589): 2015-8. [http://dx.doi.org/10.1126/science.1074196] [PMID: 12242433]

[83]   Stear MJ, Murray M. Genetic resistance to parasitic disease: particularly of resistance in ruminants to gastrointestinal nematodes. Vet Parasitol 1994; 54(1-3): 161-76. [http://dx.doi.org/10.1016/0304-4017(94)90089-2] [PMID: 7846849]

[84]   Falconer DS. Introduction to quantitative genetics. Pearson Education India 1996.

[85]   Bishop SC, Morris CA. Genetics of disease resistance in sheep and goats. Small Rumin Res 2007; 70(1): 48-59. [http://dx.doi.org/10.1016/j.smallrumres.2007.01.006]

[86]   Norris A, Foyle L, Ratcliff J. Heritability of mortality in response to a natural pancreas disease (SPDV) challenge in Atlantic salmon, *Salmo salar* L., post-smolts on a West of Ireland sea site. J Fish Dis 2008; 31(12): 913-20. [http://dx.doi.org/10.1111/j.1365-2761.2008.00982.x] [PMID: 19017068]

[87]   Kube PD, Taylor RS, Elliott NG. Genetic variation in parasite resistance of Atlantic salmon to amoebic gill disease over multiple infections. Aquaculture 2012; 364-365: 165-72. [http://dx.doi.org/10.1016/j.aquaculture.2012.08.026]

[88]   Embers ME, Narasimhan S. Vaccination against Lyme disease: past, present, and future. Front Cell Infect Microbiol 2013; 3: 6. [http://dx.doi.org/10.3389/fcimb.2013.00006] [PMID: 23407755]

[89]   Perinotto WMS, Angelo IC, Golo PS, *et al.* Susceptibility of different populations of ticks to entomopathogenic fungi. Exp Parasitol 2012; 130(3): 257-60. [http://dx.doi.org/10.1016/j.exppara.2011.12.003] [PMID: 22212684]

[90]   Plotkin SA. Need for a new Lyme disease vaccine. N Engl J Med 2016; 375(10): 911-3.
        [http://dx.doi.org/10.1056/NEJMp1607146] [PMID: 27602662]

[91]   Pichu S, Ribeiro JMC, Mather TN, Francischetti IMB. Purification of a serine protease and evidence for a protein C activator from the saliva of the tick, *Ixodes scapularis*. Toxicon 2014; 77: 32-9.
        [http://dx.doi.org/10.1016/j.toxicon.2013.10.025] [PMID: 24184517]

[92]   Assumpção TC, Mizurini DM, Ma D, *et al.* Ixonnexin from tick saliva promotes fibrinolysis by interacting with plasminogen and tissue-type plasminogen activator, and prevents arterial thrombosis. Sci Rep 2018; 8(1): 4806.
        [http://dx.doi.org/10.1038/s41598-018-22780-1] [PMID: 29555911]

[93]   Du W, Gao Z, Wang K, *et al.* Expression and function assessment of two serpin-type serine protease inhibitors from *Haemaphysalis doenitzi*. Res Vet Sci 2020; 132: 1-9.
        [http://dx.doi.org/10.1016/j.rvsc.2020.05.015] [PMID: 32464311]

[94]   Willadsen P. Anti-tick vaccines. Parasitology 2004; 129(S1) (Suppl.): S367-87.
        [http://dx.doi.org/10.1017/S0031182003004657] [PMID: 15938519]

[95]   Abbas RZ, Zaman MA, Colwell DD, Gilleard J, Iqbal Z. Acaricide resistance in cattle ticks and approaches to its management: The state of play. Vet Parasitol 2014; 203(1-2): 6-20.
        [http://dx.doi.org/10.1016/j.vetpar.2014.03.006] [PMID: 24709006]

[96]   Kongsuwan K, Josh P, Colgrave ML, *et al.* Activation of several key components of the epidermal differentiation pathway in cattle following infestation with the cattle tick, *Rhipicephalus* (Boophilus) *microplus*. Int J Parasitol 2010; 40(4): 499-507.
        [http://dx.doi.org/10.1016/j.ijpara.2009.10.013] [PMID: 19909754]

[97]   Hart BL, Hart LA. How mammals stay healthy in nature: the evolution of behaviours to avoid parasites and pathogens. Philosophical Transactions of the Royal Society B: Biological Sciences 2018; 19; 373(1751): 20170205.

[98]   Seó HLS, Pinheiro Machado Filho LC, Honorato LA, da Silva BF, do Amarante AFT, Bricarello PA. The effect of gastrointestinal nematode infection level on grazing distance from dung. PLoS One 2015; 10(6): e0126340.
        [http://dx.doi.org/10.1371/journal.pone.0126340] [PMID: 26039729]

[99]   Brambilla A, von Hardenberg A, Kristo O, Bassano B, Bogliani G. Don't spit in the soup: faecal avoidance in foraging wild Alpine ibex, Capra ibex. Anim Behav 2013; 86(1): 153-8.
        [http://dx.doi.org/10.1016/j.anbehav.2013.05.006]

[100]   Garnick SW, Elgar MA, Beveridge I, Coulson G. Foraging efficiency and parasite risk in eastern grey kangaroos (*Macropus giganteus*). Behav Ecol 2010; 21(1): 129-37.
        [http://dx.doi.org/10.1093/beheco/arp162]

[101]   Hart BL. Behavioral adaptations to pathogens and parasites: Five strategies. Neurosci Biobehav Rev 1990; 14(3): 273-94.
        [http://dx.doi.org/10.1016/S0149-7634(05)80038-7] [PMID: 2234607]

[102]   Hart BL. Behavioural defences in animals against pathogens and parasites: parallels with the pillars of medicine in humans. Philos Trans R Soc Lond B Biol Sci 2011; 366(1583): 3406-17.
        [http://dx.doi.org/10.1098/rstb.2011.0092] [PMID: 22042917]

[103]   Geiger A, Bossard G, Sereno D, *et al.* Escaping deleterious immune response in their hosts: lessons from trypanosomatids. Front Immunol 2016; 7: 212.
        [http://dx.doi.org/10.3389/fimmu.2016.00212] [PMID: 27303406]

[104]   Ribeiro JM, Walker FA. High affinity histamine-binding and antihistaminic activity of the salivary nitric oxide-carrying heme protein (nitrophorin) of *Rhodnius prolixus*. J Exp Med 1994; 180(6): 2251-7.
        [http://dx.doi.org/10.1084/jem.180.6.2251] [PMID: 7964498]

[105] Montandon CE, Barros E, Vidigal PM, *et al.* Comparative proteomic analysis of the saliva of the *Rhodnius prolixus, Triatoma lecticularia* and *Panstrongylus herreri* triatomines reveals a high interespecific functional biodiversity. Insect Biochem Mol Biol 2016; 71: 83-90. [http://dx.doi.org/10.1016/j.ibmb.2016.02.009] [PMID: 26940473]

[106] Altizer S, Bartel R, Han BA. Animal migration and infectious disease risk. Science 2011; 331(6015): 296-302.

[107] Namangala B. How the African trypanosomes evade host immune killing. Parasite Immunol 2011; 33(8): 430-7. [http://dx.doi.org/10.1111/j.1365-3024.2011.01280.x] [PMID: 21261664]

[108] Mansfield JM, Olivier M. Immune evasion by parasites. The Immune Response to Infection 2010; 30: 453-69. [http://dx.doi.org/10.1128/9781555816872.ch36]

[109] Dunn AM, Torchin ME, Hatcher MJ, *et al.* Indirect effects of parasites in invasions. Funct Ecol 2012; 26(6): 1262-74. [http://dx.doi.org/10.1111/j.1365-2435.2012.02041.x]

[110] Beckstead J, Meyer SE, Connolly BM, Huck MB, Street LE. Cheatgrass facilitates spillover of a seed bank pathogen onto native grass species. J Ecol 2010; 98(1): 168-77. [http://dx.doi.org/10.1111/j.1365-2745.2009.01599.x]

[111] De Boer RJ, Perelson AS. Towards a general function describing t cell proliferation. J Theor Biol 1995; 175(4): 567-76. [http://dx.doi.org/10.1006/jtbi.1995.0165] [PMID: 7475092]

[112] Alizon S, van Baalen M. Acute or chronic? Within-host models with immune dynamics, infection outcome, and parasite evolution. Am Nat 2008; 172(6): E244-56. [http://dx.doi.org/10.1086/592404] [PMID: 18999939]

[113] Olivier M, Gregory DJ, Forget G. Subversion mechanisms by which Leishmania parasites can escape the host immune response: a signaling point of view. Clin Microbiol Rev 2005; 18(2): 293-305. [http://dx.doi.org/10.1128/CMR.18.2.293-305.2005] [PMID: 15831826]

[114] Adamo SA. Parasites: evolution's neurobiologists. J Exp Biol 2013; 216(1): 3-10. [http://dx.doi.org/10.1242/jeb.073601] [PMID: 23225861]

[115] Damian RT. Parasite immune evasion and exploitation: reflections and projections. Parasitology 1997; 115(7) (Suppl.): 169-75. [http://dx.doi.org/10.1017/S0031182097002357] [PMID: 9571701]

[116] Foster, N., Elsheikha, H.M. The immune response to parasitic helminths of veterinary importance and its potential manipulation for future vaccine control strategies. Parasitol Res 2012; 110: 1587-99.

[117] McKeever DJ. Bovine immunity – a driver for diversity in Theileria parasites? Trends Parasitol 2009; 25(6): 269-76. [http://dx.doi.org/10.1016/j.pt.2009.03.005] [PMID: 19423397]

[118] Balmer O, Stearns SC, Schötzau A, Brun R. Intraspecific competition between co-infecting parasite strains enhances host survival in African trypanosomes. Ecology 2009; 90(12): 3367-78. [http://dx.doi.org/10.1890/08-2291.1] [PMID: 20120806]

[119] Gandon S, van Baalen M, Jansen VAA. The evolution of parasite virulence, superinfection, and host resistance. Am Nat 2002; 159(6): 658-69. [http://dx.doi.org/10.1086/339993] [PMID: 18707388]

[120] Poulin R. "Adaptive" changes in the behaviour of parasitized animals: A critical review. Int J Parasitol 1995; 25(12): 1371-83. [http://dx.doi.org/10.1016/0020-7519(95)00100-X] [PMID: 8719948]

[121] Rifkin JL, Nunn CL, Garamszegi LZ. Do animals living in larger groups experience greater

parasitism? A meta-analysis. Am Nat 2012; 180(1): 70-82.
[http://dx.doi.org/10.1086/666081] [PMID: 22673652]

[122] Vázquez DP, Poulin R, Krasnov BR, Shenbrot G. Species abundance and the distribution of specialization in host–parasite interaction networks. J Anim Ecol 2005; 74(5): 946-55.
[http://dx.doi.org/10.1111/j.1365-2656.2005.00992.x]

[123] Vázquez DP, Blüthgen N, Cagnolo L, Chacoff NP. Uniting pattern and process in plant–animal mutualistic networks: a review. Ann Bot (Lond) 2009; 103(9): 1445-57.
[http://dx.doi.org/10.1093/aob/mcp057] [PMID: 19304996]

[124] Evering T, Weiss LM. The immunology of parasite infections in immunocompromised hosts. Parasite Immunol 2006; 28(11): 549-65.
[http://dx.doi.org/10.1111/j.1365-3024.2006.00886.x] [PMID: 17042927]

[125] Milder JE, Walzer PD, Kilgore G, Rutherford I, Klein M. Clinical features of *Strongyloides stercoralis* infection in an endemic area of the United States. Gastroenterology 1981; 80(6): 1481-8.
[http://dx.doi.org/10.1016/0016-5085(81)90261-4] [PMID: 7227772]

[126] Grove DI. Strongyloidiasis in Allied ex-prisoners of war in south-east Asia. BMJ 1980; 280(6214): 598-601.
[http://dx.doi.org/10.1136/bmj.280.6214.598] [PMID: 7370602]

[127] Braga LL, Ninomiya H, McCoy JJ, *et al.* Inhibition of the complement membrane attack complex by the galactose-specific adhesin of *Entamoeba histolytica.* Arch Med Res 1992; 23(2): 133.
[PMID: 1340275]

[128] Mendez J, Sun D, Tuo W, Xiao Z. *Bovine* neutrophils form extracellular traps in response to the gastrointestinal parasite Ostertagia ostertagi. Sci Rep 2018; Dec 4;8(1): 17598.
[http://dx.doi.org/10.1038/s41598-018-36070-3]

[129] da Silva RC, Langoni H. *Toxoplasma gondii*: host–parasite interaction and behavior manipulation. Parasitol Res 2009; 105(4): 893-8.
[http://dx.doi.org/10.1007/s00436-009-1526-6] [PMID: 19548003]

[130] Thapa, B., Parajuli, R.P. & Dhakal, P. Prevalence and burden of gastrointestinal parasites in stray cattle of the Kathmandu Valley. J Parasit Dis 2022; 46, 845–853.

[131] Schimpff SC. Infections in the compromised host-an overview. Principles and practice of infectious diseases 1990; 2258-65.

CHAPTER 15

Antiparasitic Vaccines

P. Ramadevi[1,*], J. Jayalakshmi[1] and Snehil Gupta[2]

[1] *Department of Veterinary Parasitology, Sri Venkateswara Veterinary University, Tirupati-517101, India*

[2] *Department of Veterinary Parasitology, Lala Lajpat Rai University of Veterinary and Animal Sciences, Hisar, India*

Abstract: Cattle farming plays a vital role in global agriculture, providing meat and dairy products to meet the growing demand for protein. However, the industry faces significant challenges posed by parasitic infections that lead to economic losses, reduced productivity, and compromised animal welfare. To combat these issues, researchers have been exploring the development of antiparasitic vaccines for cattle. In the realm of helminths, efforts have been made to identify specific antigens from nematodes, trematodes, and cestodes that can stimulate protective immune responses in cattle. The transition from whole-organism vaccines to subunit vaccines has shown promise, with several candidates in various stages of development. Protozoal infections, including Neospora caninum and Theileria species, have been targeted with vaccines designed to reduce abortions and mortalities in cattle. Live-attenuated and subunit vaccines have been explored with varying levels of success. Achieving consistent protection across diverse parasite strains remains a challenge. Ectoparasitic arthropods like ticks and flies have also been the focus of vaccine development. Bm86-based vaccines for ticks have shown partial success but face limitations in terms of tick species and strains. Combinatorial vaccines and *in silico* approaches offer potential solutions for broader protection. Despite these advancements, several challenges persist in the development of antiparasitic vaccines for cattle. These include the need for rigorous field testing, addressing antigenic diversity, optimizing vaccine formulations, and ensuring cost-effectiveness for widespread adoption.

Keywords: Cattle, Commercialized, DNA vaccines, Killed vaccines, Lyophilization, Live vaccines, Premunitio, Subunit vaccines, Vaccine candidate.

INTRODUCTION

The ruminant world is plagued by a variety of infections, but none causes more damage to their productivity and health than parasitic infections. The majority of these infections are caused by trematodes, cestodes, nematodes, protozoans, and

---

* **Corresponding author P. Ramadevi:** Department of Veterinary Parasitology, Sri Venkateswara Veterinary University, Tirupati-517101, India; E-mail: rams.vet36@gmail.com

Tanmoy Rana (Ed.)

external parasites [1 - 4]. Both endo and ecto parasites are responsible for huge economic losses in animal production by lowering production (milk, meat, and reproduction), damaging by-products (hides), and affecting the health (treatment, control, and mortality) of animals. The estimated economic losses due to parasitic infections in cattle revealed an average reduction of 1.16 liters of milk production and a 12.95% increase in organ condemnation per animal per day [5 - 8]. Additionally, the calculated losses amounted to an average of US$50.67 per animal per year, accounting for a 17.94% decrease in financial returns [1, 2]. Traditional methods of controlling parasitic infections in cattle have often involved the use of chemotherapy, like anthelmintics, antiprotozoals, and acaricides. However, these approaches have raised concerns about the development of resistance and environmental impact [3, 4]. The emergence of drug resistance, coupled with the intricate life cycles of parasitic diseases, has posed formidable challenges to their effective control. Simultaneously, the growing demand from the public for animal products untainted by drugs has underscored the need for alternative solutions. In response to these pressing concerns, vaccination has assumed a pivotal role in the comprehensive management of parasitic diseases. The development of antiparasitic vaccines for cattle has emerged as a promising alternative, aiming to provide sustainable and effective solutions to combat parasitic infections while minimizing adverse effects [5, 6]. Vaccines have a long, successful history of preventing and controlling diseases in farm animals. Vaccines stimulate the immune response in the animal without causing disease. Immunization stands as a pivotal approach in combating infectious agents, primarily due to its potential safety, affordability, and prophylactic efficacy compared to drugs. However, the application of vaccines has mainly been successful with antimicrobial vaccines. In endeavors to create commercial vaccines targeting economically significant parasites, researchers have primarily concentrated on pinpointing specific antigen targets [9 - 12]. As a result of these endeavors, numerous potential antigens have been discovered, vaccines have been formulated using them, and their suitability and effectiveness have been assessed through testing. Despite the development of several vaccines and their subsequent testing for effectiveness, they have not been brought to the commercial market due to various technical obstacles. Consequently, only a limited number of vaccines are currently accessible for commercial utilization. While factors contributing to market failure are recognized, other influential aspects impact commercial success, such as quality, safety, efficacy, potency, consistency of production, product profile definition, onset and duration of immunity, compatibility with other products, and routes of administration [13 - 18].

Development of Parasitic Vaccines and Challenges

Vaccine development against parasites has had both successes and failures. Successful vaccines have used various technologies, including crude vaccines with irradiated nematode larvae and recombinant antigen vaccines for metazoan parasites. However, recent recombinant lungworm vaccines have not been as effective as whole organism vaccines and similar challenges exist for nematode vaccines. Subunit vaccines have been attempted, but they face obstacles such as incorrect strains, production issues, and inadequate antigen levels. Immune suppression and other factors can also hinder vaccine effectiveness. Helminth infections in cattle, particularly *Cooperia* spp and *Ostertagia ostertagi*, are increasingly resistant to antihelminthic drugs. Resistance to flukicides has also been observed in *Fasciola hepatica* [19 - 22]. To address these challenges and ensure sustainable control, alternative strategies like bioactive forages, selective breeding, nematophagous fungi, and vaccine development are needed. However, developing helminth vaccines is complex due to the parasites' intricate life cycles, diverse antigenic elements, and protein polymorphism, making it challenging to identify suitable targets. Protozoan parasites in cattle cause significant losses and pose zoonotic risks [23 - 27]. Vaccine development strategies for protozoa include using whole organisms, attenuated strains, killed organisms, subunit vaccines, and vector vaccines. Recombinant DNA technology has been used but with limited success due to the complexity and antigenic diversity of these parasites. Developing vaccines against ectoparasitic arthropods is difficult due to their size, complexity, and preference for life on the host's surface. Some research has identified immunocompetent molecules in arthropods, but challenges remain [28 - 33]. Despite these challenges, vaccination remains a promising approach for parasite control in animals, with the potential for improvement through regulatory changes and advancements in molecular techniques.

Helminth Vaccines

Fasciolosis

Liver flukes, specifically *Fasciola hepatica* and *F. gigantica*, are parasites with a wide range of hosts, and they cause significant economic losses globally. In tropical regions, fasciolosis is a prominent helminth infection in cattle, with prevalence ranging from 25% to 100% in the Middle East, Southeast Asia, and Africa. Numerous studies have explored the potential for candidate antigens from either *F. hepatica* or *F. gigantica* as vaccines for livestock (Table **1**). Prominent candidates among these antigens include fatty acid binding proteins (FABP), glutathione S-transferase (GST), Cathepsin L1 (CatL1), and Leucine aminopeptidase (LAP) [34 - 37].

Table 1. List of Some Important Commercialized Anti-parasitic Vaccines in Cattle.

Name of the Parasite	Name of the Vaccine	Antigen/Type of Vaccine	Dose and Route	Manufacturer	References
Dictylcaulus viviparus	Bovilis® Huskvac	Live attenuated	25 ml, oral route	Intervet (now MSD Animal Health)	Jarrett WF *et al.* [49],
Echinococcus granulosus	Tecnovax, EG95	Recombinant Subunit (Eg95)	1ml S/c	ProvideanHydatil	Lightowlers [59]
Theileria parva	Muguga cocktail vaccine	Sporozoites of one or more strains, Live virulent	1× SC	VetAgro Tanzania Ltd., & government-sponsored labs	Radley *et al.* [78]
Theileria annulata	Rakshavac-T, Teylovac	Macroschizonts, Live attenuated	3 mL s/c in the mid-neck region	Indian Immunologicals, Israeli company	Pipano [75]
Babesia bovis, B. bigemina	Numerous	Live attenuated	1× SC or IM in juvenile calves	Primarily government-sponsored labs	Callow *et al.* [13]; Echaide [30]
Trichomonas foetus	TrichGuard	Killed trophozoites in adjuvant,Inactivated	2×SC annually before the breeding season	Boehringer – Ingelheim,	Cobo *et al.* [17]
Neosporosis abortion in cattle	Bovillis Neogaurd	Killed tachyzoites in adjuvant	2×SC, then annually	Not available	Weston *et al.* [104]
Anaplasma marginale	Anaplaz	Killed virulent Anaplasmamarginale	S/C	Fort Dodge	Palmer [72]
Anaplasma marginale	Plazvax	Killed Anaplasmamarginale	S/c	Mallinkrodt/ Schering-Plough	Gupta *et al.* [40]
Anaplasma marginale	Anaviv	live attenuated vaccine	2 ml, I/V	*ProtaTek Int. Inc., St. Paul, USA*	Vizcaino *et al.* [100]
Rhipicephalus (Boophilus microplus)	TickGARD-plus	Recombinant subunit (Bm86)	2ml I/m in the neck	Heber Biotec S.A	Jonsson *et al.* [53]
Rhipicephalus (Boophilus) microplus	Go-Tick / Tick-Vac	Recombinant subunit (Bm86)	2ml I/m	Limor de Colombia, Bogotá, Colombia	Gupta *et al.* [40]

The native FABP found in *Fasciola*, which is a combination of several FABP isoforms, has demonstrated inconsistent and limited effectiveness in various studies against *F. gigantica* or *F. hepatica* in cattle. In these studies, efficacy is well defined for the reduction in the number of adult flukes in vaccinated animals compared to unvaccinated controls, and the observed efficacy has ranged from 31% to 55% [38 - 41].

Native *Fasciola* GST has been implicated in the evaluation of a vaccine in cattle. In trials involving *F. hepatica* GST, the average efficacy was found to be 43% across four different studies (Sexton *et al.*, 1990; Morrison *et al.*, 1996). However, when it comes to *F. gigantica*, recombinant GST (rGST) has not proven successful in providing protection to cattle. As a result, both fatty acid binding proteins and GST are not considered leading vaccine candidates for fluke infections.

Mixtures of native CatL proteases, which are liberated from the gut of adult flukes, have displayed varying levels of effectiveness in cattle against both *F. gigantica and F. hepatica*, resulting in reductions in the burden of fluke ranging from 0% to 56%. On the other hand, individual native CatL1 has demonstrated significant efficacy, ranging from 42% to 69% in cattle, according to a study [42]. Additionally, it was found that CatL1 can reduce the viability of eggs released by surviving parasites by approximately 60%. When combined with another secreted molecule called high molecular-sized haem protein, the protection against parasites was increased to 73%. In the case of recombinant CatL1, it has shown an average of 48% protection in one trial involving cattle [42]. Furthermore, inclusion bodies derived from *Escherichia coli* having the recombinant cysteine protease W (referred to as CPFhW CatL) induced a 54% protection rate in cattle [42 - 45].

Significant levels of protection, with reductions in liver fluke burdens ranging from 85% to 96%, were reported in cattle when a total adult *F. hepatica* extract was used in conjunction with alum or Freund's adjuvant [46]. Western blot analysis of the fluke extract, using immune sera, identified two major antigens with molecular weights of 200 kDa and 65 kDa as potential vaccine candidates. Various other native proteins were also tested as vaccines, including hemoglobin (Hb), peroxiredoxin (Prx), paramyosin, and a Kunitz-type trypsin inhibitor. However, significant prevention levels of 43% and 47% were only observed in cattle when Hb and paramyosin were used, respectively [47 - 49].

Several combinations of antigens have been evaluated against liver flukes *F. hepatica* and *F. gigantica* in cattle. Some antigens like cathepsin L1 and leucine aminopeptidase (LAP) induced notable prevention levels in sheep and/or cattle, both when administered as native, purified antigens and as recombinant proteins. Nevertheless, the observed protection levels were highly variable, underscoring the need to conduct multiple vaccine trials for each antigen to demonstrate consistent effectiveness. Attempts to enhance vaccine efficacy by combining different antigens, such as cathepsins with LAP or hemoglobin, or using a chimeric protein composed of leucine aminopeptidase and cathepsin L1, have not substantially improved the vaccine's efficacy. As of now, there is no commercial vaccine available against *Fasciola* infections, and the development of a commercial vaccine against liver fluke infections remains a challenging task for the future.

Schistosomiasis

There has been notable success in developing immunization strategies against schistosomiasis in cattle and sheep. In one approach, irradiated schistosomula of both *S. mattheei* and *S. bovis* were administered subcutaneously or intramuscularly to cattle or sheep, resulting in 60% protection against infection [50, 51]. Additionally, a specific molecule called rSb28GST, which is the only one cloned from *S. bovis* and has shown vaccine potential, has demonstrated efficacy in goats and cattle. This molecule was able to reduce the mean worm burden in vaccinated animals and improve their overall health. These findings highlight promising developments in the field of schistosomiasis immunization for livestock.

Echinococcus Granulosus

Echinococcus granulosus, a parasitic tapeworm found in the intestines of dogs, is responsible for causing hydatidosis in various intermediate hosts like sheep, cattle, camelids, and horses, as well as humans. This zoonotic disease poses significant economic losses and public health concerns in numerous countries, as highlighted by research [52, 53].

Effective vaccines against cysticercosis and hydatid disease caused by cestode parasites from the *Echinococcus* and *Taenia* genera have shown remarkable success. For instance, EG95, a recombinant antigen derived from the oncosphere of *E. granulosus*, serves as a vaccine against hydatid disease. It has demonstrated the ability to provide protection levels ranging from 96% to 100% in cattle against challenge infections, as evidenced by multiple trials conducted in New Zealand, Australia, Argentina, and China [54, 55]. Similarly, a vaccine targeting *Taenia ovis*, known as 45W, has achieved over 92% protection in sheep. Its homolog from *T. saginata* has been equally effective in safeguarding cattle against this parasite [56, 57]. As of now, only one recombinant vaccine for helminth parasites is available in the commercial market. This vaccine, called Providean Hidatil EG95®, developed by Tecnovax, is applied on a single antigen, EG95. It has received licensing in certain parts of South America for controlling *Echinococcus granulosus* in sheep, cattle, goats, and selected camelid species.

Oesophagostomum

Initially, successful vaccination of cattle against gastrointestinal nematodes was primarily achieved for *Oesophagostomum radiatum*. Researchers found that crude extracts and somatic antigen fractions from both the L4 and adult stages of *O. radiatum*, when combined with complete Freund's adjuvant, resulted in high levels of protection [58]. However, when calves were immunized solely with larval excretory-secretory products, they only exhibited partial protection against challenge infection [58, 59].

Surprisingly, despite the promising outcomes from early vaccine trials that showed significant protection, no further efforts were made to identify the specific antigens responsible for this protection within the partially purified somatic antigen fractions.

Ostertagia Ostertagi and Cooperia Oncophora

In regions with temperate climates, two of the most significant gastrointestinal nematodes (GIN) affecting cattle are the brown stomach worm, *O. ostertagi*, and the intestinal nematode, *C. oncophora*. Nearly all grazing cattle in these areas are co-infected with these nematode species, leading to subclinical losses. Initially, attempts were made to develop vaccines using homologues of H11, H-gal-GP, and TSBP from *O. ostertagi* and *T. circumcinta* against these non-blood-feeding nematodes, with generally positive but somewhat inconsistent results [60, 61].

Experimental native vaccines against *O. ostertagi* have included allergens like the *Ostertagia* poly-protein allergen (OPA), globin, larval gut membrane proteins, and activation-associated secreted proteins (ASPs). Among these, ASPs have shown promise as vaccine antigens. Additionally, vaccination with a fraction of adult excretory-secretory products from *O. ostertagi* obtained through thiol sepharose (ES-thiol) chromatography consistently resulted in a significant reduction in worm egg output, up to 62% [62]. The key components responsible for this protection were identified as activation-associated secreted proteins, particularly ASP1 and ASP2, with ASP1 being the most abundant. Furthermore, a double-domain ASP (dd-ASP) from *C. oncophora* has demonstrated protective effects in calves during their initial grazing season (Borloo *et al.*, 2013). However, attempts to vaccinate calves with recombinant OPA, expressed in *E. coli*, were not successful.

Haemonchus Placei and H. Similis

A vaccine containing integral membrane glycoproteins from the intestine of *Haemonchus contortus* was tested on three groups of eight 5-month-old grazing calves that were naturally infected with *Haemonchus placei, Haemonchus similis,* and other gastrointestinal nematodes. The results showed that immunization with this vaccine triggered the production of high-titer antibodies against the vaccine antigens. It also led to a significant reduction in the egg output of *Haemonchus* spp. by 85%, as well as a decrease in the numbers of *H. placei* and *H. similis* by 63% and 32%, respectively, compared to the control group [63]. In conclusion, this study demonstrated that vaccination with integral membrane glycoproteins from *H. contortus* was effective in substantially reducing the transmission of *H. placei* and *H. similis* in naturally infected cattle. This suggests that the vaccine could provide downstream protective benefits and is notable as the first successful demonstration of a vaccine protective for cattle naturally exposed to infection with any gastrointestinal nematode parasite.

Dictyocaulus Viviparus

A commercial lungworm vaccine known as Bovilis Huskvac developed decades ago (Jarrett *et al.*, 1960) consists of live irradiated third-stage (L3) *D. viviparus* larvae. The vaccination process involves administering two doses of 1000 viable irradiated larvae orally, with an interval of around 4 weeks between doses. It is recommended to complete the full vaccination schedule at least 2 weeks before turning out the vaccinated animals on pasture. Additionally, cattle that have been vaccinated should not be treated with anthelmintic medications until at least 2 weeks after the second vaccination. This vaccine is suitable for use in healthy cattle aged 8 weeks or older, including grazing young stock and adult cows. While the vaccine generally provides effective protection [64], it has certain drawbacks associated with live vaccines. These include ethical concerns related to the production of larvae in donor animals, batch-to-batch variability, and a limited shelf life (Table **2**).

Efforts have been made to address these issues by developing recombinant subunit vaccines, but these attempts have had limited success. Vaccination with recombinant proteins like acetylcholinesterase, paramyosin, or asparaginyl peptidase legumain-1, combined with various adjuvants, did not result in significant or consistent reductions in worm numbers or larval shedding.

Table 2. List of some important helminth vaccine candidates and their protection levels in cattle.

Antigen	Form	Name of the Parasite	Vaccine Protection in Animals	References
Single vaccines FABP	Native	*F. hepatica*	55%	Hillyer *et al.* [46]
-	Native	*F. gigantica*	31%	Estuningsih *et al.* [31]

(Table 2) cont.....

Antigen	Form	Name of the Parasite	Vaccine Protection in Animals	References
GST	Native	*F. hepatica*	0–69%	Morrison *et al.* [65]
-	Native	*F. hepatica*	Mean 43%: range 0–69%	Spithill *et al.* [89]
-	Native	*F. gigantica*	ns	Estuningsih *et al.* [31]
-	rGST S. bovis	*F. gigantica*	ns	De Bont *et al.* [23]
Total cathepsin L	Native	*F. gigantica*	ns	Estuningsih *et al.* [31]
Cathepsin L (CatL)	Native CatL1	*F. hepatica*	42–69%	Dalton *et al.* [22]
-	rCatL1	*F. hepatica*	48%	Golden *et al.* [38]
Cathepsin CPFhW	Recombinant Inclusion bodies	*F. hepatica*	54% (n = 3)	Wedrychowicz *et al.* [102]
Hemoglobin (Hb)	Native	*F. hepatica*	43%	Dalton *et al.* [22]
-	rHbF2	*F. hepatica*	ns	Dewilde *et al.* [26]
Paramyosin	Native	*F. hepatica*	47%	Spithill *et al.* [89]
-	Native	*F. gigantica*	ns	Estuningsih *et al.* [31]
Kunitz type molecule	Native	*F. hepatica*	ns	Spithill *et al.* [89]
Combination vaccines CatL1 + Hb	Native	*F. hepatica*	51%	Dalton *et al.* [22]
CatL2 + Hb	Native	*F. hepatica*	72% FCA/FIA	Dalton *et al.* [22], Mulcahy *et al.* [67]
CatL2 + Hb	Native	*F. hepatica*	11% FIA only	Mulcahy *et al.* [67]
CatL2 + Hb	Native	*F. hepatica*	29%	Mulcahy *et al.* [67]
CatL1 + CatL2	Native	*F. hepatica*	55%	Mulcahy *et al.* [67]
Irradiated Schistosomula	Native	*S. bovis*	60%	Agnew *et al.* [1]
EG95	Recombinant antigen	*E. granulosus*	96-100%	Larrieu *et al.* [58]
ESP	Native	*O. radiatum*	23%	Gasbarre *et al.* [35]
Soluble extract of L 4	Native	*O. radiatum*	81-99% 75-100% FEC	East *et al.* [29]
OPA, 15	Native	*O. osteortagi*	60% FEC	Vercauteren *et al.* [99]
ES-thiol	Native	*O. osteortagi*	18% 60% FEC	Geldhof *et al* [36]
O-Gal-GP	Native	*O. osteortagi*	11% 23% FEC	Smith *et al.* [87]

Antigen	Form	Name of the Parasite	Vaccine Protection in Animals	References
Globin	Native	*O. osteortagi*	28% 52%FEC	Borloo *et al.* [8]
dd- ASP	Native	*C. oncophora*	91% FEC	Vlaminck *et al.* [101]
WGH	Native	*H. placei*	53-72% >90% FEC	Siefker *et al.* [86]

Protozoal Vaccines

Neospora Caninum

Neospora caninum is an intracellular parasite that causes abortion in cattle globally. It is prevalent in various regions, with infection rates as high as 97%. Most infected cattle do not show clinical signs aside from abortion. Infected cows are at risk of repetitive abortions, leading to economic losses [65]. Various types of vaccines have been explored for *Neospora caninum*, including live vaccines like attenuated strains, genetically modified transgenic strains, and killed parasites vaccines. However, a vaccine called Bovilis Neoguard TM, based on tachyzoite lysate, was the only vaccine introduced to the market. Subsequent studies examined its effects. A study in Costa Rica found that Bovilis Neoguard TM reduced the abortion rate in dairy cows from 20% (placebo group) to 11% (vaccinated group). In New Zealand, clinical trials were conducted on five dairy cattle farms with a history of *Neospora caninum* abortions. Cows were vaccinated between days 30-60 of gestation at 4-week intervals. The study showed that in one of the herds, vaccination prevented 61% of abortions when administered after conception [66]. However, it also led to increased transplacental transmission and a potentially higher risk of early embryonic death [67]. This vaccine has now been withdrawn from the market. Several live-attenuated vaccines have been tested for *Neospora caninum* infection in cattle. The Nc-Nowra strain showed promising efficacy in preventing fetal death. Animals inoculated with Nc-Nowra tachyzoites before mating exhibited strong immune responses and protection against foetopathy upon challenge [68]. A naturally attenuated isolated, Nc-Spain1H, also demonstrated protection against fetal death and reduced vertical transmission up to 86% after challenge [69]. In a field trial, the live vaccine isolate NcIs491 was evaluated in pregnant *N. caninum* seropositive cows, resulting in a lower abortion rate compared to non-vaccinated cows, but the seropositive offspring numbers remained similar [70]. Subunit vaccines have been explored using recombinant antigens. NcGRA7 entrapped in oligomannose microsomes (M3-NcGRA7) reduced brain parasite load in non-pregnant cattle upon challenge [71]. Bacterially expressed recombinant antigens formulated with ISCOMs were administered to pregnant cattle before mating, but they did not prevent fetal infection upon challenge. The cellular immune responses were examined in pregnant heifers vaccinated with a combined recombinant antigen ISCOM formulation, live tachyzoites, or antigen extract ISCOM formulation. The immune cell infiltration differed among the groups, with animals vaccinated with live tachyzoites exhibiting milder immune responses, possibly due to a protective maternal immune response [72].

Tritrichomonas Foetus

Tritrichomonaas foetus is the major cause of reproductive failure in bovines by causing bovine trichomonosis, a sexually transmitted disease. The major losses occur in herds due to early abortions. Though these organisms do not cause symptomatic disease in males, they act as asymptomatic carriers for females. Initial attempts for immunization against bovine trichomonosis were based on subcutaneous administration of killed *T. foetus* cells in a mineral oil adjuvant to the bulls below the age of 5 years [73]. Trichguard® is a commercially available vaccine against *T. foetus* in cattle in the USA, which contains killed protozoa. Trichguard® V5L is another commercialized vaccine that reduces the shedding of *Tritrichomonas fetus* along with protection against five serovars of *Leptospira* and *Campylobacter fetus*. Commercial vaccines containing whole-cell killed *T. foetus* in oil adjuvant prevented colonization of the preputial and penile mucosa in vaccinated bulls [74].

Other types of *T. foetus* antigens, such as membrane preparations and purified membrane glycoproteins, have also demonstrated some efficacy. These antigens, when administered systemically, led to the elimination of infections in some bulls, especially when combined with a mineral oil adjuvant (Clark *et al.*, 1984). Systemic vaccination in non-pregnant heifers with immunoaffinity-purified lipophosphoglycan (LPG)/protein complex antigens (Tf1.17) induced specific antibodies and clearance of genital infections within a short timeframe [75].

Theileria

Cattle infected with *T. parva* or *T. annulata* experience an acute lymphoproliferative disease marked by symptoms like fever and enlargement of lymph nodes [76]. Anemia, resulting from the infection of red blood cells, is also observed in cases of *T. annulata* infection. Mortality rates can be as high as 90%, and death might occur within 3–4 weeks of *T. parva* infection.

Early attempts to vaccinate cattle against East coast fever using crude antigen extracts from *T.parva* parasitized leukocytes in adjuvants were unsuccessful. However, it was observed that animals recovering from clinical disease became immune to subsequent challenges [77]. Vaccination against *T. parva* using the infection and treatment method using live *T. parva* sporozoites and administering oxytetracycline offer solid protection against homologous challenge [78]. Subsequent experiments demonstrated that immunization with the Muguga cocktail (a mixture of 3 selected parasite isolates: *Muguga, Kiambu 5,* and *Serengeti*) resulted in immunity against a range of heterologous isolates [79]. This Maguga cocktail vaccine has been used successfully for field vaccination of cattle by infection and treatment at a local level in several East African countries [80, 81]. Experimental immunization with *Merikembu isolates* has shown protection against heterologous isolates [82] and has also been used successfully for the vaccination of cattle in the fields in Kenya. In the 1960s, the development of continuously growing parasitized cell lines provided a reliable *in vitro* system for producing *Theileria* parasites for vaccination against *T. annulata*. Studies showed that inoculating calves with these cell cultures resulted in the establishment of infection, with doses of at least 10^5 cells needed for consistent infection [83]. However, prolonged passage of these cultures led to a reduction in virulence, with doses of up to 10^7 cells causing only mild, transient infections. Importantly, animals immunized with these attenuated cell lines, typically with doses of 1–5 x 10^6 cells, became immune to subsequent challenges with potentially lethal doses of sporozoites [84]. Rakshavac-T is a commercial vaccine created through tissue culture attenuation of *Theileria annulata*, designed to prevent bovine tropical theileriosis in crossbred and exotic cattle. It is administered subcutaneously in the mid-neck region with a dosage of 3 mL. The vaccine is produced from around 5x 10^6 attenuated schizont-infected lymphoblast (ASIL) cells after 165 passages, a process initiated in Israel and later successfully executed in India under the All India Co-ordinated Research Project (AICRP) at multiple locations. Anand Veterinary College in Gujarat handled its commercialization, gaining clearance for large-scale production from the Indian government. Sold as "Rakshavac-T," it offers protection for 36 months in controlled settings and potentially lifelong defense with regular exposure to infection. Another vaccine, Teylovac, originating in Turkey, is created from attenuated *Theileria* schizonts carried by lymphoid cells in tissue culture. Administered subcutaneously, it provides immunity lasting a year and is suitable for all ages and breeds of cattle except calves under 3 months old [85]. Subunit vaccines for theileriosis have been developed as an alternative to live parasite-based vaccines. Novel antigens like Surface sporozoite antigen 1 (SPAG-1) and Merozoite surface antigen 1(TAMS-1) were identified as protective antigens against *T. annulata* [86], but their efficacy is still being studied. Various antigens, including polymorphic immunodominant molecule (PIM) and p67, have been evaluated as vaccine candidates, but protection levels have varied [87].

Babesia

Bovine babesiosis is a disease transmitted by ticks and caused by different species of *Babesia* parasites, primarily *Babesia bovis*, *B. bigemina*, and *B. divergens*. It is characterized by symptoms such as fever, anemia, and hemoglobinuria, with the severity varying depending on factors like the specific *Babesia* species and the age and health of the cattle. To prevent infections of *B. bigemina* and *B. bovis*, live attenuated vaccines have been developed using a traditional method known as "premunition." This process involves introducing blood from infected animals into uninfected ones, transmitting both *Babesia* and other pathogens. The attenuation process for *B. bovis* involves multiple passages around 22-25 in spleenectomized calves [88], while *B. bigemina* strains are attenuated through slower passages in intact spleen calves [89]. Vaccinated animals remain persistently infected with the vaccine strains but develop strong immune responses that protect against similar and diverse strains. Another method to attenuate parasites is using low-dose radiation, as seen in vaccines used in Mexico. These attenuated strains are expanded for vaccine production either in controlled, pathogen-free calves or *in vitro* cultures in several countries like Argentina, South Africa, and Uzbekistan, depending on the country's practices.

However, live vaccines have limitations, such as the need for a cold chain during storage, concerns about coinfections, the risk of vaccine strains regaining virulence, and the difficulty of distinguishing vaccinated from naturally infected animals [90]. Furthermore, the use of attenuated vaccines entails maintaining Babesia parasites within cattle herds, which can pose challenges, particularly if these vaccines involve strains that are transmissible through ticks.

Other vaccination strategies include subunit or inactivated vaccines, which hold promise as they have demonstrated the ability to induce immunity against *B. canis*. Inactivated vaccines are developed using specific protein fractions or secreted antigens from the parasite and have exhibited the potential to generate protective responses. Recombinant forms of these antigens can be harnessed for the creation of effective vaccines. Several *Babesia* antigens, including rhopty–associated protein-1(RAP-1), variable major surface antigens (VMSA), merozoite surface antigen-1 (MSA-1), MSA-2c, 12 D3, and the heat-shock protein 20, have been explored as potential vaccine candidates [91]. However, none of these alternatives have matched the effectiveness of live vaccines. Promisingly, efforts are also being directed towards transmission-blocking vaccine candidates (TBV) in *B. bovis* and *B. bigemina* parasites, such as members of the CCp and 6Cys families and HAP2, aiming to disrupt parasite transmission. Some kinete stage antigens like BboKSP and BbiKSP, exclusively expressed in tick stages, are also potential TBV candidates. These vaccines target antigens expressed in tick stages and have shown success in reducing transmission in various models. Developing a vaccine containing both blood-stage and tick-stage antigens could provide a comprehensive solution for controlling bovine babesiosis by reducing clinical disease and preventing transmission [92].

Eimeria

Eimeria, a genus of parasites consisting of about 200 species, infects a wide range of vertebrates globally. Although strictly host-specific, a single host can harbor multiple species simultaneously. In cattle, thirteen species of *Eimeria* are known, with *E. zuernii*, *E. bovis*, and *E. alabamensis* causing pathogenic effects [92, 93]. Young calves suffer diarrhea and anorexia, while adult cattle remain asymptomatic. Heavy *E. zuernii* infections can lead to nervous coccidiosis with neurological symptoms and high mortality. Bovine coccidiosis remains severely underexplored, which is evident from the limited research on vaccine development. Existing evidence, however, suggests the potential of using *Eimeria* species oocysts as an immunogen in vaccines against bovine coccidiosis. For instance, inoculating calves with *E. alabamensis* oocysts led to protection upon parasite exposure in the field. Another vaccine, utilizing sonicated formalin-inactivated *E. bovis* sporulated oocysts, triggered robust antibody levels and protection against challenges in calves. Additionally, experimental UV inactivation of *Eimeria* oocysts was effective in producing a protective immunogen against coccidiosis in lambs [93]. Despite these promising findings, further investigation into these research avenues remains largely unexplored.

Cryptosporidium

Cryptosporidium spp. are widespread protozoan parasites responsible for cryptosporidiosis, a gastrointestinal disease affecting various vertebrate hosts, including humans and livestock [94]. Efforts to develop a vaccine against *Cryptosporidium parvum* in cattle have taken various approaches. Initially, immunizing newborn calves with killed *C. parvum* oocysts showed promise in reducing oocyst shedding and diarrhea in controlled settings [95]. However, these vaccines did not prove effective under field conditions [96]. This challenge may be attributed to the rapid onset of cryptosporidiosis in very young calves, making it difficult to generate protective immunity through active vaccination [97]. A more promising strategy involves immunizing dams a few weeks before giving birth to produce hyperimmune colostrum containing high levels of specific antibodies [98]. This approach benefits both livestock and reduces environmental contamination with *Cryptosporidium* oocysts [99].

Several antigens have been explored as vaccine candidates for bovine cryptosporidiosis. The recombinant *C. parvum* C7 protein containing the C-terminal of the P23 antigen showed promise. Calves receiving immune colostrum from dams immunized with this protein were protected against diarrhea and showed reduced oocyst shedding [100]. Similarly, the recombinant P23 protein was investigated for passive immunization of newborn calves, resulting in over 90% inhibition of oocyst shedding when colostrum from immunized dams was administered [101]. Another study examined antibody responses in calves fed with colostrum from dams vaccinated with a recombinant *C. parvum* oocyst surface CP15/60 protein, indicating measurable quantities of specific antibodies in their serum [102]. Despite these promising results in controlled settings, none of these vaccine approaches proved effective in field conditions.

Anaplasma Marginale

Anaplasma marginale, the causative agent of bovine anaplasmosis, is a gram-negative rickettsial organism that replicates in the erythrocytes of ruminants [103]. Though they are not protozoa, they are discussed here due to their similarity in mode of transmission, clinical presentation, and vector involvement with protozoa. The history of developing vaccines for bovine anaplasmosis is marked by the significant role played by live vaccines initiated by Theiler in the early 1900s [104]. The live vaccines involve injecting blood from *A. central / A. marginale* infected carriers into susceptible animals, often combined with treatment, a technique called "premunition and chemoprophylaxis", to prevent acute anaplasmosis [105]. This method's reliability is questionable due to variations in incubation periods and infection doses, casting doubt on its effectiveness. In response to these challenges, researchers have attempted to reduce the virulence of *A. marginale* strains by passing them through unconventional hosts like sheep and deer or ^{60}Co irradiation of pathogenic strains [12, 15]. Explorations into naturally occurring low-virulence *A. marginale* strains have opened up possibilities as vaccine candidates. These strains are introduced to induce a mild clinical response. However, safety concerns have arisen due to the potential risk of transmitting other blood-borne pathogens. Attempts have been made to create inactivated vaccines using lyophilized blood containing a high concentration of infected erythrocytes or purified initial bodies [18]. Yet, earlier efforts faced practical challenges, including issues with erythrocyte stroma content and limited effectiveness [47]. These live vaccines have helped reduce the cost of cattle production. However, concerns have emerged regarding their effectiveness and safety, including reports of outbreaks caused by *A. centrale* and failures to induce immunity against *A. marginale* challenges [22].

With the advent of significant advancements in vaccine development, the recombinant proteins derived from outer membrane proteins (OMPs), major surface proteins (MSP1-5), and several type 4 secretion system (TFSS) proteins have demonstrated the potential to elicit immune responses in animal models [41]. DNA vaccines have undergone testing, and efforts have been made to cultivate *A. marginale* in tick cell lines. Genetically modified organisms, including strains with attenuated virulence, have been engineered, showing promise in stimulating immunity while reducing the severity of the disease [58].

Anaplaz, the first-ever anaplasmosis vaccine for cattle in the United States. This vaccine is composed of killed *Anaplasma marginale* organisms obtained from infected cattle. The recommended dosage involves administering 1 ml subcutaneously, with a follow-up dose after 3-4 weeks, followed by an annual revaccination consisting of a single 1 ml dose.

In California, Anavac stands as a modified live vaccine specially formulated for the safe and effective immunization of young cattle. The recommended dosage for this vaccine is 2 ml, administered intravenously, typically given when the cattle are between 6 and 12 months of age. Subsequent booster doses are recommended every 1 to 2 years, based on the herd's historical data.

On the other hand, amvaxtm contains purified initial bodies from the Florida strain of *Anaplasma marginale* [62]. It has undergone 58 serial passages and is entirely devoid of red blood cells. However, it is important to note that its use is contraindicated during pregnancy due to potential risks associated with its administration in pregnant cattle.

Plazvax® was initially introduced by Mallinckrodt and later by Schering-Plough. This vaccine contains inactivated *Anaplasma marginale* and aims to mitigate illness rather than conferring complete protection against infection. Cattle that are already infected with *Anaplasma marginale* and are subsequently vaccinated with Plazvax may continue to harbor the organism for life, essentially acting as "immune carriers". Importantly, these immune carriers can transmit the pathogen to healthy cattle through blood transfusions.

Anaviv, marketed by ProtaTek Int. Inc. in St. Paul, USA, is a live attenuated vaccine designed to combat *Anaplasma marginale* infection in cattle. It is believed to be effective in reducing parasitemia in infected animals, representing a promising approach to managing this disease (Table **3**).

Arthropod Vaccines

<u>*Horn Flies*</u>

Haematobia irritans pose a significant economic threat to cattle due to their harmful effects, causing irritation, lowered milk production, weight loss, blood loss, and hide damage. Additionally, they act as carriers for various pathogens, including the cattle parasitic nematode *Stephanofilaria stilesi* and mastitis-causing Staphylococcus spp [78]. Despite efforts to find new control methods, such as vaccines, effective targets have yet to be identified. Limited success has been achieved in cattle vaccinations against horn flies, with only two secreted salivary targets providing partial protection: an anti-thrombin peptide called thrombostasin [97] and a hematobin [72].

Table 3. List of some important protozoan vaccine candidates in cattle.

	Nc-Nowra Strain	Live Attenuated	Williams *et al.* [104]
Neospora caninum	Nc-Spain1H	Live attenuated	Mazuz *et al.* [62]
	NcIs491	Live vaccine	Mazuz *et al.* [62]
	M3-NcGRA7	Recombinant antigen	Nishimura *et al.* [70]
Tritrichomonas foetus	Tf1.17	immunoaffinity-purified lipophosphoglycan (LPG)/protein complex antigens	BonDurant *et al.* [7] Anderson *et al.* [3]
Theileria annulata	SPAG-1	Recombinant antigen	Williamson *et al.* [105]
	TAMS-1	Recombinant antigen	Dickson and Shiels [27]
Theileria parva	PIM	Recombinant antigen	Toye *et al.* [96]
	p67	Recombinant antigen	Nene *et al.* [69]
Babesia bovis	MSA-2a1, MSA-2b, MSA-2c, ribosomal phosphoprotein P0, RAP 1, BbTRAP and BboKSP	Recombinant and transmission-blocking vaccine candidates	Jerzak *et al.* [51]
Babesia bigemina	MIC-1, RAP-1, HAP2/GCS1, BbiTRAP-1, and BbiKSP	Recombinant and transmission-blocking vaccine candidates	Jerzak *et al.* [51]
Anaplasma marginale	OMP MSP1-5 TFSS	Recombinant antigen	Salinas-Estrella *et al.* [84]
Cryptosporidium parvum	Lyophilized oocysts	Attenuated strain	Harp and Goff [41]
	γ irradiated oocysts	Attenuated strain	Jenkins *et al.* [50]
	C7 protein	Recombinant protein	Perryman *et al.* [73]
	P23	Recombinant protein	Askari *et al.* [4]
	Oocysts surface CP15/60 protein	Recombinant protein	Burton *et al.* [12]

The challenge lies in the absence of rapid tools to validate promising antigens. RNA interference (RNAi) has been utilized, though its inability to directly translate a phenotype into protection has limitations. Researchers conducted an RNAi study targeting abdominal tissue transcripts of partially fed female horn flies. This study resulted in notable mortality and reduced oviposition rates for specific transcript functional groups [78]. However, the study also revealed off-target effects, impacting the obtained results. Despite these efforts, no effective candidates currently exist for managing biting flies, leaving the approach to future vaccine development strategies in need of further demonstration.

Ticks

Ticks are ectoparasites that rely on blood meals from vertebrates and are notorious vectors of diseases affecting both animals and humans. They are particularly significant as disease carriers for livestock, pets, and humans, ranking as the second most important disease vector after mosquitoes [18]. Their impact extends beyond disease transmission, as their blood-feeding behavior inflicts various harms, including damage to hides, anemia, weight loss, and secondary infections, especially in livestock.

The concept of using experimental vaccination against ticks first emerged in 1939 when William Trager demonstrated that injecting guinea pigs with extracts from *Dermanyssus gallinae* tick larvae provided partial protection against subsequent infestations [19]. Pioneering research demonstrated the feasibility of cattle vaccination against ticks, culminating in the discovery of the concealed gut antigen Bm86 found in the gut membrane of *Rhipicephalus microplus* ticks in 1986. This membrane-bound glycoprotein is localized in the tick's digestive tract and is believed to play a role in interactions between cells or pathogens and gut cells. Bm86, along with its related homolog Bm95, became the basis of the TickGARD® and TickGARD®PLUS vaccines. However, these were later discontinued due to poor returns [27]. GAVAC® and GAVAC® Plus, expressing Bm86, were successful in Latin American markets. Only one other commercial vaccine, Go-Tick or Tick-Vac, is available for the Latin American market, which claims to confer 80% protection [29].

Vaccination using Bm86-based vaccines primarily reduces the number of engorging female ticks and their reproductive capacity [86], resulting in decreased larval infestation in subsequent generations. However, these vaccines have limitations, failing to address all tick life stages, showing variable efficacy across different tick strains and species, and necessitating multiple boosts for optimal effectiveness. Research efforts have delved into combining Bm86 with other tick antigens to enhance efficacy, showcasing the potential of *combinatorial vaccines.*

A strategic approach to identifying protective antigens involves targeting proteins crucial for the parasite's biological functions and survival, encompassing tick attachment, evading host defenses, blood meal digestion, metabolism, mating, fertility, embryogenesis, and egg laying [11]. Following Bm86's success, related antigens like Hm86, Haa86, Ba86, Ree86, Dr86, Ir86, Os86, Bd86, Av86, and Ra86 were identified. Bm91, another antigen, enhanced Bm86-based vaccines' efficacy. Bm 95, sharing homology with Bm86, exhibited high efficacy in Indian trials. Additionally, Bm95 combined with *Anaplasma marginale* major surface protein showed promise. The BmA7 protein, despite its homology, did not improve Bm86's efficacy (Table **4**).

Table 4. Vaccine candidates for different ticks commonly found in cattle [40].

Protein	Tick Species
Calreticulin:	*Ambylomma americanum, Hyalomma anatolicum*
Subolesin:	*Dermacentor silvarum, Haemaphysalis longicornis, Hyalomma anatolicum, Ornithodoros moubata, Rhipicephalus microplus*
Acid Phosphatase (HL-3), Follistatin related protein, Vallocin related protein, Longistatin, Glutathione-S-transferase:	*Haemaphysalis longicornis*
Cystatin:	*Haemaphysalis longicornis, Ornithodorosmoubata, Rhipicephalus microplus*
Ferritin2:	*Hyalommaanatolicum, Rhipicephalus microplus*
Tropomyosin:	*Hyalommaanatolicum*
Cathepsin L:	*Hyalommaanatolicum, Ixodesricinus*
Hm86:	*Hyalommamarginatum*
64TRP (Tick cement protein):	*Rhipicephalusappendiculatus*
Ubiquitin, Voraxin, Bm86, Q48, Bm95+MSP1a, Subolesin+MSP1a, Cysteine endopeptidase, Yolk-Pro cathepsin,	*Rhipicephalus microplus*
Ba86	*Rhipicephalusannulatus*

A prospective vaccine candidate, Subolesin, showed potential in reducing tick egg hatching. It exhibited efficacy in various trials, suggesting its universal vaccine potential. Chimeric vaccines combining Subolesin with other antigens demonstrated high efficacy. A patent application proposed combining Bm86 and Subolesin for up to 97% efficacy. Apart from Subolesin and Bm86, multiple other vaccine candidates are under consideration. Recent studies on the acidic ribosomal protein P0 have exhibited promising results, indicating a potential vaccine antigen effective against a range of ectoparasites [34]. The availability of tick sequence databases has facilitated *in silico* vaccinology approaches, successfully identifying protective antigens, as demonstrated by the development of next-generation multi-peptide tick vaccines. Future research is crucial to pinpoint protective antigen epitopes, aiming to reduce production costs for commercially viable vaccines.

CONCLUSION

Vaccine failures are attributed to various factors, including incorrect strains or antigens, production methods, and inadequate antigen levels. Additionally, some animals fail to mount immune responses. Immune suppression, caused by factors like stress and maternal immunity in young animals, can also hinder vaccine effectiveness. Despite these challenges, vaccination remains a promising approach for controlling parasitic diseases in animals. Regulatory and pharmaceutical constraints currently limit vaccine utility, but it is expected that the harmonization of legislation and specific requirements for parasite vaccines in pharmacopeias will improve their accessibility. Advances in molecular techniques for vaccine development are also anticipated to lead to new regulations and improved vaccines in the future.

REFERENCES

[1]   Agnew AM, Murare HM, Lucas SB, Doenhoff MJ. *Schistosoma bovis* as an immunological analogue of *S. haematobium*. Parasite Immunol 1989; 11(4): 329-40.
        [http://dx.doi.org/10.1111/j.1365-3024.1989.tb00671.x] [PMID: 2506507]

[2]   Al-Nazal HA, Cooper E, Ho MF, *et al.* Pre-clinical evaluation of a whole-parasite vaccine to control human babesiosis. Cell Host Microbe 2021; 29(6): 894-903.e5.
        [http://dx.doi.org/10.1016/j.chom.2021.04.008] [PMID: 33989514]

[3]   Anderson ML, BonDurant RH, Corbeil RR, Corbeil LB. Immune and inflammatory responses to reproductive tract infection with Tritrichomonas foetus in immunized and control heifers. J Parasitol 1996; 82(4): 594-600.
        [http://dx.doi.org/10.2307/3283783] [PMID: 8691366]

[4]   Askari N, Shayan P, Mokhber-Dezfouli MR, *et al.* Evaluation of recombinant P23 protein as a vaccine for passive immunization of newborn calves against *Cryptosporidium parvum*. Parasite Immunol 2016; 38(5): 282-9.
        [http://dx.doi.org/10.1111/pim.12317] [PMID: 27012710]

[5]   Bassetto CC, Silva MRL, Newlands GFJ, *et al.* Vaccination of grazing calves with antigens from the intestinal membranes of *Haemonchus contortus*: effects against natural challenge with *Haemonchus placei* and *Haemonchus similis*. Int J Parasitol 2014; 44(10): 697-702.
        [http://dx.doi.org/10.1016/j.ijpara.2014.04.010] [PMID: 24960373]

[6]   Benitez-Usher C, Armour J, Urquhart GM. Studies on immunisation of suckling calves with dictol. Vet Parasitol 1976; 2(2): 209-22.
        [http://dx.doi.org/10.1016/0304-4017(76)90076-5]

[7]   BonDurant RH, Corbeil RR, Corbeil LB. Immunization of virgin cows with surface antigen TF1.17 of *Tritrichomonas foetus*. Infect Immun 1993; 61(4): 1385-94.
        [http://dx.doi.org/10.1128/iai.61.4.1385-1394.1993] [PMID: 8454340]

[8]   Borloo J, De Graef J, Peelaers I, *et al*. In-depth proteomic and glycomic analysis of the adult-stage *Cooperia oncophora* excretome/secretome. J Proteome Res 2013; 12(9): 3900-11.
[http://dx.doi.org/10.1021/pr400114y] [PMID: 23895670]

[9]   Breijo M, Rocha S, Ures X, *et al*. Evaluation of hematobin as a vaccine candidate to control *Haematobia irritans* (Diptera: Muscidae) Loads in Cattle. J Econ Entomol 2017; 110(3): 1390-3.
[http://dx.doi.org/10.1093/jee/tox104] [PMID: 28387808]

[10]   Brock WE, Kliewer IO, Pearson CC. A vaccine for anaplasmosis. J Am Vet Med Assoc 1965; 147: 948-51.

[11]   Brocklesby DW, Bailey KP. The immunisation of cattle against East Coast fever (Theileriaparva infection) using tetracyclines: A review of the literature and a reappraisal of the method. Bull Epizoot Dis Afr 1965; 13: 161-8.
[PMID: 14344196]

[12]   Burton AJ, Nydam DV, Jones G, *et al*. Antibody responses following administration of a Cryptosporidium parvum rCP15/60 vaccine to pregnant cattle. Vet Parasitol 2011; 175(1-2): 178-81.
[http://dx.doi.org/10.1016/j.vetpar.2010.09.013] [PMID: 20951499]

[13]   Callow LL, Dalgliesh RJ, De Vos AJ. Development of effective living vaccines against bovine babesiosis—The longest field trial? Int J Parasitol 1997; 27(7): 747-67.
[http://dx.doi.org/10.1016/S0020-7519(97)00034-9] [PMID: 9279577]

[14]   Claereabout E, Geldhof P, Raes S, Smith WD, Pettit D, Vercruysse J. Vaccination of calves against Ostertagia ostertagi with a globin-enriched protein fraction. Proceedings of the 10ᵗʰ International Congress of Parasitology.

[15]   Clark BL, Dufty JH, Parsonson IM. Immunisation of bulls against trichomoniasis. Aust Vet J 1983; 60(6): 178-9.
[http://dx.doi.org/10.1111/j.1751-0813.1983.tb05957.x] [PMID: 6626064]

[16]   Clark BL, Emery DL, Dufty JH. Therapeutic immunisation of bulls with the membranes and glycoproteins of *Trifrichomonas foetus* var. brisbane. Aust Vet J 1984; 61(2): 65-6.
[http://dx.doi.org/10.1111/j.1751-0813.1984.tb07197.x] [PMID: 6732674]

[17]   Cobo ER, Morsella C, Cano D, Cipolla A, Campero CM. Immunization in heifers with dual vaccines containing *Tritrichomonas foetus* and *Campylobacter fetus* antigens using systemic and mucosal routes. Theriogenology 2004; 62(8): 1367-82.
[http://dx.doi.org/10.1016/j.theriogenology.2003.12.034] [PMID: 15451246]

[18]   Cobo ER, Corbeil LB, Gershwin LJ, BonDurant RH. Preputial cellular and antibody responses of bulls vaccinated and/or challenged with *Tritrichomonas foetus*. Vaccine 2009; 28(2): 361-70.
[http://dx.doi.org/10.1016/j.vaccine.2009.10.039] [PMID: 19879225]

[19]   Cupp MS, Cupp EW, Navarre C, *et al*. Salivary gland thrombostasin isoforms differentially regulate blood uptake of horn flies fed on control- and thrombostasin-vaccinated cattle. J Med Entomol 2010; 47(4): 610-7.
[http://dx.doi.org/10.1093/jmedent/47.4.610] [PMID: 20695276]

[20]   Dalgliesh RJ, Callow LL, Mellors LT, McGregor W. Development of a highly infective Babesia bigemina vaccine of reduced virulence. Aust Vet J 1981; 57(1): 8-11.
[http://dx.doi.org/10.1111/j.1751-0813.1981.tb07075.x] [PMID: 7236153]

[21]   Dalimi A, Motamedi G, Hosseini M, *et al*. Echinococcosis/hydatidosis in western Iran. Vet Parasitol 2002; 105(2): 161-71.
[http://dx.doi.org/10.1016/S0304-4017(02)00005-5] [PMID: 11900930]

[22]   Dalton JP, McGonigle S, Rolph TP, Andrews SJ. Induction of protective immunity in cattle against infection with Fasciola hepatica by vaccination with cathepsin L proteinases and with hemoglobin. Infect Immun 1996; 64(12): 5066-74.
[http://dx.doi.org/10.1128/iai.64.12.5066-5074.1996] [PMID: 8945548]

[23] De Bont J, Claerebout E, Riveau G, *et al.* Failure of a recombinant *Schistosoma bovis*-derived glutathione S-transferase to protect cattle against experimental *Fasciola hepatica* infection. Vet Parasitol 2003; 113(2): 135-44.
[http://dx.doi.org/10.1016/S0304-4017(02)00450-8] [PMID: 12695038]

[24] Fuente J, Estrada-Pena A, Venzal JM, Kocan KM, Sonenshine DE. Overview: Ticks as vectors of pathogens that cause disease in humans and animals. Front Biosci 2008; Volume(13): 6938-46.
[http://dx.doi.org/10.2741/3200] [PMID: 18508706]

[25] Dennis RA, O'Hara PJ, Young MF, Dorris KD. Neonatal immunohemolytic anemia and icterus of calves. J Am Vet Med Assoc 1970; 156(12): 1861-9.
[PMID: 5464261]

[26] Dewilde S, Ioanitescu AI, Kiger L, *et al.* The hemoglobins of the trematodes *Fasciola hepatica* and *Paramphistomum epiclitum* : A molecular biological, physico-chemical, kinetic, and vaccination study. Protein Sci 2008; 17(10): 1653-62.
[http://dx.doi.org/10.1110/ps.036558.108] [PMID: 18621914]

[27] Dickson J, Shiels BR. Antigenic diversity of a major merozoite surface molecule in *Theileria annulata.* Mol Biochem Parasitol 1993; 57(1): 55-64.
[http://dx.doi.org/10.1016/0166-6851(93)90243-Q] [PMID: 8426616]

[28] Dubey J, Hemphill A, Calero-Bernal R, Schares G. Neosporosis in animals. Boca Raton (FL): CRC Press; 2017
[http://dx.doi.org/10.1201/9781315152561]

[29] East IJ, Berrie DA, Fitzgerald CJ. *Oesophagostomum radiatum:* Successful vaccination of calves with an extract of *in vitro* cultured larvae. Int J Parasitol 1988; 18(1): 125-7.
[http://dx.doi.org/10.1016/0020-7519(88)90047-1] [PMID: 3366530]

[30] Echaide IE.

[31] Estunningsih SE, Smooker PM, Wiedosari E, *et al.* Evaluation of antigens of *Fasciola gigantica* as vaccines against tropical fasciolosis in cattle. Int J Parasitol 1997; 27(11): 1419-28.
[http://dx.doi.org/10.1016/S0020-7519(97)00096-9] [PMID: 9421734]

[32] Florin-Christensen M, Schnittger L, Bastos RG, *et al.* 2021.Pursuing effective vaccines against cattle diseases caused by apicomplexan protozoa
[http://dx.doi.org/10.1079/PAVSNNR202116024]

[33] 2014.

[34] Franklin TE, Huff JW. A proposed method of premunizing cattle with minimum inocula of *Anaplasma marginale.* Res Vet Sci 1967; 8(4): 415-8.
[http://dx.doi.org/10.1016/S0034-5288(18)34600-9] [PMID: 6070724]

[35] Gasbarre LC, Douvres FW. Protection from parasite-induced weight loss by the vaccination of calves with excretory-secretory products of larval *Oesophagostomum radiatum.* Vet Parasitol 1987; 26(1-2): 95-105.
[http://dx.doi.org/10.1016/0304-4017(87)90080-X] [PMID: 3439009]

[36] Geldhof P, Claerebout E, Knox D, Vercauteren I, Looszova A, Vercruysse J. Vaccination of calves against *Ostertagia ostertagi* with cysteine proteinase enriched protein fractions. Parasite Immunol 2002; 24(5): 263-70.
[http://dx.doi.org/10.1046/j.1365-3024.2002.00461.x] [PMID: 12060320]

[37] Geldhof P, Vercauteren I, Vercruysse J, Knox DP, Van Den Broeck W, Claerebout E. Validation of the protective *Ostertagia ostertagi* ES-thiol antigens with different adjuvantia. Parasite Immunol 2004; 26(1): 37-43.
[http://dx.doi.org/10.1111/j.0141-9838.2004.00681.x] [PMID: 15198644]

[38] Golden O, Flynn RJ, Read C, *et al.* Protection of cattle against a natural infection of *Fasciola hepatica*

by vaccination with recombinant cathepsin L1 (rFhCL1). Vaccine 2010; 28(34): 5551-7. [http://dx.doi.org/10.1016/j.vaccine.2010.06.039] [PMID: 20600503]

[39]   Guasconi, L., Serradell, M.C., Borgonovo, J., Garro, A.P., Varengo, H., Caffe, G. & Masih, D.T. Immunization with crude antigens plus aluminium hydroxide protects cattle from Fasciola hepatica infection. Journal of Helminthology, 2012; 86, 64–69.

[40]   de Barros LD and Koutsodontis Cerqueira-Cézar C. Editorial: Vaccines against parasitic infections in domestic animals. Front. Vet. Sci., 2023; 1-5 10:1144700. [http://dx.doi.org/10.3389/fvets.2023.1144700]

[41]   Harp JA, Goff JP. Protection of calves with a vaccine against *Cryptosporidium parvum*. J Parasitol 1995; 81(1): 54-7. [http://dx.doi.org/10.2307/3284005] [PMID: 7876978]

[42]   Hart LT, Larson AD, Decker JL, Weeks JP, Clancy PL. Preparation of intact *Anaplasma marginale* devoid of host cell antigens. Curr Microbiol 1981; 5(2): 95-100. [http://dx.doi.org/10.1007/BF01567427]

[43]   Hatam-Nahavandi K, Ahmadpour E, Carmena D, Spotin A, Bangoura B, Xiao L. *Cryptosporidium* infections in terrestrial ungulates with focus on livestock: a systematic review and meta-analysis. Parasit Vectors 2019; 12(1): 453. [http://dx.doi.org/10.1186/s13071-019-3704-4] [PMID: 31521186]

[44]   Hecker YP, Cantón G, Regidor-Cerrillo J, *et al.* Cell mediated immune responses in the placenta following challenge of vaccinated pregnant heifers with *Neospora caninum*. Vet Parasitol 2015; 214(3-4): 247-54. [http://dx.doi.org/10.1016/j.vetpar.2015.10.015] [PMID: 26553499]

[45]   Hidalgo-Ruiz M, Mejia-López S, Pérez-Serrano RM, Zaldívar-Lelo de Larrea G, Ganzinelli S, Florin-Christensen M, Suarez CE, Hernández-Ortiz R, Mercado-Uriostegui MA, Rodríguez-Torres A, Carvajal-Gamez BI, Camacho-Nuez M, Wilkowsky SE, Mosqueda J. Babesia bovis AMA-1, MSA-2c and RAP-1 contain conserved B and T-cell epitopes, which generate neutralizing antibodies and a long-lasting Th1 immune response in vaccinated cattle. Vaccine. 2022 Feb 16;40(8):1108-1115.

[46]   Hillyer GV, Haroun ETM, Hernandez A, De Galanes MS. Acquired resistance to *Fasciola hepatica* in cattle using a purified adult worm antigen. Am J Trop Med Hyg 1987; 37(2): 362-9. [http://dx.doi.org/10.4269/ajtmh.1987.37.362] [PMID: 3661829]

[47]   Innes EA, Chalmers RM, Wells B, Pawlowic MC. A one health approach to tackle cryptosporidiosis. Trends Parasitol 2020; 36(3): 290-303. [http://dx.doi.org/10.1016/j.pt.2019.12.016] [PMID: 31983609]

[48]   Irvin AD, Morrison WI. Immunopathology, immunology and immunoprophylaxis of *Theileria* infections. In: Soulsby EJL, Ed. Immune Responses in Parasitic Infections: Immunology Immunopathology and Immunoprophylaxis. Boca Raton, Florida: CRC Press 1987; pp. 223-74.

[49]   Jarrett WF, Jennings FW, McINTYRE WI, Mulligan W, Urquhart GM. Immunological studies on *Dictyocaulus viviparus* infection; active immunization with whole worm vaccine. Immunology 1960; 3(2): 135-44. [PMID: 14406847]

[50]   Jenkins M, Higgins J, Kniel K, Trout J, Fayer R. Protection of calves against cryptosporiosis by oral inoculation with gamma-irradiated *Cryptosporidium parvum* oocysts. J Parasitol 2004; 90(5): 1178-80. [http://dx.doi.org/10.1645/GE-3333RN] [PMID: 15562625]

[51]   Jerzak M, Gandurski A, Tokaj M, Stachera W, Szuba M, Dybicz M. Advances in *Babesia* Vaccine Development: An Overview. Pathogens 2023; 12(2): 300. [http://dx.doi.org/10.3390/pathogens12020300] [PMID: 36839572]

[52]   Johnson KS, Harrison GBL, Lightowlers MW, *et al.* Vaccination against ovine cysticercosis using a defined recombinant antigen. Nature 1989; 338(6216): 585-7.

[http://dx.doi.org/10.1038/338585a0] [PMID: 2648160]

[53] Jonsson NN, Matschoss AL, Pepper P, *et al.* Evaluation of TickGARDPLUS, a novel vaccine against *Boophilus microplus*, in lactating Holstein–Friesian cows. Vet Parasitol 2000; 88(3-4): 275-85.
      [http://dx.doi.org/10.1016/S0304-4017(99)00213-7] [PMID: 10714465]

[54] Knox DP, Redmond DL. Parasite vaccines – recent progress and problems associated with their development. Parasitology 2006; 133(S2) (Suppl.): S1-8.
      [http://dx.doi.org/10.1017/S0031182006001776] [PMID: 17274842]

[55] Knox DP, Smith WD. Vaccination against gastrointestinal nematode parasites of ruminants using gut-expressed antigens. Vet Parasitol 2001; 100(1-2): 21-32.
      [http://dx.doi.org/10.1016/S0304-4017(01)00480-0] [PMID: 11522403]

[56] Kocan KM, De La Fuente J, Blouin EF, Garcia-Garcia JC. Adaptations of the tick-borne pathogen, *Anaplasma marginale*, for survival in cattle and ticks. Exp Appl Acarol 2002; 28(1-4): 9-25.
      [http://dx.doi.org/10.1023/A:1025329728269] [PMID: 14570114]

[57] Larrieu E, Mujica G, Araya D, *et al.* Pilot field trial of the EG95 vaccine against ovine cystic echinococcosis in Rio Negro, Argentina: 8 years of work. Acta Trop 2019; 191: 1-7.
      [http://dx.doi.org/10.1016/j.actatropica.2018.12.025] [PMID: 30576624]

[58] Larrieu E, Mujica G, Gauci CG, *et al.* Pilot Field Trial of the EG95 Vaccine Against Ovine Cystic Echinococcosis in Rio Negro, Argentina: Second Study of Impact. PLoS Negl Trop Dis 2015; 9(10): e0004134.
      [http://dx.doi.org/10.1371/journal.pntd.0004134] [PMID: 26517877]

[59] Lightowlers MW, Jensen O, Fernández E, *et al.* Vaccination trials in Australia and Argentina confirm the effectiveness of the EG95 hydatid vaccine in sheep. Int J Parasitol 1999; 29(4): 531-4.
      [http://dx.doi.org/10.1016/S0020-7519(99)00003-X] [PMID: 10428628]

[60] Lightowlers MW, Flisser A, Gauci CG, Heath DD, Jensen O, Rolfe R. Vaccination against cysticercosis and hydatid disease. Parasitol Today 2000; 16(5): 191-6.
      [http://dx.doi.org/10.1016/S0169-4758(99)01633-6] [PMID: 10782077]

[61] Lightowlers MW, Lawrence SB, Gauci CG, *et al.* Vaccination against hydatidosis using a defined recombinant antigen. Parasite Immunol 1996; 18(9): 457-62.
      [http://dx.doi.org/10.1111/j.1365-3024.1996.tb01029.x] [PMID: 9226681]

[62] Mazuz ML, Fish L, Wolkomirsky R, *et al.* The effect of a live *Neospora caninum* tachyzoite vaccine in naturally infected pregnant dairy cows. Prev Vet Med 2015; 120(2): 232-5.
      [http://dx.doi.org/10.1016/j.prevetmed.2015.03.020] [PMID: 25890821]

[63] Meyvis Y, Geldhof P, Gevaert K, Timmerman E, Vercruysse J, Claerebout E. Vaccination against *Ostertagia ostertagi* with subfractions of the protective ES-thiol fraction. Vet Parasitol 2007; 149(3-4): 239-45.
      [http://dx.doi.org/10.1016/j.vetpar.2007.08.014] [PMID: 17881131]

[64] Morgoglione ME, Bosco A, Maurelli MP, *et al.* A 10-year surveillance of *Eimeria* spp. In cattle and buffaloes in a Mediterranean area. Front Vet Sci 2020; 7: 410.
      [http://dx.doi.org/10.3389/fvets.2020.00410] [PMID: 32851006]

[65] Morrison C, Colin T, Sexton JL, *et al.* Protection of cattle against *Fasciola hepatica* infection by vaccination with glutathione S-transferase. Vaccine 1996; 14(17-18): 1603-12.
      [http://dx.doi.org/10.1016/S0264-410X(96)00147-8] [PMID: 9032888]

[66] Morzaria SP, Irvin AD, Taracha E, *et al.* Immunization against east coast fever: The use of selected stocks of *Theileria parva* for immunization of cattle exposed to field challenge. Vet Parasitol 1987; 23(1-2): 23-41.
      [http://dx.doi.org/10.1016/0304-4017(87)90022-7] [PMID: 3105160]

[67] Mulcahy G, O'Connor F, McGonigle S, *et al.* Correlation of specific antibody titre and avidity with protection in cattle immunized against *Fasciola hepatica*. Vaccine 1998; 16(9-10): 932-9.

[http://dx.doi.org/10.1016/S0264-410X(97)00289-2] [PMID: 9682340]

[68]   Mulcahy G, O'Connor F, Clery D, *et al.* Immune responses of cattle to experimental anti-Fasciola hepaticavaccines. Res Vet Sci 1999; 67(1): 27-33.
[http://dx.doi.org/10.1053/rvsc.1998.0270] [PMID: 10425237]

[69]   Nene V, Iams KP, Gobright E, Musoke AJ. Characterisation of the gene encoding a candidate vaccine antigen of *Theileria parva* sporozoites. Mol Biochem Parasitol 1992; 51(1): 17-27.
[http://dx.doi.org/10.1016/0166-6851(92)90196-Q] [PMID: 1565135]

[70]   Nishimura M, Kohara J, Kuroda Y, *et al.* Oligomannose-coated liposome-entrapped dense granule protein 7 induces protective immune response to *Neospora caninum* in cattle. Vaccine 2013; 31(35): 3528-35.
[http://dx.doi.org/10.1016/j.vaccine.2013.05.083] [PMID: 23742998]

[71]   Ortega-Mora LM, Sánchez-Sánchez R, Rojo-Montejo S, *et al.* A new inactivated *Tritrichomonas foetus* vaccine that improves genital clearance of the infection and calving intervals in cattle. Front Vet Sci 2022; 9: 1005556.
[http://dx.doi.org/10.3389/fvets.2022.1005556] [PMID: 36277069]

[72]   Palmer GH. Anaplasmo vaccines. In: Wright LG, Ed. Veterinary Protozoan and Hemoparasite Vaccines. Boca Raton: CRC Press 1989; p. I-30.

[73]   Perryman LE, Kapil SJ, Jones ML, Hunt EL. Protection of calves against cryptosporidiosis with immune bovine colostrum induced by a *Cryptosporidium parvum* recombinant protein. Vaccine 1999; 17(17): 2142-9.
[http://dx.doi.org/10.1016/S0264-410X(98)00477-0] [PMID: 10367947]

[74]   Pipano E. Schizonts and tick stages in immunization against *Theileria annulata* infection. In: Irvin AD, Cunningham MP, Young AS, Eds. Advances in the Control of Theileriosis. The Hague: Martinus Nijhoff 1981; pp. 242-52.
[http://dx.doi.org/10.1007/978-94-009-8346-5_43]

[75]   Pipano E. Vaccines against hemoparasitic diseases in Israel with special reference to quality assurance. Trop Anim Health Prod 1997; 29(S4) (Suppl.): 86S-90S.
[http://dx.doi.org/10.1007/BF02632940] [PMID: 9512751]

[76]   Pipano E, Tsur I. Experimental immunization against *Theileria annulata* with a tissue culture vaccine. Lab Trials Refuah Vet 1966; 23: 186-94.

[77]   Pipano E. Vaccination against *Theileria annulata* theileriosis. In: Wright IG, Ed. Veterinary Protozoan and Hemoparasite Vaccines. Boca Raton, FL: CRC Press 1989; pp. 203-34.

[78]   Radley DE, Brown CGD, Cunningham MP, *et al.* East coast fever: 3. Chemoprophylactic immunization of cattle using oxytetracycline and a combination of theilerial strains. Vet Parasitol 1975; 1(1): 51-60.
[http://dx.doi.org/10.1016/0304-4017(75)90007-2]

[79]   Rashid M, Rashid MI, Akbar H, et al. A systematic review on modelling approaches for economic losses studies caused by parasites and their associated diseases in cattle. Parasitology. 2018;146(2):129-141.
[http://dx.doi.org/10.1017/S0031182018001282] [PMID: 30068403]

[80]   Ristic M, Carson CA. Methods of immunoprophylaxis against bovine anaplasmosis with emphasis on use of the attenuated *Anaplasma marginale* vaccine. Adv Exp Med Biol 1977; 93: 151-88.
[http://dx.doi.org/10.1007/978-1-4615-8855-9_10] [PMID: 596296]

[81]   Rodríguez M, Rubiera R, Penichet M, *et al.* High level expression of the B. microplus Bm86 antigen in the yeast *Pichia pastoris* forming highly immunogenic particles for cattle. J Biotechnol 1994; 33(2): 135-46.
[http://dx.doi.org/10.1016/0168-1656(94)90106-6] [PMID: 7764729]

[82]   Rodríguez-Mallon A, Encinosa PE, Méndez-Pérez L, *et al.* High efficacy of a 20 amino acid peptide of

the acidic ribosomal protein P0 against the cattle tick, *Rhipicephalus microplus*. Ticks Tick Borne Dis 2015; 6(4): 530-7.
[http://dx.doi.org/10.1016/j.ttbdis.2015.04.007] [PMID: 25958782]

[83]   Rojo-Montejo S, Collantes-Fernández E, López-Pérez I, Risco-Castillo V, Prenafeta A, Ortega-Mora LM. Evaluation of the protection conferred by a naturally attenuated *Neospora caninum* isolate against congenital and cerebral neosporosis in mice. Vet Res 2012; 43(1): 62.
[http://dx.doi.org/10.1186/1297-9716-43-62] [PMID: 22913428]

[84]   Salinas-Estrella E, Amaro-Estrada I, Cobaxin-Cárdenas ME, Preciado de la Torre JF, Rodríguez SD. Bovine Anaplasmosis: Will there ever be an almighty effective vaccine? Front Vet Sci 2022; 9: 946545.
[http://dx.doi.org/10.3389/fvets.2022.946545] [PMID: 36277070]

[85]   Sexton JL, Milner AR, Panaccio M, *et al.* Glutathione S-transferase. Novel vaccine against *Fasciola hepatica* infection in sheep. J Immunol 1990; 145(11): 3905-10.
[http://dx.doi.org/10.4049/jimmunol.145.11.3905] [PMID: 1978849]

[86]   Siefker C, Rickard LG. Vaccination of calves with *Haemonchus placei* intestinal homogenate. Vet Parasitol 2000; 88(3-4): 249-60.
[http://dx.doi.org/10.1016/S0304-4017(99)00208-3] [PMID: 10714462]

[87]   Smith WD, Smith SK, Pettit D, Newlands GF, Skuce PJ. Relative protective properties of three membrane glycoprotein fractions from *Haemonchus contortus*. Parasite Immunol 2000; 22(2): 63-71. b
[http://dx.doi.org/10.1046/j.1365-3024.2000.00277.x] [PMID: 10652118]

[88]   Smith WD, Smith SK, Pettit D. Evaluation of immunization with gut membrane glycoproteins of *Ostertagia ostertagi* against homologous challenge in calves and against *Haemonchus contortus* in sheep. Parasite Immunol 2000; 22(5): 239-47. a
[http://dx.doi.org/10.1046/j.1365-3024.2000.00303.x] [PMID: 10792763]

[89]   Spithill TW, Smooker PM, Sexton JL, Bozas E, Morrison CA, Parsons JC. The development of vaccines against fasciolosis. In: Dalton JP, Ed. Fasciolosis. Oxon: CABI Publishing 1999; pp. 377-410.

[90]   Spreull J. East Coast Fever Inoculation in the Transkeian Territories, South Africa. J Comp Pathol Ther 1914; 27: 299-304.
[http://dx.doi.org/10.1016/S0368-1742(14)80052-0]

[91]   Stahl P, Poinsignon Y, Pouedras P, *et al.* Case report of the patient source of the *Babesia microti* R1 reference strain and implications for travelers. J Travel Med 2018; 25(1): tax073.
[http://dx.doi.org/10.1093/jtm/tax073] [PMID: 29394381]

[92]   Stutzer C, Richards SA, Ferreira M, Baron S, Maritz-Olivier C. Metazoan parasite vaccines: present status and future prospects. Front Cell Infect Microbiol 2018; 8: 67.
[http://dx.doi.org/10.3389/fcimb.2018.00067] [PMID: 29594064]

[93]   Theiler A. 1911.

[94]   Todorovic RA, Lopez LA, Lopez AG, Gonzalez EF. Bovine babesiosis and anaplasmosis: Control by premunition and chemoprophylaxis. Exp Parasitol 1975; 37(1): 92-104.
[http://dx.doi.org/10.1016/0014-4894(75)90056-9] [PMID: 1116519]

[95]   Torres L, Almazán C, Ayllón N, *et al.* Functional genomics of the horn fly, *Haematobia irritans* (Linnaeus, 1758). BMC Genomics 2011; 12(1): 105.
[http://dx.doi.org/10.1186/1471-2164-12-105] [PMID: 21310032]

[96]   Toye PG, Goddeeris BM, Iams K, Musoke AJ, Morrison WI. Characterization of a polymorphic immunodominant molecule in sporozoites and schizonts of *Theileria parva*. Parasite Immunol 1991; 13(1): 49-62.
[http://dx.doi.org/10.1111/j.1365-3024.1991.tb00262.x] [PMID: 1901640]

[97]   Trager W. Acquired immunity to ticks. J Parasitol 1939; 25(1): 57-81.
       [http://dx.doi.org/10.2307/3272160]

[98]   Uilenberg G. Immunization against diseases caused by *Theileria parva* : a review. Trop Med Int
       Health 1999; 4(9): A12-20.
       [http://dx.doi.org/10.1046/j.1365-3156.1999.00446.x] [PMID: 10540307]

[99]   Vercauteren I, Geldhof P, Vercruysse J, *et al.* Vaccination with an *Ostertagia ostertagi* polyprotein
       allergen protects calves against homologous challenge infection. Infect Immun 2004; 72(5): 2995-
       3001.
       [http://dx.doi.org/10.1128/IAI.72.5.2995-3001.2004] [PMID: 15102812]

[100] Vizcaino O, Carson CA, Lee AJ, Ristic M. Efficacy of attenuated *Anaplasma marginale* vaccine under
       laboratory and field conditions in Colombia. Am J Vet Res 1978; 39(2): 229-33.
       [PMID: 629456]

[101] Vlaminck J, Borloo J, Vercruysse J, Geldhof P, Claerebout E. Vaccination of calves against *Cooperia
       oncophora* with a double-domain activation-associated secreted protein reduces parasite egg output
       and pasture contamination. Int J Parasitol 2015; 45(4): 209-13.
       [http://dx.doi.org/10.1016/j.ijpara.2014.11.001] [PMID: 25513963]

[102] Wedrychowicz H, Kesik M, Kaliniak M, *et al.* Vaccine potential of inclusion bodies containing
       cysteine proteinase of *Fasciola hepatica* in calves and lambs experimentally challenged with
       metacercariae of the fluke. Vet Parasitol 2007; 147(1-2): 77-88.
       [http://dx.doi.org/10.1016/j.vetpar.2007.03.023] [PMID: 17481823]

[103] Weston JF, Heuer C, Williamson NB. Efficacy of a *Neospora caninum* killed tachyzoite vaccine in
       preventing abortion and vertical transmission in dairy cattle. Prev Vet Med 2012; 103(2-3): 136-44.
       [http://dx.doi.org/10.1016/j.prevetmed.2011.08.010] [PMID: 21925752]

[104] Williams DJL, Guy CS, Smith RF, *et al.* Immunization of cattle with live tachyzoites of *Neospora
       caninum* confers protection against fetal death. Infect Immun 2007; 75(3): 1343-8.
       [http://dx.doi.org/10.1128/IAI.00777-06] [PMID: 17145943]

[105] Williamson S, Tait A, Brown D, *et al. Theileria annulata* sporozoite surface antigen expressed in
       Escherichia coli elicits neutralizing antibody. Proc Natl Acad Sci USA 1989; 86(12): 4639-43.
       [http://dx.doi.org/10.1073/pnas.86.12.4639] [PMID: 2499888]

CHAPTER 16

Preventive Measures and Control of Parasites

Muhammad Tahir Aleem[1,2,*], **Fakiha Kalim**[3], **Azka Kalim**[4], **Furqan Munir**[3] and **Jazib Hussain**[5]

[1] *MOE Joint International Research Laboratory of Animal Health and Food Safety, College of Veterinary Medicine, Nanjing Agricultural University, Nanjing 210095, China*

[2] *Center for Gene Regulation in Health and Disease, Department of Biological, Geological, and Environmental Sciences, College of Sciences and Health Professions, Cleveland State University, Cleveland, OH 44115, USA*

[3] *Department of Parasitology, Faculty of Veterinary Science, University of Agriculture, Faisalabad 38040, Pakistan*

[4] *Faculty of Medical Sciences, Government College University, Faisalabad-38000, Pakistan*

[5] *DNRF Center for Chromosome Stability, Department of Cellular and Molecular Medicine, Faculty of Health and Medical Sciences, University of Copenhagen, Denmark*

Abstract: Parasitism is one of the greatest challenges faced by the cattle industry worldwide. Parasites and parasite-borne infections not only pose various adverse impacts on the health of cattle but also affect the marketing and import-export of animals and their products, which lead to the loss of billions of dollars on an annual basis. Therefore, devising appropriate preventive measures and control strategies is direly needed in order to fight against these devils that affect cattle health. As the kinds of parasites and the degree of their impacts on cattle vary significantly according to climatic conditions, geography, genotype of cattle, production environment, cattle age, and management approaches, precise and suitable preventive and control measures must be adopted according to faced factors and situations. Nowadays, many approaches are extensively utilized for parasitic control, like pasture management, waste management, deworming, grazing management, nutritional management, management of dwelling places or sheds, immunization, and biological control. It is not possible to issue general guidelines and recommendations for parasitic control in cattle due to diverse geo-climatic conditions and methods opted for rearing the cattle. Due to the increasing incidence of anti-parasitic drug resistance in animals, it is crucial to design a sustainable parasite control approach, which must involve the host as well as the host control measures to achieve maximum productivity from cattle for an indefinite time period.

*** Corresponding author Muhammad Tahir Aleem:** MOE Joint International Research Laboratory of Animal Health and Food Safety, College of Veterinary Medicine, Nanjing Agricultural University, Nanjing 210095, China; Center for Gene Regulation in Health and Disease, Department of Biological, Geological, and Environmental Sciences, College of Sciences and Health Professions, Cleveland State University, Cleveland, OH 44115, USA; E-mail: dr.tahir1990@gmail.com

Keywords: Biological control, Cattle, Control, Endoparasites, Ectoparasites, Economic losses, Management, Parasites, Prevention.

INTRODUCTION

Parasitism is one of the biggest challenges faced by the cattle industry globally [1, 2]. Parasites and parasite-borne infections not only pose various adverse impacts on cattle health but also affect the marketing and import-export of animals and their products [3]. The cattle industry faces the loss of billions of dollars on an annual basis due to parasitism [4]. Parasitic diseases cause a reduction in weight, feed utilization efficiency, and milk production [5 - 8]. These are also considered one of the main causes of liver rejections in abattoirs and mortality in young and adult cattle [9 - 16]. The reproduction and defense response of animal's body to immunization and infection are also affected badly due to parasitic infestations [17 - 23]. Additionally, some cattle parasites are also zoonotic in nature, which may threaten human health [4]. The health and welfare of the cattle kept on farms are also compromised because of parasitic infestation. According to the definition proposed by the World Organization for Animal Health, "good animal welfare is considered when an animal is in good health condition, well fed, safe, comfortable, is not suffering from discomforting conditions like pain, fear, and distress, and is able to manifest behaviors that are essential for its physical and mental well-being". Suitable veterinary care, management, shelter, nutrition, and prevention of disease are the basic requirements of good animal welfare [24]. Cattle infected with gastrointestinal nematodes and liver fluke may contribute to increased greenhouse gas emissions compared to uninfected ones [25, 26].

Enormous production and economic losses associated with parasitic infections in cattle provide ground for the application of strategies to control the key parasites affecting the cattle in order to ensure profitability, improve animal welfare, and potentially play a part in minimizing greenhouse gas emissions. Still, cattle operations face limited operating margins [27, 28], so the methods used to alleviate losses arose due to parasitism need to be cost-efficient. Effective, cost-efficient, profit-generating management of parasitic diseases depends upon the comprehension of various variables impacting the level of disease. The kinds of parasites, the degree of their impacts on cattle, and the steps taken for their control vary according to climatic conditions, geography, genotype of cattle, production environment, cattle age, and management approaches (Fig. **1**). For instance, the environmental conditions in the tropical and sub-tropical regions are generally favorable for the developmental stages of many parasites. For this reason, the prevalence and diversity of parasitic infections present in those regions are significantly greater as compared to those in temperate climate regions [3, 29 - 32]. As a result, the control strategies developed for parasite control in temperate regions will not be effective in other climates [31]. Cattle genotypes vary in their vulnerability to different parasites. For example, *Bos taurus* cattle are often seen to be more susceptible to tick infestation than *Bos indicus* breeds [12, 33, 34]. *Bos taurus* cattle have also been suggested to exhibit resistance against the gastrointestinal nematodes as compared to *Bos indicus* breeds [35]. Young cattle, particularly those grazing on the pasture for the first time, are seen to have a higher chance of acquiring gastrointestinal nematode infection than adult cattle [35 - 37]. Cattle grazing on pastures have increased exposure to helminths than cattle feeding in feedlots [38 - 40]. Moreover, nutritional status and seasonality also influence the exposure of cattle and response to parasitic activity [41].

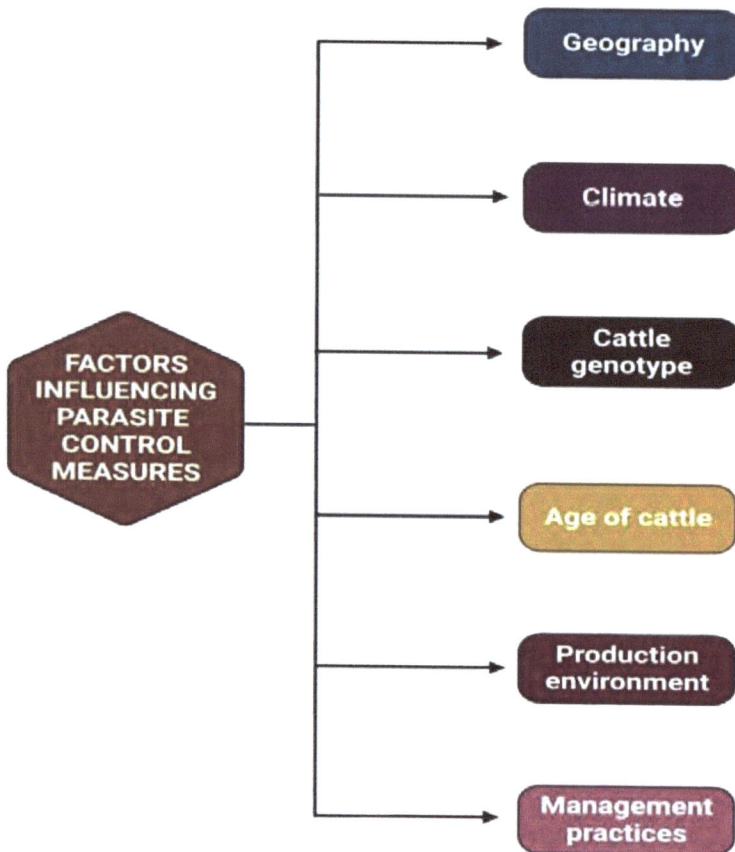

Fig. (1). Various factors affecting the parasite control measures.

Therapeutic control of parasitic diseases commonly involves the administration of parasiticides to enhance reproductive performance, prevent future diseases, and achieve production gains [42]. However, the rational use of parasiticides has given rise to the problem of parasitic resistance [43 - 47]. Due to alterations in the sensitivity of parasites towards acaricides and anthelmintics, cost-efficient treatments should be developed that positively return the investment, keeping in view all the input costs. The objectives of treating parasites in cattle vary depending on the goals of the producer. In some parts of the world, the aim is merely the prevention of mortality. In other parts of the world, where controls essential for maximizing survival have already been implemented by the producers, the key aim is to optimize productivity. Resources for alleviating the impacts of parasitism also vary according to region and type of production. Even within a delimited territory, no single parasite control approach is appropriate for all the herds [48]. This chapter puts a spotlight on the preventive measures and control strategies opted against the parasites of cattle. Fig. (**2**) describes the different impacts of parasites on animal and human health. As these parasites cause remarkable production and financial losses, devising and choosing a suitable prevention and control approach is direly needed.

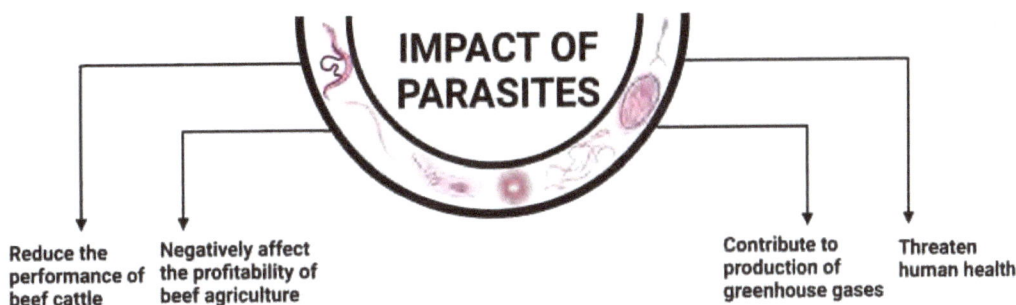

IMPACT OF PARASITES

| Reduce the performance of beef cattle | Negatively affect the profitability of beef agriculture | Contribute to production of greenhouse gases | Threaten human health |

Fig. (2). Different impacts of parasites on animal and human health.

COMPREHENDING CATTLE PARASITES

The parasites found in cattle may be present within the body *i.e.*, endoparasites, or outside the body of the animal *i.e.*, ectoparasites. The endoparasites affecting the cattle include helminths [49] and protozoa [50], whereas the ectoparasites include insects, ticks, and mites [16, 51, 52]. The presence of parasites and their possible impacts depend upon a variety of factors, such as climatic conditions, geography, genotype of cattle, production environment, cattle age, and management approaches. The mode of transmission of parasites also varies [53, 54]. Tables **1** and **2** describe the mode of transmission of different endoparasites and ectoparasites, along with their effects on cattle.

Table 1. Mode of transmission and effects of different endoparasites in cattle

Endoparasites commonly found in catle			
Parasite name	**Mode of transmission**	**Effect on cattle**	**References**
Bunostomum phlebotomum	Ingestion of virulent larvae found on contaminated pastures or direct contact of cattle's skin with the infective larvae, leading to penetration of larvae into the animal body.	Anemia, weight loss, blackish stool, intermittent diarrhea, hypoproteinemia, altered growth and development.	[55, 56]
Cooperia species	Consumption of infective larvae found on contaminated grasslands or water bodies or physical contact with virulent animals and contaminated food or water.	Reduction in weight gain, loss of appetite, and decrease in feed intake.	[57, 58]
Dictyocaulus viviparus	Consumption of infective grass.	Reduced milk production, respiratory distress, inappetence, weakness.	[59 - 61]
Fasciola gigantica	Consumption of grass or water contaminated with parasite eggs or larvae.	Reduced milk and meat production, reduced fertility, hepatic seizures, and even mortality.	[62 - 64]
Fasciola hepatica	Accidental ingestion of parasite, either by consumption of contaminated feed or water.	Retarded growth, reduced fertility, anemia, low body weight, and even death	[62, 65 - 68]
Haemonchus placei	Ingestion of virulent larvae found on contaminated pastures	Decreased levels of proteins, anemia, loss of weight, malaise.	[55, 69, 70]
Nematodirus helvetianus	Contact with virulent larvae found on contaminated pastures or water.	Hypoproteinemia, loss of weight, diarrhea (greenish stool), loss of appetite.	[71 - 73]
Oesophagostomum radiatum	Consumption of virulent larvae found on contaminated grasslands or water bodies or physical contact with contaminated feces.	Loss of appetite, anemia, raised levels of proteins, and excessive blood clotting leading to hemorrhage.	[55, 71]
Ostertagia ostertagi	Ingestion of virulent larvae found on contaminated grazing lands.	Altered feeding and grazing behavior, changes in posture, reduction in weight gain.	[74, 75]

(Table 1) cont.....

Endoparasites commonly found in catle			
Parasite name	**Mode of transmission**	**Effect on cattle**	**References**
Paramphistomatidae spp.	Consumption of infective pastures with parasite eggs.	Less milk production, hemorrhage, loss of appetite, low body weight, hypoproteinemia, diarrhea, edema, and even death if not diagnosed and treated timely.	[76 - 81]
Trichostrongylus axei and Trichostrongylus colubriformi	Ingestion of virulent larvae found on contaminated pastures.	Immunopathological changes leading to apathy, malaise, and reduced weight.	[82, 83]

Table 2. Mode of transmission and effects of different ectoparasites in cattle.

Ectoparasites commonly found in cattle			
Parasite name	**Mode of transmission**	**Effect on cattle**	**References**
Rhipicephalus (Boophilus) microplus	Direct physical contact.	Anemia, adverse decreased milk and meat production, reduced productivity, loss of blood, deterioration of animal hides, may lead to other fatal diseases.	[84 - 88]
Rhipicephalus appendiculatus	Direct skin contact	Lymphadenopathy, anemia, deformity in the affected ears, low PCV (Packed Cell Volume).	[89 - 91]
Amblyomma hebraeum	Direct contact	Adverse effects on udder, lameness, animal hide damage.	[92 - 94]
Amblyomma americanum	Close contact with the parasite or parasite-infected animal.	Skin wounds, transmission of heartwater.	[95 - 97]
Amblyomma cajannense	Direct physical contact	Reduced meat production, inflammation, decreased body weight gain, compromised animal hides.	[4, 98 - 100]
Ixodes ricinus	Close contact with the parasite-infected animal, animal migration.	Fever, lameness, inflammation of lymph nodes, loss of appetite.	[101, 102]
Haematobia irritans	Physical contact, relocating the cattle from one place to another, sharing the shed with the infected animals.	Reduced meat and milk production, decreased weight gain.	[103 - 106]
Stomoxys calcitrans	Physical contact, flying from one infected animal to another.	Reactionary behaviors to flies (skin twitches, head throws, leg stamps, *etc*), reduced meat and milk production.	[107, 108]
Musca autumnalis	Sharing resting or grazing places, close contact.	Eye irritation, reduced milk production, adversely affected DMI (Dry Matter Intake), fly-repelling behaviors (skin twitches, head throws, leg stamps, *etc*).	[109 - 111]

(Table 2) cont.....

Ectoparasites commonly found in cattle			
Parasite name	**Mode of transmission**	**Effect on cattle**	**References**
Culicidae	Flying and biting one infected animal to another.	Reduced body weight gains, altered milk production Sudden attack of several mosquitoes may suffocate the animal and ultimately lead to death.	[112, 113]
Cochliomyia hominivorax	Dumping eggs in the wounds of animals which hatch and get nourishment from body tissues.	Itching, sharp pain, myiasis.	[114, 115]
Linognathus vituli	Feeding on the same grazing land, having close contact with the infected animals.	Irritation, malnutrition, anemia, decreased body weight gain, carelessness.	[116 - 120]
Culicoides sonorensis	Direct contact	Engorgement, hypersensivity, dry skin.	[121 - 124]
Hypoderma bovis	Eggs are dumped in the host's epidermis, and larvae breach into the skin.	Decreased milk and meat production, hides damage, ataxia, malaise, stiffness.	[125 - 127]
Melophagus ovinus	Direct physical contact with parasite-infected animal.	Stunted growth, irritation, anemia, decreased production and may lead to mortality.	[128 - 130]

PASTURE MANAGEMENT APPROACH FOR EFFECTIVE PARASITIC CONTROL

Pasture management is an efficacious approach to control the endoparasites in cattle [131, 132], as cattle may ingest parasitic larvae while grazing. Generally, cattle are allowed to graze clean pastures for maximal production. Clean pastures are pastures that have not been grazed for almost six to twelve months [131]. These pastures do not have any hay or silage crops. As these pastures have minimal contamination, there is much less risk of getting infected [133].

Pasture Rotation

Pasture rotation is a method that is commonly used nowadays for attaining the objective of parasite-free grazing lands [134]. It is a technique in which the larger paddocks are distributed into smaller paddocks, and cattle are easily moved from one small paddock to another [131, 135, 136]. The primary goal of this technique is that the animals should not be allowed to graze the same pasture until the infection risk is minimized. The number of paddocks has an indirect relation with parasitism. If the number of paddocks and time of rotation are raised, parasitism is minimized [131]. Usually, grazing must be avoided when the light strength (intensity of light) is poor. At sunrise, sunset, or hazy sky, there is a high risk of transmission of parasites as the parasite's larvae move freely on the plants. In the rainy season, the concentration of parasites usually increases, and it decreases in the summer or winter season. Grazing should be restricted to the summer and winter seasons as the possibility of larval ingestion decreases in these seasons. More infective larvae are present on the parts of the plant near the ground. The cattle should be allowed to graze up to ten centimeters from the ground in a pasture [137]. This diminishes the risk of parasitic infection [131].

Pasture Resting Period

The pasture rest period is also as essential as pasture rotation. It is a feasible strategy for the growth and enrichment of grazing lands [138]. It is necessary for better management of pastures. The pasture resting period is the time period in which the grazing land (pasture) rests, not used for grazing, for replenishment of the pasture after the grazing period is over [131]. Enough pasture resting period is necessary to enhance the quality of forage, production, and resilience. The duration of the grazing period generally depends on the pasture state, stocking density, and quantity of the forage. The grazing period is advised to be short because it is more advantageous to cattle than long grazing periods (Fig. 3). The recommended duration of the grazing period is a few days to a few weeks [139]. The pasture resting period is determined by the time period required for the replenishment of forages, pasture quality, pasture management, and weather. Its recommended duration is around two to seven weeks [140]. Rest should be given during the growing period as it provides a faster enhancement in the quantity of grasses in the grazing lands [138].

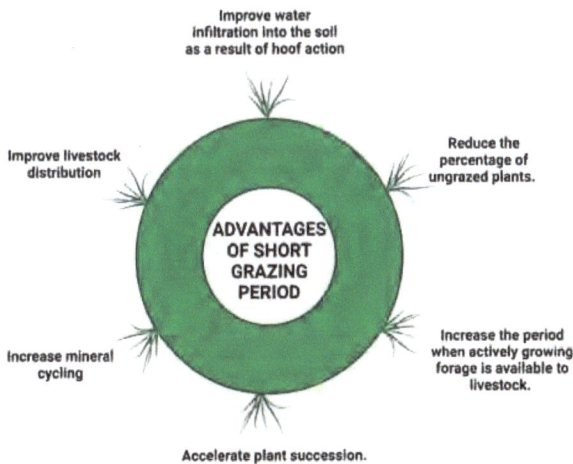

Fig. (3). Some general advantages of short grazing period.

Waste Management and Removal

Fecal wastes and other wastes (Fig. **4**) usually contain high proportions of various parasites [141]. A proper waste management system is necessary for handling and disposing of the wastes to establish a healthy and hygienic environment. It is essential to avoid the transmission of parasites. Thus, it decreases the risk of parasite invasion as cattle grazing on pastures with fecal and other wastes are prone to parasitic infection.

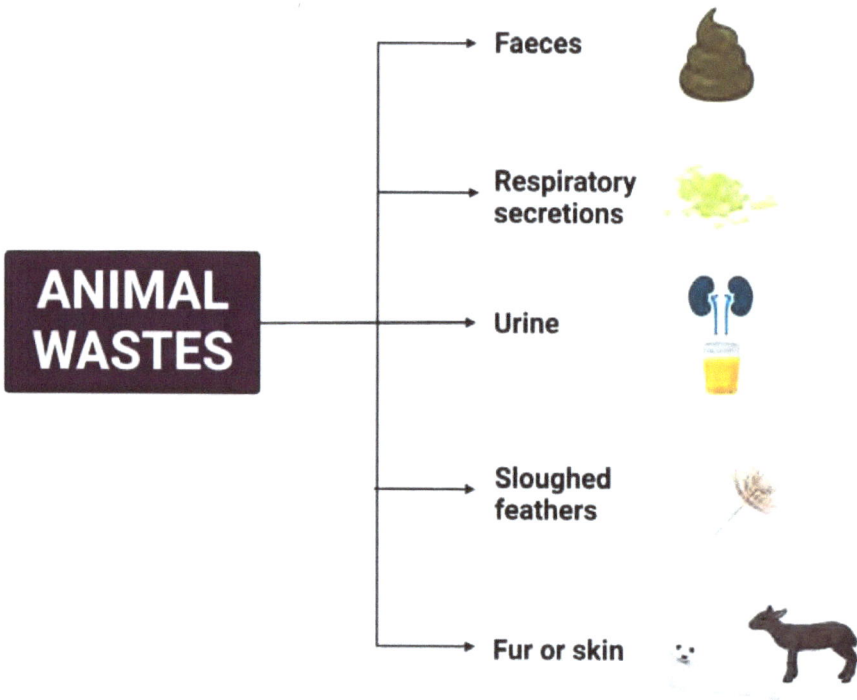

Fig. (4). Different forms of animal wastes.

Various approaches and principles (Fig. (**5**) have been adopted lately for waste management. Fecal wastes and other wastes must be collected from grazing lands or pastures to minimize the growth and accumulation of the eggs and larvae of different parasites. Other approaches may include compositing, treating the wastes, or dumping the wastes in the allotted places, usually far away from the pastures [142].

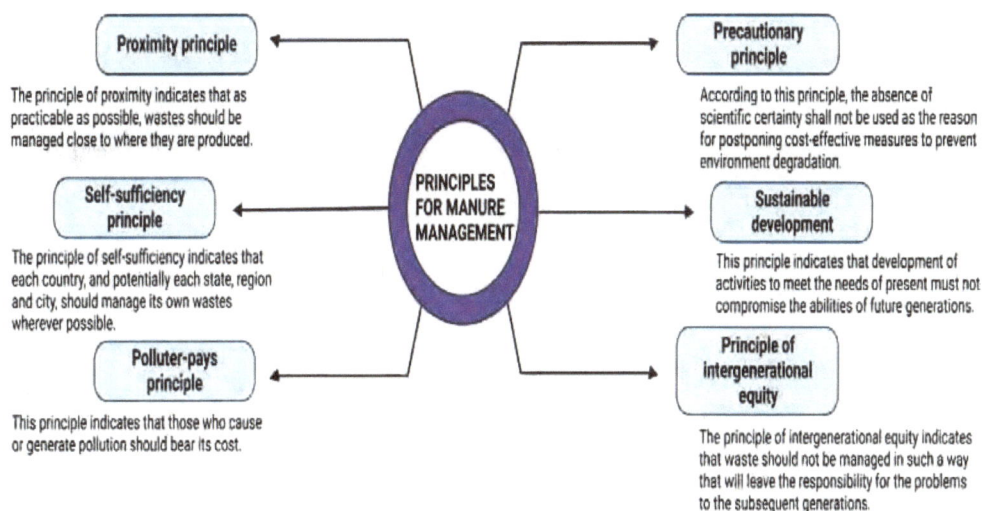

Fig. (5). Some basic principles for manure management.

Fecal Examination and Deworming Practices

Fecal examination plays a vital role in determining the presence of parasites and is a widely used practice in both medical and veterinary fields [143, 144]. It can indicate the presence of helminths (nematodes, trematodes, cestodes) and protozoal species [145, 146]. A fecal exam must be performed at regular intervals in order to detect parasitic infections timely in the animals. This approach is significant in the prevention and control of infectious and zoonotic parasitic diseases. The fecal examination also aids in keeping track of the success of treatment administered against the parasites by estimating the parasitic burden. The fecal exam also aids in devising selective treatment against the parasites. The conventional use of anti-parasitic drugs has given rise to the issue of parasitic resistance in cattle [147, 148]. Due to this, parasites tend to show insensitivity towards many anti-parasitic drugs. A lot of studies are being conducted in order to find possible solutions to this problem. One of the suggested solutions is targeted selective therapy (TST), which involves the treatment of only selected animals that require anti-parasitic treatment [149 - 152]. The potential advantages and disadvantages of TST are described in Fig. (**6** and **7**), respectively.

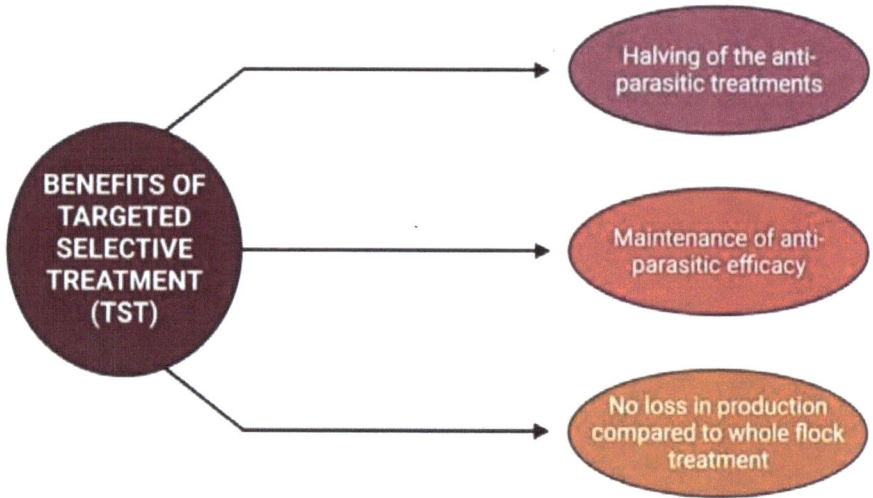

Fig. (6). Potential advantages of TST.

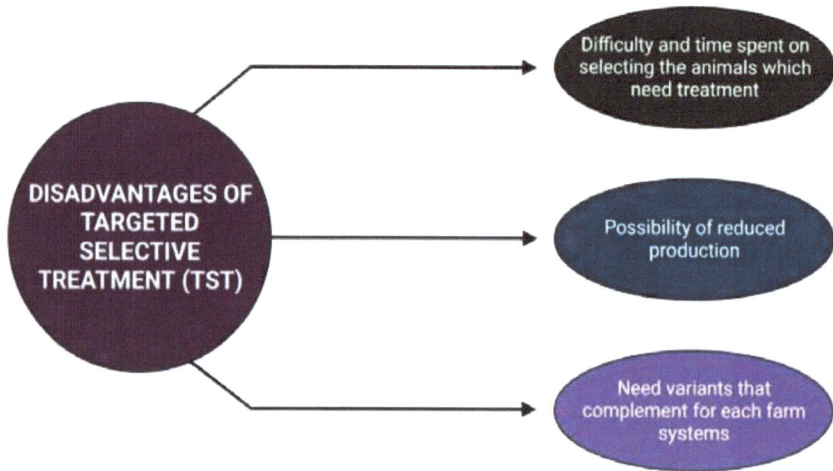

Fig. (7). Potential disadvantages of TST.

The TST relies on the concept of refugia, which means the portion of the parasitic population that is unexposed to anti-parasitic drugs. The objective of a refugia-based strategy is to minimize the utilization of anti-parasitics, which will reduce the selection of resistant parasite alleles and ultimately increase the effectiveness of anti-parasitic drugs for a longer period of time [153]. Deworming, as the name indicates, is a term used for the process of administering drug formulations in order to get rid of parasite (worm) load. A rotational administration approach may be used regarding dewormers in cattle to address resistance issues. Fig. (8) illustrates the general deworming protocol for the cattle present in the tropical and subtropical regions.

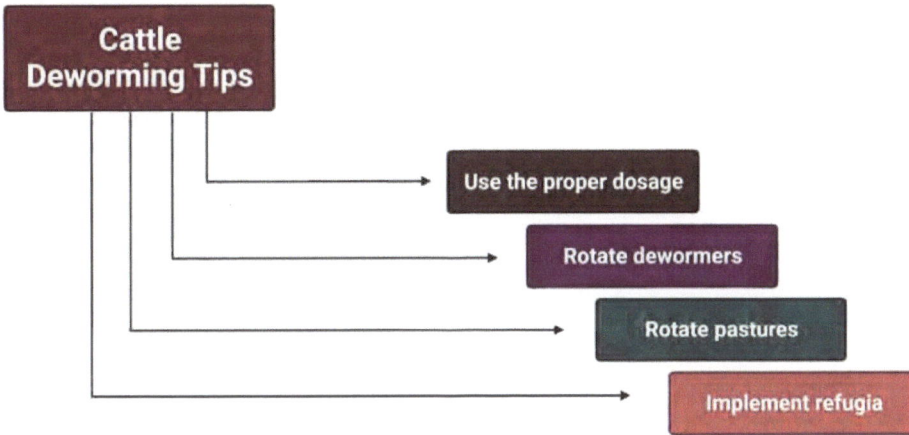

Fig. (8). General deworming protocols for cattle.

The anti-parasitic properties of many natural products have been recognized and are considered "alternative dewormers". These natural products can be utilized as an alternative to the chemicals employed for the control of parasites in cattle and include diatomaceous earth, herbal formulations, and charcoal. Moreover, copper oxide particles, which are administered as a bolus, have been observed to minimize worm infections in ruminants [154]. Garlic [155], wild ginger or snakeroot, conifers, wormwood (*Artemisia* spp.), goosefoot, pumpkin seeds, pyrethrum (plant extract from *Chrysanthemum*) [156], carrot and fennel seeds, mustard and castor oil [157], *etc.* are some examples of botanical dewormers. Different methods for the administration of dewormers against parasites are available in the market. Fig. (9) shows some commonly available forms of dewormers used against ecto and endoparasites in cattle.

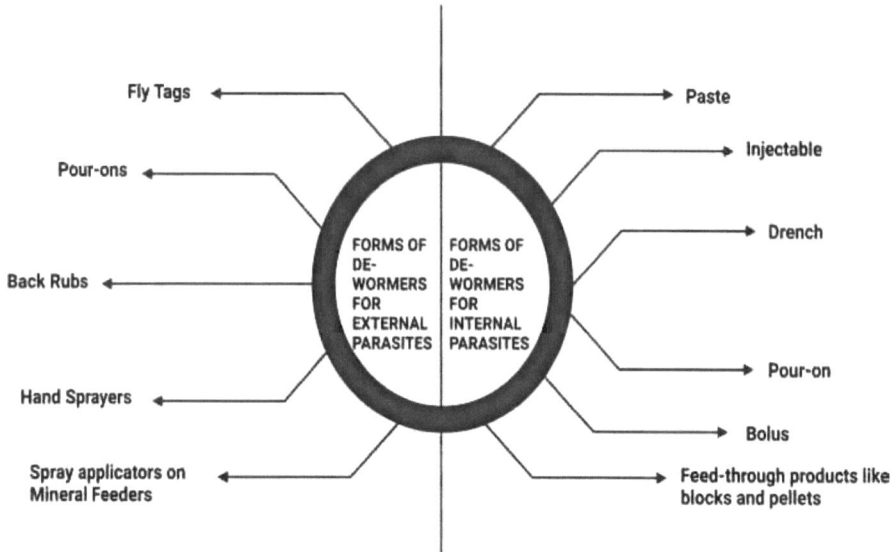

Fig. (9). Different forms of dewormers used against external and internal parasites causing infection in cattle.

It is necessary to know the active constituent of parasiticides used for deworming. Fig. (**10**) illustrates some commonly used parasiticides for deworming.

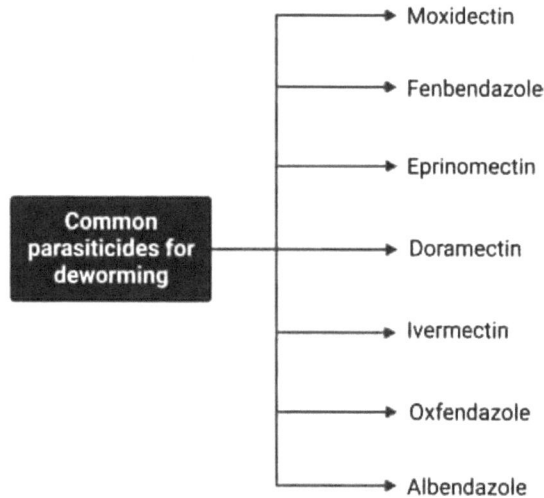

Fig. (10). Some commonly used parasiticides for the purpose of deworming.

GRAZING MANAGEMENT STRATEGIES

Grazing management is the practice of altering grazing methods to attain particular goals [158], including getting rid of parasites. Grazing management strategies contribute significantly to the prevention and control of parasites in cattle [159, 160]. Following are some common tools used to manage the grazing system.

Grazing Intensity or Stocking Rate

Grazing intensity, stocking rate, or stocking intensity is the overall impact of grazing animals on a pasture at a particular time [161, 162]. Grazing intensity increases with the increase in the grazing period [163]. It influences the parasite burden on the pastures. Overcrowding of cattle leads to more animal waste, and there is more risk of ingestion of parasites on grazing [164, 165]. By lowering grazing intensity, there will be fewer contaminated pastures and, ultimately, less contact with fecal deposits. This will eventually lessen the load of parasites in the cattle [138, 164].

Age Group Distribution for Grazing

Cattle are divided into groups on the basis of their age while grazing in order to avoid the possibility of parasite transmission. The susceptibility of cattle against parasite attack differs from one age group to another. So, it is advised to let a certain age group of animals graze in a certain pasture [131, 166]. Young calves and heifers are more prone to parasites than older animals. They should be kept in different places from older cattle. It is recommended to let young cattle graze before the older ones because parasites generally reside in the lower parts of grasses. Older animals have generally attained immunity to parasites over the grazing period, so they will be less affected by the eggs or larvae on the grazing land after the young calves and heifers have grazed.

Multi-species Grazing

Different types of parasites affect different species of animals. The parasites infecting cattle do not survive in goats and sheep [167], and the same goes for horses. This is why the grazing lands on which the horses and large ruminants (buffalo, cattle, yak, ponies, mules, and donkeys) graze arc safe for goats [168] and sheep [167, 169, 170] and *vice versa*. The grazing lands can be rotated between sheep, goats, horses, and cattle to disrupt the life cycle of parasites. Each kind of animal have a different grazing pattern that works in favor of the other animal; for instance, sheep eat short grasses and weeds [171], whereas cattle have an inclination towards taller grasses [38].

Zero Grazing

Zero grazing can be defined as a practice in which the animals are captivated in a specific area and cannot graze openly in the grazing lands [172] in order to lessen the burden of parasites in a pasture. During their captivity, the cattle are fed on the fodder or barn [173], and water containers must be devoid of fecal or other waste matters [38].

MANAGEMENT OF DWELLING PLACES OR SHEDS

Proper environmental control strategies influence the populations of parasites [174], including flies on the pastures [175]. A clean and hygienic environment must be maintained in the housing places of the cattle. The cattle residing in the uncontaminated and healthy environment tend to have better resistance or tolerance against parasitic attacks as compared to those living in unsatisfactory and nasty conditions [38]. The dwelling places or sheds of the cattle must be airy, well-ventilated, and luminous for the passage of air, light, and moisture [131, 176]. The populations of parasites increase at a higher rate in a dark and humid place [131, 177]. Overcrowding of animals at a place provides an ideal environment where parasites can grow freely [178, 179]. In such cases, animals should not be fed on open pastures; they must be given fodders in their specific shed without the contamination of feces or other waste matters. Water should be pure and free from fecal matter, and watering areas must be made of cement with proper drainage systems in order to avoid any contaminants [180]. The presence of proper drainage systems decreases the chances of parasite survival. The animals that are newly added to the sheds must be quarantined for around four to six weeks. Anti-parasitic drugs should be administered to these newly introduced animals [181, 182]. Animal manure should be piled up on one side. In this way, the eggs or larvae of the parasites would be destroyed because of the heat produced by composting [183]. It is advised to let the bedding material disintegrate alongside the animal manure. This is beneficial for parasite control because the bedding material is a major source of several infections caused by parasites. Nitrogenous fertilizers [38, 184] (such as urea, *etc.*), sodium hypochlorite solutions [185, 186], and lime solutions [187, 188] are said to be effective against parasitic eggs or larvae. Their application to the surface of animal dung or wastes may contribute to the destruction of parasites [189].

MANAGEMENT OF NUTRITION AND DEVELOPING IMMUNITY

Maintaining the good condition of the animal body and fulfilling the nutritional requirements are beneficial in minimizing the effects of both endoparasites and ectoparasites [190]. The animals suffering from malnutrition are more prone to parasitic infections [191]. That is why it is seen that animals get infected in longer cold seasons or in conditions of drought because nutritional requirements cannot be met in these situations. Consumption of a healthy diet and all essential nutrients will lead to the development of immunity in cattle against parasitic infections [190]. Fig. (**11**) depicts a few common advantages of taking a healthy and hygienic diet.

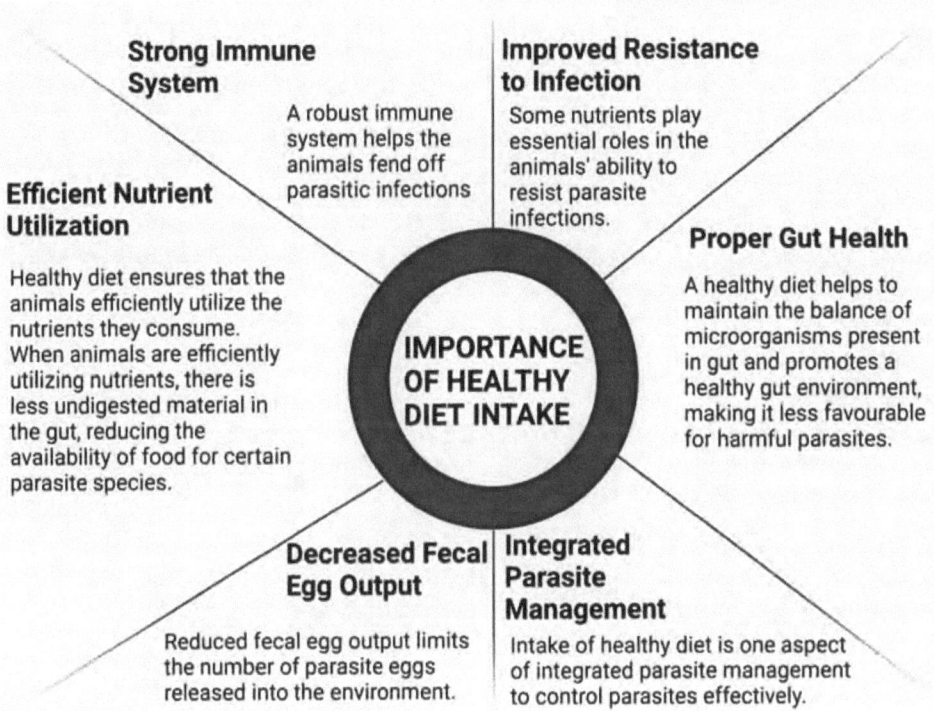

Strong Immune System
A robust immune system helps the animals fend off parasitic infections

Improved Resistance to Infection
Some nutrients play essential roles in the animals' ability to resist parasite infections.

Efficient Nutrient Utilization
Healthy diet ensures that the animals efficiently utilize the nutrients they consume. When animals are efficiently utilizing nutrients, there is less undigested material in the gut, reducing the availability of food for certain parasite species.

IMPORTANCE OF HEALTHY DIET INTAKE

Proper Gut Health
A healthy diet helps to maintain the balance of microorganisms present in gut and promotes a healthy gut environment, making it less favourable for harmful parasites.

Decreased Fecal Egg Output
Reduced fecal egg output limits the number of parasite eggs released into the environment.

Integrated Parasite Management
Intake of healthy diet is one aspect of integrated parasite management to control parasites effectively.

Fig. (11). Some benefits of taking a healthy diet.

Intake of Vitamin Supplements

Vitamins A, B, and D are necessary for the development of immunity against the eggs or larvae of the parasites [192]. Vitamin A or retinol [193, 194] is a fundamental vitamin to boost the coherence of the epithelium of animal intestines [195]. The deficiency of vitamin A disrupts the immunological responses in the intestines of cattle [196]. This tempers the immunity of hosts against the parasites [197]. Vitamin A deficiency also alters the production of cytokines by lymphocytes and macrophages. This alteration results in significant changes in the general actions of the immune cells of animals [38]. Vitamin A disrupts the immune system mechanisms regarding T helper 2 (Th2) cells [198, 199] by managing retinoic acid as it is the primary metabolite generated on oxidation

[131]. Sufficient vitamin supplements must be advised for animals suffering from certain vitamin deficiencies [200].

Consumption of Mineral Supplements

Iron, sodium, zinc, phosphorus, cobalt, potassium, *etc.*, are some minerals found to be important for the adequate working of animal immune system responses to enhance the immunity of hosts against parasites [192]. The deficiency of zinc affects the function of T helper cells [201]. It was declared by Scott and Koski [202] that the hosts suffering from zinc deficiency are more susceptible to parasitic infestation as compared to those that are well-nourished [203]. They used zinc deficient micewith parasitic infections [202]. They noticed that there is a suppressed production of interleukin 4 (IL-4). This decreased level of IL-4 results in lowered concentrations of IgG1, IgE, and eosinophiles. This zinc deficiency also alters the normal functioning of T cells and APCs (antigen-presenting cells). Cook-Mills and his colleagues [204] found that animals with zinc deficiency suffer from altered functioning of natural killer cells (NK cells) and changes in the phagocytosis pattern by macrophages. These changes can be the result of lowered capacity of oxidative burst or respiratory burst. CD4 to CD8 ratio lowers because there is significant reduction in the concentration of thymulin in blood due to zinc deficiency. The deficiency of zinc decreases the production of Th1 cytokines IFN-γ and IL 2. This does not affect the synthesis of Th2 (T helper 2 cells) cytokines IL 4, IL 6, and IL10 [205]. Cobalt is necessary for the production of vitamin B_{12} [206 - 209]. Its deficiency makes the animals prone to infections [210, 211], especially parasitic infections. If hosts are under the influence of hematophagous parasites such as *Bunostomum* spp [212, 213], *Haemonchus* spp [214, 215], *etc.*, then iron-enriched supplements should given in order to overcome anemia [38, 55, 213].

Immunization

Immunization is said to be the most reliable, efficacious, and eco-friendly way for parasite control. Because of this reason, it is also called Green Solutions. This method makes animals rely less on pesticides and other anti-parasitic drugs [216]. The use of vaccines against various parasites boosts animal well-being, enhances public health, and solves issues related to anthelmintic resistance. Vaccines control the sources of food-borne pathogens and zoonoses. This increases the productivity of animals and benefits the economy [217, 218].

BIOLOGICAL CONTROL

Biological control involves the utilization of living organisms (Fig. **12**) for the control of targeted organisms such as parasites, thus diminishing the pathogen population below a threshold level where it cannot cause clinical issues and production and financial losses [131]. The natural presence of various nematode-feeding fungi like *Paecilomyces lilacinus, Duddingtonia flagrans, Arthrobotrys oligospora, Drechmeria coniospora, Verticillium chlamydosporium,* and *Harposporium anguillulae* in the feces of ruminants has been described [219]. These nematophagous fungi possess the ability to infect and deteriorate the parasitic ova, thus preventing the development of the infective larval stage from eggs on pasture. *Duddingtonia flagrans* is extensively applied to control parasites of grazing animals that are found in the gastrointestinal region by lowering the parasite load as it is considered comparatively easy to culture and release in the environment against the targeted parasitic organisms in a controlled manner [220, 221].

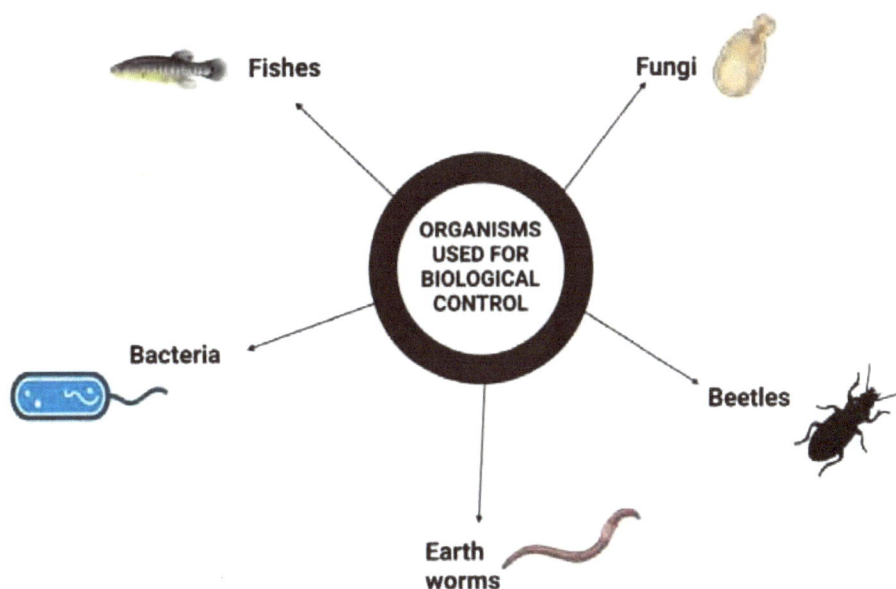

Fig. (12). Some commonly used organisms for biological control of parasites in cattle.

According to a study, the parasitic burden can be substantially reduced by the intake of 5,00,000 spores of the fungi/kg body weight of the cattle as a bolus [222]. Despite all the mentioned benefits of using fungi as biological control agents against cattle parasites (Fig. **13**), the major hurdles in the utilization of fungi for this purpose include a lack of appropriate application systems, evaluation of long-term ecological effects, and acceptance of this method by the farmers. Earthworms are considered natural plough as they can ingest the eggs and larvae of worms while feeding, thus damaging the ova in the gut or carting them below the surface of the soil. Dung beetles are also employed as biological control agents as they can kill the eggs and larvae of many parasites by ingesting manure. Mosquitoes act as vectors for a variety of diseases in cattle. Poeicila and Gambusia can be used for the biological control of mosquitoes. Furthermore, bacteria such as *Bacillus sphaericus* and *Bacillus thuringiensis* israelensis are also widely utilized as effective agents for the biological control of mosquito larvae.

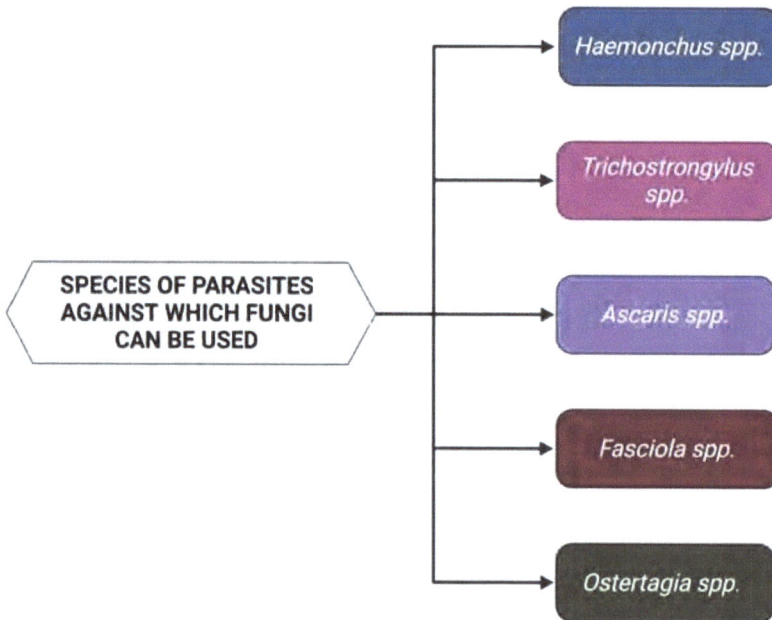

Fig. (13). Species of cattle parasites against which fungi can be used.

CONCLUSION

Parasitism in cattle causes significant production losses and thus impedes profitable cattle farming. As a matter of fact, the financial losses in most parasitic infections are due to the loss of productivity and not because of mortality. Proper preventive and control measures should be adopted for the effective management of parasites in cattle in order to sustain profitability in cattle farming. A variety of preventive and control strategies have been discussed in this chapter, including pasture management, waste management, deworming, grazing management, nutritional management, management of dwelling places or sheds, immunization, and biological control. None of the single control strategies will give long-term solutions to the burning problem of parasite control. A combination of more than one approach is important to accomplish sustainable control of the parasites in cattle.

REFERENCES

[1]   Fitzpatrick JJVp. Global food security: the impact of veterinary parasites and parasitologists 2013.
        [http://dx.doi.org/10.1016/j.vetpar.2013.04.005]

[2]   Gazzonis AL, *et al.* Gastrointestinal parasitic infections in intensive dairy cattle breeding: Update on the epidemiology and associated risk factors in northern Italy 2022.
        [http://dx.doi.org/10.1016/j.parint.2022.102641]

[3]   Food and AOotU Nations, Guidelines resistance management and integrated parasite control in ruminants. Italy: Food and Agriculture Organization of the United Nations Rome 2004.

[4]   Strydom T, Lavan RP, Torres S, Heaney K. The Economic Impact of Parasitism from Nematodes, Trematodes and Ticks on Beef Cattle Production. Animals (Basel) 2023; 13(10): 1599.
        [http://dx.doi.org/10.3390/ani13101599] [PMID: 37238028]

[5]   Jittapalapong S, *et al.* Prevalence of gastro-intestinal parasites of dairy cows in Thailand 2011.

[6]   Huang C-C, *et al.* Investigation of gastrointestinal parasites of dairy cattle around Taiwan 2014.
        [http://dx.doi.org/10.1016/j.jmii.2012.10.004]

[7]   Squire SA, Amafu-Dey H, Beyuo JJLRfRD. Epidemiology of gastrointestinal parasites of cattle from selected locations in Southern Ghana 2013.

[8]   Vanisri V, *et al.* Prevalence of gastrointestinal parasites in cattle in and around Cheyyar taluk, Thiruvannamalai district 2016.

[9]   Corwin RMJVp. Economics of gastrointestinal parasitism of cattle 1997.
        [http://dx.doi.org/10.1016/S0304-4017(97)00110-6]

[10]   Sanchez J, Dohoo IJTCVJ. A bulk tank milk survey of Ostertagia ostertagi antibodies in dairy herds in Prince Edward Island and their relationship with herd management factors and milk yield 2002.

[11]   Kivaria, F.M., Kapaga, A.M., Mbassa, G.K., Mtui, P.F. & Wani, R.J., 'Epidemiological perspectives of ticks and tick-borne diseases in South Sudan: Cross-sectional survey results. Onderstepoort Journal of Veterinary Research 2012; 79(1): 400.
        [http://dx.doi.org/10.4102/ojvr.v79i1.400]

[12]   Bianchin, I., Catto, J.B., Kichel, A.N. et al. The effect of the control of endo- and ectoparasites on weight gains in crossbred cattle (Bos taurus taurus ×Bos taurus indicus) in the central region of Brazil. Trop Anim Health Prod 2007; 39: 287-96.
        [http://dx.doi.org/10.1007/s11250-007-9017-1]

[13]   Strydom T, Lavan RP, Torres S, Heaney K. The Economic Impact of Parasitism from Nematodes, Trematodes and Ticks on Beef Cattle Production. Animals (Basel) 2023; May 10; 13(10): 1599.

[14]   Rodríguez-Vivas RI, *et al.* Potential economic impact assessment for cattle parasites in Mexico. RE:view 2017; 8(1): 61-74.

[15]   Rashid M, *et al.* A systematic review on modelling approaches for economic losses studies caused by parasites and their associated diseases in cattle 2019.
        [http://dx.doi.org/10.1017/S0031182018001282]

[16]   De León AAP, Mitchell RD III, Watson DWJVCoNAFAP. Ectoparasites of cattle 2020.

[17]   Gasbarre LCJVp. Effects of gastrointestinal nematode infection on the ruminant immune system 1997.
        [http://dx.doi.org/10.1016/S0304-4017(97)00104-0]

[18]   Stromberg BE, Averbeck GA. The role of parasite epidemiology in the management of grazing cattle. Int J Parasitol 1999; Jan; 29(1): 33-9.

[19]   Loyacano A, *et al.* Effect of gastrointestinal nematode and liver fluke infections on weight gain and reproductive performance of beef heifers 2002.
[http://dx.doi.org/10.1016/S0304-4017(02)00130-9]

[20]   Charlier J, *et al.* Recent advances in the diagnosis, impact on production and prediction of Fasciola hepatica in cattle 2014.

[21]   McNeilly TN, Nisbet AJJP. Immune modulation by helminth parasites of ruminants: implications for vaccine development and host immune competence 2014.
[http://dx.doi.org/10.1051/parasite/2014051]

[22]   Johnson J, *et al.* Reduced gastrointestinal worm burden following long term parasite control improves body condition and fertility in beef cows 2020.
[http://dx.doi.org/10.1016/j.vetpar.2020.109259]

[23]   Backes E, *et al.* Evaluation of postweaning performance and reproductive measurements in fall-born replacement beef heifers treated with different anthelmintic regimens 2021.
[http://dx.doi.org/10.15232/aas.2020-02125]

[24]   Dimander SO, Höglund J, Uggla A, Spörndly E, Waller PJ. Evaluation of gastro-intestinal nematode parasite control strategies for first-season grazing cattle in Sweden. Vet Parasitol 2003; Feb 13;111(2-3): 193-209.

[25]   Jonsson N, *et al.* Liver fluke in beef cattle–Impact on production efficiency and associated greenhouse gas emissions estimated using causal inference methods 2022.
[http://dx.doi.org/10.1016/j.prevetmed.2022.105579]

[26]   Fox NJ, Smith LA, Houdijk JGM, Athanasiadou S, Hutchings MR. Ubiquitous parasites drive a 33% increase in methane yield from livestock. Int J Parasitol 2018; Nov;48(13): 1017-21.

[27]   Thanasuwan S, Piratae S, Tankrathok A. Prevalence of gastrointestinal parasites in cattle in Kalasin Province, Thailand. Vet World 2021; Aug;14(8): 2091-6.
[http://dx.doi.org/10.14202/vetworld.2021.2091-2096]

[28]   Lopes LB, *et al.* Economic impacts of parasitic diseases in cattle 2016.
[http://dx.doi.org/10.1079/PAVSNNR201510051]

[29]   Baihaqi Z.A, Widiyono I, Nurcahyo W. Prevalence of gastrointestinal worms in Wonosobo and thin-tailed sheep on the slope of Mount Sumbing, Central Java, Indonesia. Vet World 2019; 12(11): 1866-71.

[30]   Navarre, C. B., New era of parasite control—BMPs for beef cattle. In AABP Proceedings of the Annual Conference 2019; 52(2): 103-9.
[http://dx.doi.org/10.21423/aabppro20197105]

[31]   Navarre CBJVCFAP. Epidemiology and control of gastrointestinal nematodes of cattle in southern climates 2020.
[http://dx.doi.org/10.1016/j.cvfa.2019.11.006]

[32]   Hildreth MB, McKenzie JBJVCFAP. Epidemiology and control of gastrointestinal nematodes of cattle in northern climates 2020.
[http://dx.doi.org/10.1016/j.cvfa.2019.11.008]

[33]   Yessinou RE, Adoligbe C, Akpo Y, Adinci J, Youssao Abdou Karim I, Farougou S. Sensitivity of Different Cattle Breeds to the Infestation of Cattle Ticks Amblyomma variegatum, Rhipicephalus microplus, and Hyalomma spp. on the Natural Pastures of Opkara Farm, Benin. J Parasitol Res 2018; Mar 25(2018): 2570940.

[34]   Oliveira M, *et al.* Resistance of beef cattle of two genetic groups to ectoparasites and gastrointestinal nematodes in the state of São Paulo, Brazil 2013.
[http://dx.doi.org/10.1016/j.vetpar.2013.06.021]

[35]   Riley D, Sawyer J, Craig TJVP. Shedding and characterization of gastrointestinal nematodes of

growing beef heifers in Central Texas 2020.
[http://dx.doi.org/10.1016/j.vpoa.2020.100024]

[36] Smith HJCJoCM. On the development of gastrointestinal parasitism in bovine yearlings 1970.

[37] Ciordia HJAjovr. Occurrence of gastrointestinal parasites in Georgia cattle 1975.

[38] Kumar N, *et al.* Internal parasite management in grazing livestock 2013.
[http://dx.doi.org/10.1007/s12639-012-0215-z]

[39] Yazwinski TA, *et al.* Current status of parasite control at the feed yard 2015.
[http://dx.doi.org/10.1016/j.cvfa.2015.03.005]

[40] Hayward AD, Skuce PJ, McNeilly TNJIJfP. The influence of liver fluke infection on production in sheep and cattle: a meta-analysis 2021.
[http://dx.doi.org/10.1016/j.ijpara.2021.02.006]

[41] Nicaretta JE, *et al.* Rhipicephalus microplus seasonal dynamic in a Cerrado biome, Brazil: An update data considering the global warming 2021.
[http://dx.doi.org/10.1016/j.vetpar.2021.109506]

[42] Vercruysse J, Claerebout EJVp. Treatment vs non-treatment of helminth infections in cattle: defining the threshold 2001.
[http://dx.doi.org/10.1016/S0304-4017(01)00431-9]

[43] Abbas RZ, *et al.* Acaricide resistance in cattle ticks and approaches to its management: the state of play 2014.
[http://dx.doi.org/10.1016/j.vetpar.2014.03.006]

[44] Kumar R, Sharma AK, Ghosh SJVp. Menace of acaricide resistance in cattle tick, Rhipicephalus microplus in India: Status and possible mitigation strategies 2020.
[http://dx.doi.org/10.1016/j.vetpar.2019.108993]

[45] Dzemo WD, Thekisoe O, Vudriko PJH. Development of acaricide resistance in tick populations of cattle: A systematic review and meta-analysis 2022.
[http://dx.doi.org/10.1016/j.heliyon.2022.e08718]

[46] Kaplan RM, Vidyashankar ANJVp. An inconvenient truth: global worming and anthelmintic resistance 2012.
[http://dx.doi.org/10.1016/j.vetpar.2011.11.048]

[47] Coles G, Stafford K, MacKay PJTVR. Ivermectin-resistant Cooperia species from calves on a farm in Somer 1998.

[48] Craig TMJVCFAP. Gastrointestinal nematodes, diagnosis and control 2018.
[http://dx.doi.org/10.1016/j.cvfa.2017.10.008]

[49] Hotez, P., Bethony, J., Diemert, D. *et al.* Developing vaccines to combat hookworm infection and intestinal schistosomiasis. Nat Rev Microbiol 2010; 8: 814-26.
[http://dx.doi.org/10.1016/B978-0-7020-3935-5.00116-6]

[50] Soulsby, E.J.L. Helminths, Arthropods and Protozoa of Domesticated Animals (6th Edition of Monnig's Veterinary Helminthology & Entomology). Baillière Tindall & Cassell Ltd 1968; 176-325.

[51] Yacob H, Ataklty H, Kumsa BJER. Major ectoparasites of cattle in and around Mekelle, northern Ethiopia 2008.
[http://dx.doi.org/10.1111/j.1748-5967.2008.00148.x]

[52] Iqbal A, *et al.* Epizootiology of Ectoparasitic Fauna Infesting Selected Domestic Cattle Population of Punjab, Pakistan. 2014.

[53] Poulin R, Krasnov BR, Mouillot DJTip. Host specificity in phylogenetic and geographic space 2011.
[http://dx.doi.org/10.1016/j.pt.2011.05.003]

[54] Kumar P, Kumar P, Mandal D, Velayutham R. The emerging role of Deubiquitinases (DUBs) in

parasites: A foresight review. Front Cell Infect Microbiol 2022; Sep 27(12): 985178.

[55]   Craig TM. Helminth Parasites of the Ruminant Gastrointestinal Tract 2009.
       [http://dx.doi.org/10.1016/B978-141603591-6.10022-3]

[56]   Jex AR, *et al.* The mitochondrial genomes of Ancylostoma caninum and Bunostomum
       phlebotomum–two hookworms of animal health and zoonotic importance 2009.
       [http://dx.doi.org/10.1186/1471-2164-10-79]

[57]   Stromberg BE, Gasbarre LC, Waite A, *et al.* Cooperia punctata: Effect on cattle productivity? Vet
       Parasitol 2012; 183(3-4): 284-91.
       [http://dx.doi.org/10.1016/j.vetpar.2011.07.030] [PMID: 21821358]

[58]   Barone CD, *et al.* Wild ruminants as reservoirs of domestic livestock gastrointestinal nematodes 2020.
       [http://dx.doi.org/10.1016/j.vetpar.2020.109041]

[59]   Pinilla León JC, Delgado NU, Florez AA. Prevalence of gastrointestinal parasites in cattle and sheep
       in three municipalities in the Colombian Northeastern Mountain. Vet World 2019; Jan;12(1): 48-54.

[60]   Dank M, *et al.* Association between Dictyocaulus viviparus status and milk production parameters in
       Dutch dairy herds 2015.
       [http://dx.doi.org/10.3168/jds.2015-9408]

[61]   Hagberg M. Immune cell responses to the cattle lungworm, Dictyocaulus viviparus. 2008.

[62]   Vázquez A., Alda P., Lounnas M., Sabourin É., Alba A., Pointier J. Lymnaeid snails hosts of fasciola
       hepatica and fasciola gigantica (trematoda: digenea): a worldwide review. CABI Reviews 2019; 1-15.
       [http://dx.doi.org/10.1079/pavsnnr201813062]

[63]   Acha PN, Szyfres B. Zoonosis y enfermedades transmisibles comunes al hombre ya los animales:
       clamidiosis, rickettsiosis y virosis 3. Pan American Health Organization 2003.

[64]   Rizwan M, *et al.* Prevalence of fascioliasis in livestock and humans in Pakistan: A systematic review
       and meta-analysis 2022.
       [http://dx.doi.org/10.3390/tropicalmed7070126]

[65]   Garcia-Campos A, Power C, O'Shaughnessy J, Browne C, Lawlor A, McCarthy G, O'Neill EJ, de
       Waal T. One-year parasitological screening of stray dogs and cats in County Dublin, Ireland.
       Parasitology 2019; May;146(6): 746-52.

[66]   Mitchell GJIP. Update on fasciolosis in cattle and sheep 2002.
       [http://dx.doi.org/10.1136/inpract.24.7.378]

[67]   Kaplan RMJVT. Fasciola hepatica: a review of the economic impact in cattle and considerations for
       control 2001.

[68]   da Costa RA, Corbellini LG, Castro-Janer E, Riet-Correa F. Evaluation of losses in carcasses of cattle
       naturally infected with Fasciola hepatica: effects on weight by age range and on carcass quality
       parameters. Int J Parasitol 2019; 49(11): 867-72.
       [http://dx.doi.org/10.1016/j.ijpara.2019.06.005] [PMID: 31545963]

[69]   Ballweber LR. PARASITES | Internal. In: Jensen WK, Ed. Encyclopedia of Meat Sciences. Elsevier
       2004; pp. 983-9.
       [http://dx.doi.org/10.1016/B0-12-464970-X/00040-4]

[70]   Arsenopoulos KV, *et al.* Haemonchosis: A challenging parasitic infection of sheep and goats 2021.
       [http://dx.doi.org/10.3390/ani11020363]

[71]   Gelberg HB. Alimentary System and the Peritoneum, Omentum, Mesentery, and Peritoneal Cavity1.
       In: Zachary JF, Ed. Pathologic Basis of Veterinary Disease. Mosby 2017; pp. 324-411.e1.
       [http://dx.doi.org/10.1016/B978-0-323-35775-3.00007-2]

[72]   Alhaboubi AR, Fadhil AI, Feidhel SRJVW. Prevalence and molecular identification of Nematodirus
       helvetianus in camels in Iraq 2021.

[http://dx.doi.org/10.14202/vetworld.2021.1299-1302]

[73]   James E. Miller, R.M.K., D.G. Pugh, *Internal Parasites*. In: Pugh ANBDG, Ed. Sheep and Goat Medicine. W.B. Saunders 2012; pp. 106-25.

[74]   Szyszka O, *et al.* Do the changes in the behaviours of cattle during parasitism with Ostertagia ostertagi have a potential diagnostic value? 2013.
         [http://dx.doi.org/10.1016/j.vetpar.2012.10.023]

[75]   Lützelschwab CM, Fiel CA, Pedonesse SI, Najle R, Rodríguez E, Steffan PE, Saumell C, Fusé L, Iglesias L. Arrested development of Ostertagia ostertagi: effect of the exposure of infective larvae to natural spring conditions of the humid pampa (Argentina). Vet Parasitol 2005; Feb 28;127(3-4): 253-62.

[76]   Mason C, *et al.* Disease associated with immature paramphistome infection in sheep 2012.
         [http://dx.doi.org/10.1136/vr.e2368]

[77]   Devos J, *et al.* Paramphistomosis in sheep; natural infection of lambs by Calicophoron daubneyi 2013.

[78]   Rangel-Ruiz L, Albores-Brahms S, Gamboa-Aguilar JJVp. Seasonal trends of Paramphistomum cervi in Tabasco, Mexico 2003.

[79]   Delafosse A. Rumen fluke infections (Paramphistomidae) in diarrhoeal cattle in western France and association with production parameters. Vet Parasitol Reg Stud Reports 2022; Apr;29: 100694.
         [http://dx.doi.org/10.1016/j.vprsr.2022.100694]

[80]   Khedri J, Radfar MH, Nikbakht B, Zahedi R, Hosseini M, Azizzadeh M, Borji H. Parasitic causes of meat and organs in cattle at four slaughterhouses in Sistan-Baluchestan Province, Southeastern Iran between 2008 and 2016. Vet Med Sci 2021; Jul;7(4): 1230-6.

[81]   Chowdhury T, *et al.* Coproscopic and slaughter house study of paramphistomiasis in cattle at sylhet division of Bangladesh 2019.

[82]   Mondal MM-H, *et al.* Examination of gastrointestinal helminth in livestock grazing in grassland of Bangladesh 2000.
         [http://dx.doi.org/10.3347/kjp.2000.38.3.187]

[83]   Cardia DFF, Rocha-Oliveira RA, Tsunemi MH, Amarante AFT. Immune response and performance of growing Santa Ines lambs to artificial *Trichostrongylus colubriformis* infections. Vet Parasitol 2011; 182(2-4): 248-58.
         [http://dx.doi.org/10.1016/j.vetpar.2011.05.017] [PMID: 21641720]

[84]   de Miranda RL, de Castro JR, Olegário MMM, *et al.* Oocysts of Hepatozoon canis in *Rhipicephalus* (Boophilus) *microplus* collected from a naturally infected dog. Vet Parasitol 2011; 177(3-4): 392-6.
         [http://dx.doi.org/10.1016/j.vetpar.2011.01.044] [PMID: 21324597]

[85]   Miraballes C, Riet-Correa F. A review of the history of research and control of *Rhipicephalus* (Boophilus) *microplus*, babesiosis and anaplasmosis in Uruguay. Exp Appl Acarol 2018; 75(4): 383-98.
         [http://dx.doi.org/10.1007/s10493-018-0278-3] [PMID: 30083875]

[86]   Rodríguez-Vivas RI. P.-C.L., Rosado-Aguilar JA, Ojeda-Chi MM, Trinidad-Martinez I, Miller RJ, Li AY, de León AP, Guerrero F, Klafke G., *Rhipicephalus* (Boophilus) microplus resistant to acaricides and ivermectin in cattle farms of Mexico. Rev Bras Parasitol Vet 2014; 113(22)

[87]   Guerrero FD, Andreotti R, Bendele KG, *et al. Rhipicephalus* (Boophilus) *microplus* aquaporin as an effective vaccine antigen to protect against cattle tick infestations. Parasit Vectors 2014; 7(1): 475.
         [PMID: 25306139]

[88]   Jain P, Satapathy T, Pandey RK. *Rhipicephalus microplus*: A parasite threatening cattle health and consequences of herbal acaricides for upliftment of livelihood of cattle rearing communities in Chhattisgarh. Biocatal Agric Biotechnol 2020; 26: 101611.
         [http://dx.doi.org/10.1016/j.bcab.2020.101611]

[89] Tuppurainen ESM, Lubinga JC, Stoltsz WH, *et al.* Mechanical transmission of lumpy skin disease virus by *Rhipicephalus appendiculatus* male ticks. Epidemiol Infect 2013; 141(2): 425-30.
[http://dx.doi.org/10.1017/S0950268812000805] [PMID: 22717050]

[90] Castro J, Cunningham M, Dolan T, Dransfield R, Newson R, Young A. Effects on cattle of artificial infestations with the tick Rhipicephalus appendiculatus 1985.
[http://dx.doi.org/10.1017/S0031182000048988]

[91] Njaa BL. The Ear1. In: Zachary JF, Ed. Pathologic Basis of Veterinary Disease. Mosby 2017; pp. 1223-1264.e1.
[http://dx.doi.org/10.1016/B978-0-323-35775-3.00020-5]

[92] Norval R, *et al.* The effects of the bont tick, Amblyomma hebraeum, on milk production of Sanga and Sanga x Brahman cattle 1997.
[http://dx.doi.org/10.1111/j.1365-2915.1997.tb00304.x]

[93] Bryson NR, Horak IG, Venter EH, Yunker CE. Collection of free-living nymphs and adults of Amblyomma hebraeum (Acari: Ixodidae) with pheromone/carbon dioxide traps at 5 different ecological sites in heartwater endemic regions of South Africa. Exp Appl Acarol 2000; 24(12): 971-82.

[94] Jongejan F, *et al.* Amblyomma hebraeum is the predominant tick species on goats in the Mnisi Community Area of Mpumalanga Province South Africa and is co-infected with Ehrlichia ruminantium and Rickettsia africae 2020.
[http://dx.doi.org/10.1186/s13071-020-04059-5]

[95] Rodrigues V, *et al.* Immunomodulatory effects of Amblyomma variegatum saliva on bovine cells: characterization of cellular responses and identification of molecular determinants 2018.
[http://dx.doi.org/10.3389/fcimb.2017.00521]

[96] Tolleson DR, Teel PD, Stuth JW, Strey OF, Welsh TH Jr, Carstens GE, Longnecker MT, Banik KK, Prince SD. Effects of a lone star tick (Amblyomma americanum) burden on performance and metabolic indicators in growing beef steers. Vet Parasitol 2010; Oct 11;173(1-2): 99-106.

[97] Tolleson D.R. Tolleson, J.W. Stuth, P.D. Teel, G. Carstens, T.H. Welsh Effects of a Lone Star tick (Amblyomma americanum) burden on growing beef steers: Near infrared spectra of feces. Abstract J Anim Sci 2004; 2004: 82.

[98] Gilbert LJAroe. The impacts of climate change on ticks and tick-borne disease risk 2021.
[http://dx.doi.org/10.1146/annurev-ento-052720-094533]

[99] Carvalho-Costa TM, *et al.* Immunosuppressive effects of Amblyomma cajennense tick saliva on murine bone marrow-derived dendritic cells 2015.
[http://dx.doi.org/10.1186/s13071-015-0634-7]

[100] Ndlovhu DN. Alternative methods used by small-holder farmers to control ticks and bovine dermatophilosis and the impact of a changing interface of Amblyomma ticks on dermatophilosis in Zimbabwe. University of Fort Hare 2014.

[101] Goddard J, Varela-Stokes AS.Role of the lone star tick, Amblyomma americanum (L.), in human and animal diseases. Vet Parasitol 2009; Mar 9;160(1-2): 1-12.

[102] Černý J, *et al.* Management options for Ixodes ricinus-associated pathogens: a review of prevention strategies 2020.

[103] Boland H, Scaglia G, Umemura KJTPAS. 2008.

[104] Jensen KM, *et al.* Variation in the load of the horn fly, Haematobia irritans, in cattle herds is determined by the presence or absence of individual heifers 2004.
[http://dx.doi.org/10.1111/j.0269-283X.2004.00506.x]

[105] Schafaschek ALL, Portugal TB, Filus A, de Moraes A, Guaraldo AC, Pritsch IC, Molento MB. Transient Threshold Abundance of Haematobia Irritans (Linnaeus, 1758) In Cattle Under Integrated

Farming Systems. International Journal of Plant, Animal and Environmental Sciences 2021; 11: 322-41.

[106] Oyarzún-Ruiz P, Cifuentes-Castro C, Varas F, Grandón-Ojeda A, Cicchino A, Mironov S, et al. Helminth and ectoparasitic faunas of the Harris's hawk, Parabuteo unicinctus (Accipitriformes: Accipitridae), in Chile: new data on host-parasite associations for Neotropical raptors. Braz J Vet Parasitol 2022; 31(3): e007522.
[http://dx.doi.org/10.1590/S1984-29612022046]

[107] Showler AJ, Kubofcik J, Ricciardi A, Nutman TB. Differences in the Clinical and Laboratory Features of Imported Onchocerciasis in Endemic Individuals and Temporary Residents. Am J Trop Med Hyg 2019; May;100(5): 1216-22.

[108] Shea-Donohue T, Qin B, Smith A. Parasites, nutrition, immune responses and biology of metabolic tissues. Parasite Immunol 2017; May;39(5): 12422.

[109] Lymbery AJ, Smit NJ. Conservation of parasites: A primer. Int J Parasitol Parasites Wildl 2023; Jul 3(21): 255-63.
[http://dx.doi.org/10.1016/j.ijppaw.2023.07.001] [PMID: 37483309]

[110] Perttu R, *et al.* Effects of mesh leggings on fly pressure and fly avoidance behaviors of pastured dairy cows 2020.
[http://dx.doi.org/10.3168/jds.2019-17267]

[111] Robertson, Lucy Jane, Solveig Jore, Vidar Lund and Danica Grahek□Ogden. Risk assessment of parasites in Norwegian drinking water: opportunities and challenges. Food and Waterborne Parasitology 2021; 22: e00112.

[112] Pérez de León AA, Mitchell RD III, Watson DW. Ectoparasites of Cattle. Vet Clin North Am Food Anim Pract 2020; 36(1): 173-85.
[http://dx.doi.org/10.1016/j.cvfa.2019.12.004] [PMID: 32029183]

[113] Frisch JE, O'Neill CJ, Kelly MJ. Using genetics to control cattle parasites-the Rockhampton experience. Int J Parasitol 2000; Mar;30(3): 253-64.

[114] Costa-Junior LM, Chaudhry UN, Silva CR, Sousa DM, Silva NC, Cutrim-Júnior JAA, Brito DRB, Sargison ND. Nemabiome metabarcoding reveals differences between gastrointestinal nematode species infecting co-grazed sheep and goats. Vet Parasitol 2021; Jan;289: 109339.

[115] Osorio J, *et al.* Role of ivermectin in the treatment of severe orbital myiasis due to Cochliomyia hominivorax 2006.
[http://dx.doi.org/10.1086/507038]

[116] Nafstad O, Grønstøl H. G.H., *Eradication of lice in cattle.* Acta Vet Scand 2001; 42(1): 81.
[http://dx.doi.org/10.1186/1751-0147-42-81] [PMID: 11455889]

[117] Hornok, S., Fedák, A., Baska, F. et al. Bovine besnoitiosis emerging in Central-Eastern Europe, Hungary. Parasites Vectors 2014; 7: 20.
[http://dx.doi.org/10.1186/1756-3305-7-20]

[118] Holdsworth P, Rehbein S, Jonsson NN, Peter R, Vercruysse J, Fourie J. World Association for the Advancement of Veterinary Parasitology (WAAVP) second edition: Guideline for evaluating the efficacy of parasiticides against ectoparasites of ruminants. Vet Parasitol 2022; Feb;302: 109613.
[http://dx.doi.org/10.1016/j.vetpar.2021.109613]

[119] Iritani R, Sato T. Host-Manipulation by Trophically Transmitted Parasites: The Switcher-Paradigm. Trends Parasitol 2018; Nov;34(11): 934-44.

[120] Rony S, *et al.* Epidemiology of ectoparasitic infestations in cattle at Bhawal forest area. Gazipur 2010; 8(1): 27-33.

[121] Mullens B, *et al.* Feeding and survival of Culicoides sonorensis on cattle treated with permethrin or pirimiphos-methyl 2000.

[http://dx.doi.org/10.1046/j.1365-2915.2000.00243.x]

[122]   Mullen G.R., Murphree C.S. Medical and Veterinary Entomology. Elsevier; San Diego, CA, USA Biting midges (Ceratopogonidae) 2019; 213-36.

[123]   Riglar DT, Richard D, Wilson DW, Boyle MJ, Dekiwadia C, Turnbull L, Angrisano F, Marapana DS, Rogers KL, Whitchurch CB, Beeson JG, Cowman AF, Ralph SA, Baum J. Super-resolution dissection of coordinated events during malaria parasite invasion of the human erythrocyte. Cell Host Microbe 2011; Jan 20;9(1): 9-20.

[124]   Lehiy CJ, *et al.* Physiological and immunological responses to Culicoides sonorensis blood-feeding: a murine model 2018.
[http://dx.doi.org/10.1186/s13071-018-2935-0]

[125]   Mia MM, Hasan M, Chowdhury MR. A systematic review and meta-analysis on prevalence and epidemiological risk factors of zoonotic Fascioliasis infection among the ruminants in Bangladesh. Heliyon 2021; Nov 27;7(12): e08479.
[http://dx.doi.org/10.1016/j.heliyon.2021.e08479]

[126]   Francesconi F, Lupi O. Myiasis. Clin Microbiol Rev 2012; Jan;25(1): 79-105.
[http://dx.doi.org/10.1128/CMR.00010-11]

[127]   Marcogliese DJ, Pietrock M. Combined effects of parasites and contaminants on animal health: parasites do matter. Trends Parasitol 2011; Mar;27(3): 123-30.

[128]   Rashidi S, Mansouri R, Ali-Hassanzadeh M, Ghani E, Barazesh A, Karimazar M, Nguewa P, Carrera Silva EA. Highlighting the interplay of microRNAs from Leishmania parasites and infected-host cells. Parasitology 2021; Oct;148(12): 1434-46.

[129]   Wang, N., Wang K, Liu Y, Zhang X, Zhao J, Zhang S, & Zhang L. Molecular characterization of Cryptosporidium spp., Enterocytozoon bieneusi and Giardia duodenalis in laboratory rodents in China. Parasite 2022; 29: 46.

[130]   Tachikawa, Hiroyuki, Grygier, Mark J., and Cairns, Stephen D. Live specimens of the parasite Petrarca madreporae (Crustacea: Ascothoracida) from the deep-water coral Madrepora oculata in Japan, with remarks on the structure of its spectacular galls. Journal of Marine Science and Technology 2020; 28(1): 58-64.

[131]   Kumar N, Rao TKS, Varghese A, Rathor VS. Internal parasite management in grazing livestock. J Parasit Dis 2013; 37(2): 151-7.
[http://dx.doi.org/10.1007/s12639-012-0215-z] [PMID: 24431559]

[132]   Stuedemann J, *et al.* Bermudagrass management in the Southern Piedmont USA: V: Gastrointestinal parasite control in cattle 2004.

[133]   Younie D, *et al.* Grassland management and parasite control. Wallingford, Oxon, UK: CABI Publishing 2004; pp. 308-28.

[134]   Bork EW, *et al.* Comparative pasture management on Canadian cattle ranches with and without adaptive multipaddock grazing 2021.
[http://dx.doi.org/10.1016/j.rama.2021.04.010]

[135]   Johnson PT, Hoverman JT. Heterogeneous hosts: how variation in host size, behaviour and immunity affects parasite aggregation. J Anim Ecol 2014; Sep;83(5): 1103-2.

[136]   Lambert MG, Clark DA, Litherland AJ. Advances in pasture management for animal productivity and health. N Z Vet J 2004; 52(6): 311-9.
[http://dx.doi.org/10.1080/00480169.2004.36447] [PMID: 15768131]

[137]   Hejcmanová P, *et al.* Behavioural patterns of heifers under intensive and extensive continuous grazing on species-rich pasture in the Czech Republic 2009.
[http://dx.doi.org/10.1016/j.applanim.2009.01.003]

[138]   Scanlan JC, McIvor JG, Bray SG, *et al.* Resting pastures to improve land condition in northern

Australia: guidelines based on the literature and simulation modelling. Rangeland J 2014; 36(5): 429-43.
[http://dx.doi.org/10.1071/RJ14071]

[139] Holechek JL, *et al.* Short-duration grazing: the facts in 1999-2000. Rangelands. 2000;22(1):19-23.
[http://dx.doi.org/10.2458/azu_rangelands_v22i1_holechek]

[140] Colvin AF, *et al.* Intensive rotational grazing assists control of gastrointestinal nematodosis of sheep in a cool temperate environment with summer-dominant rainfall 2008.
[http://dx.doi.org/10.1016/j.vetpar.2008.01.014]

[141] Sobsey DM, *et al.* Pathogens in animal wastes and the impacts of waste management practices on their survival, transport, and fate. In: Animal Agriculture and the Environment, National Center for Manure & Animal Waste Management White Papers. St. Joseph (MI): ASABE; 2006.

[142] Malomo GA, *et al.* Sustainable animal manure management strategies and practices 2018.
[http://dx.doi.org/10.5772/intechopen.78645]

[143] McHardy IH, *et al.* Detection of intestinal protozoa in the clinical laboratory 2014.
[http://dx.doi.org/10.1128/JCM.02877-13]

[144] Das M, *et al.* Gastrointestinal parasitic infections in cattle and swamp buffalo of Guwahati, Assam, India 2018.
[http://dx.doi.org/10.18805/ijar.B-3427]

[145] Income N, *et al.* Helminth infections in cattle and goats in Kanchanaburi, Thailand, with focus on strongyle nematode infections 2021.
[http://dx.doi.org/10.3390/vetsci8120324]

[146] Hastutiek P, *et al.* Prevalence and diversity of gastrointestinal protozoa in Madura cattle at Bangkalan Regency, East Java, Indonesia 2019.
[http://dx.doi.org/10.14202/vetworld.2019.198-204]

[147] Stafford K, Coles GJVR. Nematode control practices and anthelmintic resistance in dairy calves in the south west of England 1999.
[http://dx.doi.org/10.1136/vr.144.24.659]

[148] Pomroy WJNZvj. Anthelmintic resistance in New Zealand: a perspective on recent findings and options for the future 2006.
[http://dx.doi.org/10.1080/00480169.2006.36709]

[149] Charlier J, Vercruysse J, Morgan E, van Dijk J, Williams DJ. Recent advances in the diagnosis, impact on production and prediction of Fasciola hepatica in cattle. Parasitology 2014; Mar;141(3): 326-5.

[150] Högberg N, Hessle A, Lidfors L, Baltrušis P, Claerebout E, Höglund J. Subclinical nematode parasitism affects activity and rumination patterns in first-season grazing cattle. Animal 2021; Jun;15(6): 100237.

[151] Cabaret JJP. Pro and cons of targeted selective treatment against digestive-tract strongyles of ruminants 2008.
[http://dx.doi.org/10.1051/parasite/2008153506]

[152] Cooke AS, *et al.* Modelling the impact of targeted anthelmintic treatment of cattle on dung fauna 2017.
[http://dx.doi.org/10.1016/j.etap.2017.07.012]

[153] Van Wyk JA, Hoste H, Kaplan RM, Besier RB. Targeted selective treatment for worm management--how do we sell rational programs to farmers? Vet Parasitol 2006; Jul 31;139(4): 336-46.

[154] Burke J, *et al.* Interaction between copper oxide wire particles and Duddingtonia flagrans in lambs 2005.
[http://dx.doi.org/10.1016/j.vetpar.2005.06.018]

[155] Worku M, Franco R, Baldwin KJAoBS. Efficacy of garlic as an anthelmintic in adult Boer goats 2009.

[http://dx.doi.org/10.2298/ABS0901135W]

[156] Athanasiadou S, Githiori J, Kyriazakis IJA. Medicinal plants for helminth parasite control: facts and fiction 2007.
[http://dx.doi.org/10.1017/S1751731107000730]

[157] Manthri S, Sravanthi KC, Sidagonde SJJP. Anthelmintic activity of castor oil and mustard oil 2011.

[158] Lynn E. Sollenberger, G.E.A., Marcelo O. Wallau, Managing grazing in forage–livestock systems. In: Monte Rouquette GEA, Ed. Management Strategies for Sustainable Cattle Production in Southern Pastures. Academic Press 2020; pp. 77-100.

[159] Myers GH. Strategies to control internal parasites in cattle and swine. J Anim Sci 1988; Jun;66(6): 1555-64.

[160] Veronika Maurer PH. Hubertus Hertzberg, Reducing anthelmintic use for the control of internal parasites in organic livestock systems. In: Cooper UNJ, Leifert C, Eds. In Woodhead Publishing Series in Food Science, Technology and Nutrition, Handbook of Organic Food Safety and Quality. Woodhead Publishing 2007; pp. 221-40.
[http://dx.doi.org/10.1533/9781845693411.2.221]

[161] Holechek JL. G.H., Molinar F, Galt D., Grazing intensity: critique and approach. Rangelands Archives 1998; 20(5): 15-8.

[162] Fenetahun Y, *et al.* Impact of Grazing Intensity on Soil Properties in Teltele Rangeland. Ethiopia 2021; p. 9.

[163] Sobsey DM, *et al.* Pathogens in animal wastes and the impacts of waste management practices on their survival, transport, and fate. In: Animal Agriculture and the Environment, National Center for Manure & Animal Waste Management White Papers. St. Joseph (MI): ASABE; 2006.

[164] Hedberg-Alm Y, Penell J, Riihimäki M, Osterman-Lind E, Nielsen MK, Tydén E. Parasite Occurrence and Parasite Management in Swedish Horses Presenting with Gastrointestinal Disease—A Case–Control Study. Animals 2020; 10(4): 638.

[165] Proudman C, Matthews JJIP. Control of intestinal parasites in horses 2000.
[http://dx.doi.org/10.1136/inpract.22.2.90]

[166] Thamsborg SM, Roepstorff A, Larsen MJVp. Integrated and biological control of parasites in organic and conventional production systems 1999.
[http://dx.doi.org/10.1016/S0304-4017(99)00035-7]

[167] Christensen KJSA, Illustration O. Internal parasites of the goat 2005.

[168] Luginbuhl JJNCSU. Gastrointestinal parasite management of meat goats. Raleigh 1998.

[169] Mohamed AE, Ghandour ZM, Al-Karawi MA, Yasawy MI, Sammak B. Gastrointestinal parasites presentations and histological diagnosis from endoscopic biopsies and surgical specimens. Saudi Med J 2000; Jul;21(7): 629-34.

[170] Shadbolt T, Pocknell A, Sainsbury AW, Egerton-Read S, Blake DP. Molecular identification of Sarcocystis wobeseri-like parasites in a new intermediate host species, the white-tailed sea eagle (Haliaeetus albicilla). Parasitol Res 2021; May;120(5): 1845-50.

[171] Whittier WD, Zajac AM, Umberger SH. Control of internal parasites in sheep 2009.

[172] Haskell M, *et al.* Housing system, milk production, and zero-grazing effects on lameness and leg injury in dairy cows 2006.
[http://dx.doi.org/10.3168/jds.S0022-0302(06)72472-9]

[173] Mohammed R, *et al.* Grazing cows are more efficient than zero-grazed and grass silage-fed cows in milk rumenic acid production 2009.
[http://dx.doi.org/10.3168/jds.2008-1613]

[174] Rosenzweig C, *et al.* Climate change and extreme weather events-Implications for food production,

plant diseases, and pests 2001.

[175] Stromberg BE, Moon RD. Parasite control in calves and growing heifers. Vet Clin North Am Food Anim Pract 2008; 24(1): 105-16.
[http://dx.doi.org/10.1016/j.cvfa.2007.12.003] [PMID: 18299034]

[176] Madke P, *et al.* Study of behavioural and physiological changes of crossbred cows under different shelter management practices 2010.

[177] Pedreira J, *et al.* Prevalences of gastrointestinal parasites in sheep and parasite-control practices in NW Spain 2006.
[http://dx.doi.org/10.1016/j.prevetmed.2006.01.011]

[178] Malan F, *et al.* Wildlife parasites: lessons for parasite control in livestock 1997.
[http://dx.doi.org/10.1016/S0304-4017(97)00030-7]

[179] Raza A, Rand J, Qamar AG, Jabbar A, Kopp S. Gastrointestinal Parasites in Shelter Dogs: Occurrence, Pathology, Treatment and Risk to Shelter Workers. Animals (Basel) 2018; 8(7): 108.
[http://dx.doi.org/10.3390/ani8070108] [PMID: 30004469]

[180] Willms WD, *et al.* Effects of water quality on cattle performance 2002.

[181] Geary TG, Conder GA, Bishop BJTip. The changing landscape of antiparasitic drug discovery for veterinary medicine 2004.
[http://dx.doi.org/10.1016/j.pt.2004.08.003]

[182] Vercruysse J, Rew RS. Macrocyclic lactones in antiparasitic therapy. CAB International 2002.
[http://dx.doi.org/10.1079/9780851996172.0000]

[183] Maqbool I, Wani ZA, Shahardar RA, Allaie IM, Shah MM. Integrated parasite management with special reference to gastro-intestinal nematodes. J Parasit Dis 2017; Mar;41(1): 1-8.

[184] McKenzie VJ, Townsend AR. Parasitic and Infectious Disease Responses to Changing Global Nutrient Cycles. EcoHealth 2007; 4(4): 384-96.
[http://dx.doi.org/10.1007/s10393-007-0131-3]

[185] Conder G, Johnson SJTJop. Viability of infective larvae of Haemonchus contortus, Ostertagia ostertagi, and Trichostrongylus colubriformis following exsheathment by various techniques 1996.
[http://dx.doi.org/10.2307/3284123]

[186] Perry BD, Randolph TF. Improving the assessment of the economic impact of parasitic diseases and of their control in production animals. Vet Parasitol 1999; 84(): 145-68.

[187] Gupta O, *et al.* Calcium oxide as grain protectant. Note 1980. India

[188] Mukerjee RJIvj. Toxicity of certain chemicals on the larval stages of some amphistomes of domesticated animals 1973.

[189] Howell J, *et al.* Control of gastrointestinal parasite larvae of ruminant using nitrogen fertilizer, limestone and sodium hypochlorite solutions 1999.
[http://dx.doi.org/10.1016/S0921-4488(98)00186-2]

[190] Ingale S, *et al.* Nutrition-parasite interaction-a review 2010.

[191] Spears JWJPotns. Micronutrients and immune function in cattle 2000.
[http://dx.doi.org/10.1017/S0029665100000835]

[192] Hughes S, Kelly PJPi. Interactions of malnutrition and immune impairment, with specific reference to immunity against parasites 2006.
[http://dx.doi.org/10.1111/j.1365-3024.2006.00897.x]

[193] Rahmati-Holasoo, H., Azizzadeh, M., Ebrahimzadeh Mousavi, H. Histopathological, morphological, and molecular characterization of fish-borne zoonotic parasite Eustrongylides Excisus infecting Northern pike (Esox lucius) in Iran. BMC Vet Res 2024; 20: 291.

[194] McGill JL, Kelly SM, Guerra-Maupome M, *et al.* Vitamin A deficiency impairs the immune response to intranasal vaccination and RSV infection in neonatal calves. Sci Rep 2019; 9(1): 15157.
[http://dx.doi.org/10.1038/s41598-019-51684-x] [PMID: 31641172]

[195] Villamor E, Fawzi WWJCmr. Effects of vitamin A supplementation on immune responses and correlation with clinical outcomes 2005.
[http://dx.doi.org/10.1128/CMR.18.3.446-464.2005]

[196] Amimo JO, *et al.* Immune impairment associated with vitamin a deficiency: Insights from clinical studies and animal model research 2022.
[http://dx.doi.org/10.3390/nu14235038]

[197] Coop R, Kyriazakis IJVp. Nutrition–parasite interaction 1999.
[http://dx.doi.org/10.1016/S0304-4017(99)00070-9]

[198] Stephensen CBJAron. Vitamin A, infection, and immune function 2001.

[199] Stephensen CB, *et al.* Vitamin A enhances *in vitro* Th2 development *via* retinoid X receptor pathway. 2002.
[http://dx.doi.org/10.4049/jimmunol.168.9.4495]

[200] Herdt TH, Stowe HDJVCoNAFAP. Fat-soluble vitamin nutrition for dairy cattle 1991.
[http://dx.doi.org/10.1016/S0749-0720(15)30796-9]

[201] Cunningham-Rundles S, *et al.* Mechanisms of nutrient modulation of the immune response 2005.
[http://dx.doi.org/10.1016/j.jaci.2005.04.036]

[202] Scott ME, Koski KGJTJon. Zinc deficiency impairs immune responses against parasitic nematode infections at intestinal and systemic sites 2000.
[http://dx.doi.org/10.1093/jn/130.5.1412S]

[203] Miller WJJJoDS. Zinc nutrition of cattle: a review 1970.
[http://dx.doi.org/10.3168/jds.S0022-0302(70)86355-X]

[204] Cook-Mills J, *et al.* Possible roles for zinc in destruction of Trypanosoma cruzi by toxic oxygen metabolites produced by mononuclear phagocytes 1990.
[http://dx.doi.org/10.1007/978-1-4613-0553-8_10]

[205] Rink L, Kirchner HJTJon. Zinc-altered immune function and cytokine production 2000.
[http://dx.doi.org/10.1093/jn/130.5.1407S]

[206] Hokama S, Toda T, Kusano N, Nakamura H, Nakasone I, Nagamine T, Urasaki H, Chinen S, Kinjoh N, Sakiyama K, Yohena K, Taira S, Kyan T, Ohshiro M. [Recent features of parasites detected from clinical specimens]. Rinsho Byori 1996; Apr;44(4): 379-83. Japanese.

[207] Osman D, *et al.* The requirement for cobalt in vitamin B12: A paradigm for protein metalation 2021.
[http://dx.doi.org/10.1016/j.bbamcr.2020.118896]

[208] Rickes EL, *et al.* Vitamin B12, a cobalt complex 1948.
[http://dx.doi.org/10.1126/science.108.2797.134]

[209] Stangl G, *et al.* Cobalt–deficiency–induced hyperhomocysteinaemia and oxidative status of cattle 2000.
[http://dx.doi.org/10.1017/S0007114500000027]

[210] Vellema P, *et al.* The effect of cobalt supplementation on the immune response in vitamin B12 deficient Texel lambs 1996.
[http://dx.doi.org/10.1016/S0165-2427(96)05560-2]

[211] Marley C, Fraser M, Davies D, Rees M, Vale J, Forbes A. The effect of mixed or sequential grazing of cattle and sheep on the faecal egg counts and growth rates of weaned lambs when treated with anthelmintics. Vet Parasitol 2006; 142: 134-41.

[212] Gao J-F, *et al.* Comparative analyses of the complete mitochondrial genomes of the two ruminant

hookworms Bunostomum trigonocephalum and Bunostomum phlebotomum 2014.
[http://dx.doi.org/10.1016/j.gene.2014.03.017]

[213] Jex AR, Waeschenbach A, Hu M, *et al.* The mitochondrial genomes of *Ancylostoma caninum* and *Bunostomum phlebotomum* – two hookworms of animal health and zoonotic importance. BMC Genomics 2009; 10(1): 79.
[http://dx.doi.org/10.1186/1471-2164-10-79] [PMID: 19210793]

[214] Amarante AFTdJRBdPV. Why is it important to correctly identify Haemonchus species? 2011.
[http://dx.doi.org/10.1590/S1984-29612011000400002]

[215] Liu L, Zhang Z, Liu H, *et al.* Identification and characterisation of the haemozoin of *Haemonchus contortus*. Parasit Vectors 2023; 16(1): 88.
[http://dx.doi.org/10.1186/s13071-023-05714-3] [PMID: 36879311]

[216] Kalyanasundaram RJJoVP. Role of parasite vaccines in sustained animal health and production 2015.

[217] Sander VA, *et al.* Use of Veterinary Vaccines for Livestock as a Strategy to Control Foodborne Parasitic Diseases 2020.
[http://dx.doi.org/10.3389/fcimb.2020.00288]

[218] Innes EA, *et al.* Developing vaccines to control protozoan parasites in ruminants: dead or alive? 2011.
[http://dx.doi.org/10.1016/j.vetpar.2011.05.036]

[219] Larsen MJIJfP. Biological control of helminths 1999.
[http://dx.doi.org/10.1016/S0020-7519(98)00185-4]

[220] Waller PJ, Thamsborg SMJTiP. 2004.

[221] Perry BD, Randolph TF. Improving the assessment of the economic impact of parasitic diseases and of their control in production animals. Vet Parasitol 1999; 84: 145-68.

[222] Sanyal P, Chauhan J, Mukhopadhyaya PJVrc. Implications of fungicidal effects of benzimidazole compounds on Duddingtonia flagrans in integrated nematode parasite management in livestock 2004.
[http://dx.doi.org/10.1023/B:VERC.0000034997.50332.77]

SUBJECT INDEX

A

Air drying 229
Allergic reactions 233
Alveolar echinococcosis 151, 153
Amphistomiasis 234
Amphistomosis 173
Anaemia 57, 59, 60, 61, 62, 63, 65, 82, 83, 84, 167, 168, 179, 181, 182
Anaplasmosis 10, 12, 14, 15, 20, 64, 83, 181, 182, 183, 273, 312
  acute 312
  bovine 64, 181, 182, 312
Ancylostoma 3
Anemia 2, 4, 30, 31, 32, 33, 34, 109, 148, 149, 150, 151, 183, 329, 330, 331
  erythrophagocytosis-induced 183
Animal 2, 65, 73, 79, 80, 209, 330, 333, 338, 339, 340
  disease transmission 79
  grub infestation 80
  intestines 209, 340
  manure 339
  migration 330
  mortality 65
  productivity 2
  skin 73
  wastes 333, 338
Anthelmintic(s) 22, 23, 32, 29, 33, 36, 39, 42, 96, 99, 101, 104, 106, 115, 118, 138, 145, 146, 149, 151, 249, 252, 253, 257, 264
  activity 252, 257
  commercial 145
  drugs 32, 36, 39, 42, 96, 99, 101, 104, 106, 118, 149
  therapies 146, 169
  treatment 29, 33
Anthiomaline injection 141
Anti-infective prophylaxis 153
Anti-parasitic properties 336
Anti-protozoal drugs 253

Anti-thrombin peptide 314
Antimicrobial properties 256
Antiparasitic drugs 96, 220, 252, 253, 254, 262, 263, 264
Aorta, thoracic 60
Asthma 142, 144
Attenuated schizont-infected lymphoblast (ASIL) 309

B

Babesia transmission 11
Babesiosis 10, 11, 62, 63, 64, 65, 178, 179, 180, 253, 255, 279, 280
Bacteria 83, 88, 263, 283, 343
  pathogenic 88
Bacterial infections 107, 138, 232, 278
Beef industries 69, 182
Bile duct 168, 174
  hyperplasia 174
  hypertrophy 168
Blood 12, 13, 14, 17, 18, 19, 20, 22, 42, 49, 73, 75, 76, 77, 78, 82, 108, 316
  meal digestion 316
  parasites 22
  transport 73
  trypomastigotes 49
Bloodstream infection 50
Bovis infestation 107
Bradycardia 261
Breast lesions 71
Bronchi, infected 136
Bronchiolitis 209
Bronchitis 136
Bronchoscope 144
Bronchoscopy 138

C

Cattle 2, 41, 43, 48, 65, 132, 133, 134, 148, 150, 156, 178, 180, 308, 313, 325, 326, 338

husbandry 132, 133
industries 2, 65, 178, 180, 325, 326
infections 134, 148, 150
parasites infecting 338
pregnant 156, 308, 313
ranching, contemporary 48
reproduction 41, 43
trypanosomes 65
Chemoprophylactic medicines 66
Chemotherapy 64, 250, 253, 299
Cholestasis 173
CNS tissues 97
Coagulative necrosis 233
Coccidiosis 8, 94, 253, 254, 255, 256, 257,
    263, 311
  bovine 311
  intestinal 94
  treatment of 253, 254, 255, 256, 257
Coelomyarian 236, 237
Comprehensive parasite management 37
Computed tomography (CT) 51, 201
Consumption of grass 329
Contaminated pastures 6, 30, 32, 33, 45, 135,
    150, 329, 330, 338
Cryptosporidium 8, 229, 244, 311
  infection 8, 229, 244
  oocysts 229, 311
Cyst(s) 98, 107, 152, 197
  development 98, 107
  maturation 197
  microscopic 152
Cystic echinococcosis 151, 174, 175, 176
Cysticercoids 32
Cysticercosis 71, 192, 194, 196, 303
  bovine 196

D

Diarrhea 2, 4, 8, 9, 30, 31, 32, 33, 34, 146,
    261, 311, 312, 329, 330
  hemorrhagic watery 8
  malabsorptive 9
  neonatal 8
Diseases 59, 90, 94, 132, 133, 137, 161, 230,
    281, 308, 311
  autoimmune 281
  chronic liver 161
  deficiency 230
  gastrointestinal 311
  immunological 59

neurological 94
respiratory 132, 133, 137
transboundary 90
transmitted 308
Disorders 79, 80, 97, 116, 123, 124, 163, 192,
    201, 256
  gastrointestinal 79
  immunological 192
  inflammatory 201
  metabolic 256
  neurological 80
DNA vaccines 298, 313
Drug resistance, anti-parasitic 325

E

Ear infections 115, 119, 120
Ectoparasites 68, 73, 74, 260, 264, 278, 315,
    316, 326, 328, 330, 331
Epidemiology, disease's 182, 200
Erythrocytes 11, 22, 60, 64, 179, 182, 263,
    312
  infected 11, 182, 312
  parasite-containing 263
Eurytrematosis 169, 170

F

Fasciolosis, chronic 163
Fat necrosis 80, 207
Fatty acid binding proteins (FABP) 300, 302,
    305
Fecal 32, 46, 333
  flotation 32
  inspection 46
  wastes 333
Feces 7, 8, 9, 10, 21, 33, 34, 133, 134, 135,
    144, 146, 150, 151, 283, 329
  contaminated 329
Fertility, reduced 35, 44, 329
Fetal death 307
Fetus's autolysis 205
Fibrinoid necrotic vascular lesions 89, 202
Fibroblasts 59, 202, 204, 232
Fibrogenesis 175
Fibrosis 58, 59, 140, 168, 174, 203, 209, 232
Fly control techniques 122
Food 8, 9, 86, 132, 143, 193, 198, 204, 250,
    278, 288, 329
  consuming 193

contaminated 143, 204, 329
disease-free 250
hygienic 288
Freund's adjuvant 302
Fungi, nematophagous 300, 342

G

GABA-mediated neurotransmission 258
Gastrointestinal nematode infection 327
Genetic 24, 29, 36, 52, 72, 273, 282, 283
mutations 72
selection 24, 29, 36, 52, 273, 282, 283
Giardia infection 9
Giardiasis 9, 253
GIN infections 21
Glutathione *S*-transferase (GST) 300, 302, 306
Grazing intensity 338

H

Haematocrit centrifugation technique (HCT) 66
Haemoglobinaemia 63
Haemolytic anaemia 179
Haemoprotozoan 10, 57, 231
diseases 10
parasites 10, 57, 231
Haemorrhagic ulcerations 174
Hair follicles 19, 86, 107, 243
Head shaking 103, 106, 118, 120
Helminth 231, 241, 242, 300, 303
parasites 231, 241, 242, 303
vaccines 300
Hepatic 59, 166, 260
fibrosis 166
microsome 260
syndrome 59
Homeostasis 68
Human 9, 66
immunodeficiency virus (HIV) 9
trypanosome 66
Hydatid cysts, sterile 236
Hydatidosis neosporosis 192
Hyperkalemia 63
Hyperkeratosis 71, 243
Hyperplasia 172, 173, 209

I

Illnesses 40, 41, 58, 59, 60, 68, 71, 72, 73, 84, 108, 109, 110, 116, 117, 140, 151, 192, 211
chronic 84, 192
inflammatory 72
respiratory 140
Immature heartworm 258
Immune 276, 278, 280, 281, 286
memory 278
-neural network 286
response, innate 276, 280, 281
Immunity 23, 133, 134, 139, 140, 272, 274, 275, 276, 277, 278, 280, 281, 282, 286, 288, 309
innate 281, 286
nematodes 272
Immunohistochemical method 247
Immunological reactions 109, 247
Infection-induced neuroinflammation 95
Infections 100, 103, 133, 157, 279, 308
fungal 100, 103
gastrointestinal 279
genital 308
respiratory 133, 157
Infiltration 72, 282, 308
immune cell 282, 308
inflammatory 72
Inflammation 40, 41, 80, 100, 103, 105, 106, 107, 109, 118, 121, 122, 123, 136, 144, 207, 232, 330
bronchial 136, 144
granulomatous 232
Inflammatory response 44, 59, 98, 100, 105, 211, 232, 273, 279
Injury 95, 173
hepatic 173
neuronal 95
Integral membrane glycoproteins 305
Intestinal syndrome 58
Intestine 196, 197
enterocytes 197
sarcocystosis 196

K

Kidney 42, 45, 51
damage 51
dysfunction 42, 45

L

Lesions 90, 181, 196, 211, 232
  fibrotic 196, 211
  hyperplastic-neoplastic 232
  inflammatory 232
  necropsy 181
  necrotic 90
Liver 160, 163, 165, 166, 168, 170
  cirrhosis 168
  damage 166, 170
  destruction 168
  parasite infections 160
  parenchyma 163, 165, 166

M

Meat 26, 66
  consuming cattle 26
  infected 66
Mechanisms 52, 253, 256, 271, 273, 276, 279,
    281, 283, 284, 286, 288, 289
  host resistance 283
  immune 276
  medication resistance 52
Metabolism 252, 255, 256, 264, 316
  carbohydrate 264
  nucleic acid 255
Microscopy, electron 197
Microtomy 245
Mitochondrial reductase 264
Molecular techniques 21, 109, 300, 317
Muscle(s) 8, 70, 194, 195, 196, 197, 198, 202,
    207, 208, 235, 239, 242
  cardiac 8, 195, 196, 197, 202
  sarcocystosis 196

N

Nematode parasites 134, 145, 147, 305
  gastrointestinal 305
Nematodes, metastrongyloidea 157
Neospora 48, 205, 206, 274, 307
  agglutination test (NAT) 205
  caninum infections 48, 274, 307
  immunohistochemistry 206
  infections 206
Neosporosis 9, 203, 204, 205, 274, 301
  abortion 301
  lesions 205

Neurofibromatosis 71
Neurological 94, 95, 99
  abnormalities 99
  architecture 94
  dysfunction 95
Neurotransmission 264
Neutrophils 105
Next-generation sequencing (NGS) 52
Nitrogenous fertilizers 339
Non-invasive intestinal infection 197

O

Obstruction, bronchiole 136
Oesophagus, muscular 238
Oil 68, 229, 336
  castor 336
  immersion magnification 229
Onchocerciasis 60, 70, 78
Oocysts 9, 177, 178, 197, 202, 204, 218, 220,
    223, 224, 225, 229, 244, 311
  alabamensis 311
  resistant 177
Organophosphate insecticide 79, 96, 252
Osteomyelitis 80, 201, 207
Outer membrane proteins (OMPs) 312, 314

P

Pancreatitis 261
Parafilaria 69, 70
  infection 69
  lesions 70
Parasite(s) 40, 52, 94, 95, 97, 133, 160, 167,
    175, 218, 253, 276, 330, 331, 341
  agent 133
  cysts 175, 218
  hematophagous 341
  illness 167
  -infected animal 330, 331
  infectious 253
  neurotropic 94, 95, 97
  pancreas-associated 160
  respiratory 133
  urinary system 40, 52
  vector-transmitted 276
Parasite infections 2, 29, 34, 35, 39, 41, 50,
    52, 72, 110, 116, 117, 125, 127, 192
  economic implications of 29, 39
  gastrointestinal 2, 34

Parasitic 4, 6, 12, 17, 65, 103, 107, 116, 230, 271, 274, 288, 303, 326, 341
  bronchitis 6
  defense 274
  diseases, infectious 12
  infestations 103, 116, 271, 326, 341
  invasion 107, 288
  tapeworm 303
Parasitophorous vacuole membrane (PVM) 202
Pathognomonic tissue cysts 89, 202
Pneumonitis 89, 144, 209
  interstitial 209
Polymerase chain reaction (PCR) 42, 44, 48, 49, 63, 66, 96, 148, 205
Polymorphic immunodominant molecule (PIM) 309
Postmortem lesions 61
Processes 80, 211, 225, 237, 239, 273, 285
  cytoplasmic 239
  ecological 285
  flotation 225
  immune system-mediated 211
  modulatory 80
  natural evolutionary 273
  worms transmit 237
Procyclic trypomastigote transformation 108
Protein(s) 76, 255, 256, 284, 298, 300, 303, 308, 310, 312, 314, 316, 329
  binding 255
  chimeric 303
  heat-shock 310
  polymorphism 300
  salivary gland 284
Proteolytic enzymes 171
Protozoal 298, 307
  infections 298
  vaccines 307
Protozoan 8, 9, 40, 88, 97, 243, 274, 285, 311
  infections 8
  parasites 9, 40, 88, 97, 243, 274, 285, 311

R

Ramifications 52
Reproduction, asexual 7, 153
Resistance 36, 52, 126, 220, 260, 263, 264, 270, 271, 272, 276, 277, 278, 279, 280, 282, 288, 289, 341
  age-related 279

anthelmintic 220, 341
genetic 126
medication 52
natural 36
phenotypes 263
Respiratory 133, 146, 148, 149, 152, 157
  disorders 146, 148, 149, 152
  system of cattle 133, 157
Response, immunohistochemistry 247
RNA interference (RNAi) 315

S

Salivary glands 49, 62, 179
Sarcocystis 153, 154, 196, 231
Sarcocystosis 153, 156, 157, 192, 196
Sarcocysts 153, 154, 197
Schizogony 61, 154, 197
Sexual reproduction 47, 62, 143, 154
Signaling 96, 103
  molecules 103
  pathways 96
Signals, genetic 272
Skin, auricular 73
Systems 49, 100, 101, 103, 110, 134, 157, 198, 210, 254, 263, 277
  cell-mediated immune 277
  cytochrome 254, 263
  lymphatic 49, 134
  neurological 100, 101, 103, 110, 198
  pulmonary 157, 210

T

Targeted selective therapy (TST) 334, 335
Techniques 51, 96, 99, 126, 230, 243, 247
  histopathological 230, 243
  imaging 51, 99
  immunochemical 247
  immunomodulatory 96, 126
Therapeutic control of parasitic diseases 328
Therapy 50, 70, 79, 81, 108, 109, 110, 138, 152, 153, 157, 180, 183, 286
  anti-infective drug 153
  antibiotic 138
  immunosuppressive 286
  protracted medication 152
Threats, significant economic 313
Thrombosis 89, 202
Tick-borne diseases (TBD) 10, 11, 20, 180

Transmission 8, 10, 66, 67, 144, 145, 146,
        147, 193, 194, 204, 208, 274, 330, 331
    methods 66, 193, 274
    techniques 193
Trichomonas infections 45
Trypanosomatids 284
Trypanosomiasis 10, 21, 65, 66, 263
Tumor development 260

U

Ulcers, abomasal 181
Urinary tract infections 41, 49, 50, 53

V

Vaccines 298, 299, 303, 308, 309, 315
    antimicrobial 299
    combinatorial 298, 315
    commercial 299, 303, 308, 309, 315
Variable 109, 310
    major surface antigens (VMSA) 310
    surface glycoproteins (VSGs) 109

W

Waste management 325, 333, 343
Water, consuming 195
Western blot analysis 302
Worms 3, 20, 21, 33, 45, 50, 88, 97, 102, 103,
        104, 105, 106, 120, 121, 122, 123, 124,
        125, 144, 150, 241, 258, 259
    abomasum 3
    brain 97
    filariasis 241
    gastrointestinal 3
    gulosa 102
    hermaphroditic 88
    intestinal 258, 259
    kidney 45, 50
    nematode 122
    parasitic trematode 33

Z

Zinc deficiency 341

www.ingramcontent.com/pod-product-compliance
Lightning Source LLC
Chambersburg PA
CBHW050803220326
41598CB00006B/101